Public Health Law

California/Milbank Series on Health and the Public

Public Health Law

Power, Duty, Restraint

Lawrence O. Gostin

UNIVERSITY OF CALIFORNIA PRESS
Berkeley · Los Angeles · London

THE MILBANK MEMORIAL FUND
New York

University of California Press
Berkeley and Los Angeles, California

University of California Press, Ltd.
London, England

© 2000 by
Lawrence O. Gostin

Library of Congress Cataloging-in-Publication Data
Gostin, Larry O. (Larry Ogalthorpe)
    Public health law : power, duty, restraint /
    Lawrence O. Gostin.
        p. cm. — (California/Milbank series on health
    and the public; 3)
    "A copublication with the Milbank Memorial
    Fund."
    Includes bibliographical references and index.
    ISBN 0-520-22646-1 (cloth : alk. paper)—
    ISBN 0-520-22648-8 (pbk. : alk. paper)
    1. Public health laws—United States. I. Title.
    II. Series.
    KF3775. G67   2000
    344.73'04—dc21

                                    00-037773

Printed and bound in Canada

08 07 06 05 04 03 02 01 00
10 9 8 7 6 5 4 3 2 1

The paper used in this publication is both acid-free
and totally chlorine-free (TCF). It meets the minimum requirements of ANSI/NISO Z39.48-1992
(R 1997) (*Permanence of Paper*).

Contents

List of Illustrations

List of Tables

Abbreviations

ACIP	Advisory Committee on Immunization Practices
ACTG	AIDS Clinic Trials Group
ADA	Americans with Disabilities Act
AIDS	Acquired Immunodeficiency Syndrome
ALI	American Law Institute
AMA	American Medical Association
APHA	American Public Health Association
BRACA	Genetic test for propensity to breast cancer
CDC	Centers for Disease Control and Prevention
CIOMS	Council of International Organizations of Medical Sciences
CSTE	Council of State and Territorial Epidemiologists
DES	Diethylstilbestrol
DHHS	Department of Health and Human Services
DOL	Department of Labor
FDA	Food and Drug Administration
FOIA	Freedom of Information Act

FTC	Federal Trade Commission
GBS	Guillain-Barré syndrome
HCWs	Health care workers
HEDIS	Health Plan Employer Data and Information Sets
HEW	Department of Health, Education, and Welfare
HHS	Department of Health and Human Services
HIV	Human immunodeficiency virus
HMO	Health maintenance organization
IOM	Institute of Medicine
IRB	Institutional Review Board
M.TB	*Mycobacterium* tuberculosis
NCVIA	National Childhood Vaccine Injury Act
NEISS	National Electronic Injury Examination Survey
NHANES	National Health and Nutrition Examination Survey
OSHA	Occupational Safety and Health Administration
PKU	Phenylketonuria
PPD	Skin test for diagnosis of tuberculosis infection
PV	Predictive value
rBST	Recombinant bovine somatotropin
STD	Sexually transmitted disease
TB	Tuberculosis
USDA	United States Department of Agriculture
USMHS	United States Marine Hospital Service
USPHS	United States Public Health Service
VMI	Virginia Military Institute

Foreword

The Milbank Memorial Fund is an endowed national foundation that engages in nonpartisan analysis, study, research, and communication on significant issues in health care and public health. The Fund makes available the results of its work in meetings with decision-makers, reports, articles, and books.

The purpose of the Fund's publishing partnership with the University of California Press is to encourage the synthesis and communication of findings from research and experience that could contribute to more effective health policy. Larry Gostin's book achieves this goal.

Gostin brings to this book vast experience as a lawyer and legal scholar on public health issues. For many years, in both the United Kingdom and the United States, Gostin has been a lawyer's lawyer as well as an adviser to policymakers on the most controversial issues in public health law. This combination of scholarship and experience leads Gostin to propose that public health law should be an instrument for developing as well as implementing public policy. He offers a critical analysis and synthesis of law and science that promises to improve the effectiveness of public policy in enhancing the health of populations.

The Fund and the University of California Press solicit written reviews for the books in this series from both academic experts and persons who make and implement policy. Then the reviewers meet with the author to discuss the manuscript. The academic reviewers of Gostin's manuscript strongly advised the publication of a *Reader*, for use in conjuction with this volume in courses on public health, law, and ethics. This *Reader* is now in preparation by the University of California Press.

Daniel M. Fox
President

Samuel L. Milbank
Chairman

Preface

Good health is fundamentally important because it is essential to happiness, livelihood, political participation, and many of the other elements necessary for a life full of contentment and achievement. Certainly, health is not the only important social value and, on occasion, public health aspirations may have to yield to other values. Additionally, elected officials are not obligated to spend inordinate amounts of tax dollars on a single public good such as health when there are many competing political claims for limited resources. Nevertheless, I think it is important that any book purporting to examine carefully the interface between law and health begin by emphasizing the powerful collective benefits afforded by assuring the conditions for a healthy population.

Libraries throughout the United States are replete with books on the general subject of law and health. Why then offer a book on public health law? The reason is that the vast majority of these books are concerned principally with medicine and personal health care services—clinical decision-making, delivery, organization, and finance. Personal medical services are an important part of what makes a community healthy. Yet medicine is only one contributor to health, and probably a relatively small one at that. Virtually all of the national health expenditures (excluding environmental funding) are devoted to medical care; only a tiny fraction is allocated to population-based public health initiatives.

In this book, I offer a systematic definition and theory of public health law. The definition is based on a broad notion of the government's inherent responsibility to advance the population's health and well-being:

The legal powers and duties of the state to assure the conditions for people to be healthy (e.g., to identify, prevent, and ameliorate risks to health in the population) and the limitations on the power of the state to constrain the autonomy, privacy, liberty, proprietary, or other legally protected interests of individuals for protection or promotion of community health.

I explain why public health law is a coherent field, distinct from other intellectual activities at the intersection of law and health. In particular, I offer five characteristics that help distinguish public health law from the vast literature on law and medicine (see Figure 1):

The government's responsibility to advance the public's health

The population-based perspective

The relationship between the people and the state

The discrete set of services and scientific methodologies

The role of coercion

This book, therefore, is about the complex problems that arise when government regulates to prevent injury and disease or to promote the public's health. The government possesses the authority and responsibility to persuade, create incentives, or even compel individuals and businesses to conform to health and safety standards for the collective good. This power and obligation forms the essence of what we call public health law.

In addition to offering a definition and theory, I examine the analytical methods and tools of public health law, principally *constitutional law*, which empowers government to act for the community's health and limits that power; *statutory and administrative law*, which provide the vast regulatory structure at the federal, state, and local levels for responding to health threats; and *tort law*, which affords a civil remedy against individuals and businesses whose unreasonably risky conduct causes injury or disease.

Accordingly, much of the book discusses the extensive body of legal doctrine that informs the field of public health law. A book on public

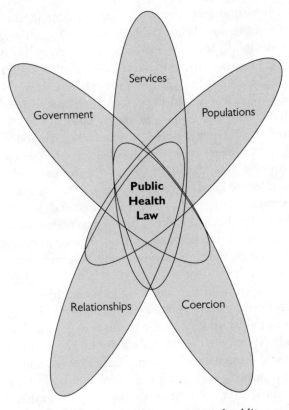

Figure 1.   The essential characteristics of public
health law.

health law, intended for a broad audience, cannot consider all of the
nuances and complexities of legal doctrine. For the sake of succinctness
and clarity, the text sometimes may imply that the law is more mono-
lithic and predictable than it really is. Subsequent chapters often present some of the subtleties of the law as applied to particular problems
in public health. Nevertheless, a much more careful examination of
statutes, administrative rules, and policies is essential in resolving specific legal problems facing public health authorities.

    I often return to two themes in this book: the trade-offs between
public goods and private rights, and the dilemma of whether to use coercive or voluntary public health measures. As to the first theme, I emphasize the collective goods that are achieved, or achievable, through
legal and regulatory approaches. Seen in this way, the law is a potent
tool for the realization of healthier and safer populations. At the same

time, I closely examine the complexity of, and conundrums posed by, public health regulation. While public health regulation is intended to achieve public goods, it often does so at the expense of private rights and interests. Consequently, in thinking about public health regulation, we have to take a hard look at the trade-offs—between the common welfare, on the one hand, and the personal burdens and economic interests of individuals and businesses, on the other.

Characterizing these trade-offs between collective goods and individual rights is only one of several possible ways to conceptualize the problem. Another way would be to characterize the trade-off as between two collective goods—the good of public health and the good of limited government. After all, society gains a great deal of benefit from the protection of individual liberties through a constitutional system of limited governmental interference. Still, an analysis of collective goods versus individual rights captures at least one important way of thinking about public health.

Another problem with characterizing public health law as a series of trade-offs between private rights and public goods is that often the most effective public health policy is to *enhance* private rights to attain public goods. My friend, the late Jonathan Mann, was particularly eloquent in urging the conclusion that public health and human rights are synergistic; preserving and promoting individual rights most often advances human well-being. Certainly, coercive policies may have unintended effects on group behaviors (e.g., driving people away from health care services). Furthermore, antidiscrimination, privacy, and other legal safeguards have public health, as well as intrinsic, value. Nevertheless, sometimes public health authorities confront hard choices between public goods and private rights, and many of the chapters in this book explore these complex choices.

The trade-offs between individual and population-based perspectives lead to a second, related theme. Public health scholars and practitioners, for as long as people have organized societies to defend their health and security, have grappled with the decision of whether to use voluntary or coercive approaches in achieving collective benefits. Is it always, or almost always, better to persuade individuals to change their behavior, to provide the means for behavioral change, and to restructure environments to promote the public's health? Alternatively, should public health authorities resort to compulsion of individuals and businesses? And, if compulsion is warranted, under what circumstances should public health authorities wield their power? In this book, I propose a systematic evaluation of public health regulation that helps balance private rights and public goods. The model I propose is intended to assess the circumstances when government rightfully should be able to demand conformance with public standards.

In writing this book, I learned a great deal about myself. I come from a strong civil liberties background. As a young Fulbright scholar at the Universities of Oxford and London in the mid-1970s, I went on to become the Legal Director of the National Association of Mental Health (MIND) (where my colleagues and I brought a series of well-known cases before the European Court of Human Rights) and, later, the head of the National Council of Civil Liberties (the United Kingdom equivalent to the American Civil Liberties Union). After returning to the United States in the late 1980s, I served on the ACLU's National Board of Directors and National Executive Committee, and in the early 1990s, I chaired its Privacy Committee. During all those years, I subscribed to the dominant liberal position that individual freedom is, by far, the preferred value to guide ethical and legal analysis in matters of physical and mental health.

Despite my background as a civil libertarian, in this book I question the primacy of individual freedom (and its associated concepts—autonomy, privacy, and liberty) as the prevailing social norm. Freedom is a powerful and important idea, but I think scholars have given insufficient attention to equally strong values that are captured by the notions of partnership, citizenship, and community. As members of a society in which we all share a common bond, our responsibility is not simply to defend our own right to be free from economic or personal restraint. We also have an obligation to protect and defend the community as a whole against threats to health, safety, and security. Each member of society owes a duty—one to another—to promote the common good. And each member benefits from participating in a well-regulated society that reduces risks that are common to all.

In summary, this book offers a theory and definition of public health law, an examination of its principal analytical methods, and an exploration of its dominant themes, such as the trade-offs between individual rights and public benefits and between voluntary and coercive public health approaches. In this book, I aspire to create a record of the field of public health law at the turn of the millennium. The transition from the nineteenth to the twentieth century marked, perhaps, the golden age of public health, and several influential treatises were written on public health law. I learned a great deal from these works, and I hope that scholars in future generations may benefit from observing the field of public health law through the lens of this book. Although it, to be sure, falls far short of the task required to resolve the profoundly complicated problems that have long perplexed scholars of public health law, the book at least tries to provide an honest account of the doctrine and the controversies facing the field in the year 2000.

I have in mind diverse audiences for this book. Most important, it is designed for scholars and practitioners in public health generally and public health law particularly. It is intended to be useful for legislators as well as officials in the executive and judicial branches at the federal, state, and local levels. I have also designed this book for teachers and students of public health law and hope that it provides a useful and systematic method of instruction for courses in schools of law, public health, medicine, health administration, and other fields. For pedagogic purposes, this book is accompanied by a *Reader in Public Health, Law, and Ethics*, comprising the major scholarly articles and judicial cases in the field. This *Reader* will be periodically updated on the Internet to ensure its timeliness. I welcome the guidance of my colleagues in making the book and supplemental readings clearer and more informative.

I hope that this book will also be read by the informed lay public. Public health law fundamentally concerns the relationships among political representatives and their constituents. As such, the field is one that every informed citizen should study and understand. The subject is fascinating and nuanced, taking the reader into constitutional history and design, theories of democracy and political participation, and the rights and obligations of individuals and businesses.

ORGANIZATION OF THE BOOK

The book is organized into three major sections: Part One, Conceptual Foundations of Public Health Law; Part Two, Public Health and Civil Liberties in Conflict; and Part Three, The Future of Public Health Law.

Part One covers the conceptual foundations of public health law in four chapters:

A theory and a definition of public health law

Public health in the constitutional design

Constitutional limits on the exercise of public health powers

A systematic evaluation of public health regulation

Part One, and particularly chapters 2 and 3, contain considerable discussion of doctrine that may, at once, be insufficiently detailed for legal scholars and overly pedantic for students of public health. Despite the unavoidable difficulties of addressing multiple audiences, I felt it important to develop a common understanding of the constitutional basis for the exercise of public health powers and the limits on those powers. I decided not to examine the rich constitutional history and structures at the state level, which are equally important to the field of public health but whose inclusion would have made the book too diverse and detailed.

Part Two, consisting of six chapters, explores the major substantive areas of public health practice as well as the conflicts with individual rights and interests that arise. By constructing the chapters in this way, I was able both to explain a doctrinal area in public health law and to show its effects on individuals and businesses. This method of development also allowed me to investigate the paradoxes of public health law (i.e., the fact that regulation has a beneficial effect on the population's health, but often an adverse effect on personal and economic interests). In Part Two, I do not cover the full range of public health practice, but I do attempt to provide a representative survey:

The public health information infrastructure (surveillance, reporting, partner notification, and population-based research) and the conflict with personal privacy

Health, communication, and behavior (health education campaigns, restraints on commercial speech, and compelled commercial speech) and the conflict with the freedom of expression

Immunization, testing, and screening and the conflict with bodily integrity

Restrictions of the person (quarantine, isolation, civil commitment, compulsory physical examination, medical treatment, and criminal penalties for knowing or willful exposure to an infectious condition) and the conflict with autonomy, liberty, and bodily integrity

Regulatory powers of public health agencies (e.g., licenses, inspections, nuisance abatements) and the conflict with professional, property, and business interests (examining economic due process, freedom of contract, and regulatory "takings")

Tort law (negligence and strict liability) and the conflict with professional, property, and business interests

In many of these chapters, I include cases studies of important public health problems that illustrate the conflicts (e.g., perinatal transmission of HIV, swine flu immunization, cigarette advertising, and firearms
litigation).

Part Three, consisting of chapter 11 only, envisions the future of
public health law. In this chapter, I return to some of the important
themes in public health law presented in this book, examine the inade-
quacies of extant public health statutes, and present guidelines for public health law reform in America.

CONVENTION

This book was written for scholars and practitioners in both law and
public health. In an attempt to make this material as widely accessible
as possible, *The Chicago Manual of Style* (14th edition) was used for
the bibliography format and *The Bluebook: A Uniform System of
Citation* (16th edition) was used for the end notes.

Acknowledgments

I am indebted to so many people for their vital contributions to this book that I hardly know where to begin. Most important, Daniel M. Fox, President of the Milbank Memorial Fund, supported, organized, and persistently encouraged this enterprise from its very beginnings. Lynne Withey, Associate Director of the University of California Press, has been Dan Fox's partner in this venture and has similarly encouraged and promoted this undertaking.

My academic institutions, Georgetown University Law Center and the Johns Hopkins University School of Hygiene and Public Health, have been intellectual homes for this project, and many other related projects, on public health law. Among the many people at these institutions who have contributed richly to my thinking are, foremost, Dean Judith Areen and Dean Alfred Sommer, both of whom have devoted themselves personally to this book. I presented papers from this book at dean's lectures and faculty research workshops at these and other academic institutions. At Georgetown, my valued colleagues who have been most closely involved include M. Gregg Bloche; David D. Cole; David C. Vladeck; William N. Eskridge, Jr. (now at Yale); Chai R. Feldblum; Heidi L. Feldman; Steven Goldberg; Lisa Heinzerling; Patricia A. King; Richard Lazarus; Louis M. Seidman; and Mark M. Tushnet. At Johns Hopkins, my valued colleagues who have been close collaborators with me in exploring the field of public health law and ethics for many years include Ruth Faden, Stephen Teret, and Jon Vernick.

I also want to thank the staff at the Georgetown University Law Library (notably Robert L. Oakley, Vivian L. Campbell, Joan Marshall, and Karen Summerhill), the William H. Welch Library of Medicine at the Johns Hopkins University, the Centre for Socio-Legal Research (notably Dennis Gallaghan) of the University of Oxford, and the Bodleian Library of the University of Oxford.

I also had exceptional editorial and research assistance at Georgetown. William Naugle, and his successor, Anna Selden, spent endless hours reading and editing the manuscript and graphics in this book. Equally important, James G. Hodge, Jr., spearheaded a substantial research effort over several years. Among the students participating in the research team under Prof. Hodge's direction were Mira Burghardt, Heather Butts, Brant Campbell, Aimee Doyle, K. Sarah Galbraith, Kevin Greaney, Jeffrey S. Huang, Tyng Loh, Mark Lowry, Bradley Malin, David Maria, Lee Matovcik, Charles J. Muhl, Monique V. Nolan, Jennifer Phelps, Ethan Preston, Debra Reichman, Julia M. Rothstein, Ahren S. Tryon, Jennifer Vinson, Joseph Wang, and Ruqaiijah Yearby. I want to especially thank two students in the Georgetown/Johns Hopkins University Program on Law and Public Health: Lance Gable and Bill Tarantino.

Outside my own academic institutions I have found close colleagues and friends with whom to share enduring interests in public health law and ethics. Among my closest colleagues, whose work always inspires me, are Ronald Bayer (Columbia), Richard J. Bonnie (Virginia), Allan M. Brandt (Harvard), James Curran (Emory), the late William Curran (Harvard), Nancy Neveloff Dubler (Albert Einstein), Kristine M. Gebbie (Columbia), Frank Grad (Columbia), the Hon. Justice Michael Kirby (High Court of Australia), Wendy Parmet (Northeastern), Marjorie Shultz (Berkeley), and David W. Webber.

I want to mention especially Scott Burris (Temple) and Zita Lazzarini (Connecticut), with whom I have worked closely on public health law writing projects. I also want to thank particularly my close colleagues at Johns Hopkins, Stephen Teret and Jon Vernick, at the University of Michigan, Peter D. Jacobson, and at Arizona State University, Daniel S. Strouse, who test-piloted this book with their students. I have learned a great deal from these colleagues.

The Milbank Memorial Fund facilitated meetings, conversations, and written reviews on the content of the book with many of the most insightful and experienced scholars and practitioners in the fields of

public health and law: Christopher Atchison, Mark Barnes, Barbara
DeBuono, Mary desVignes-Kendrick, David Fidler, Richard A.
Goodman, Mark Hall, Thomas A. LaVeist, Paul W. Nannis, Lloyd F.
Novick, Terry O'Brien, Carol Roddy, William L. Roper, Mark
Rothstein, Leonard S. Rubenstein, Ciro V. Sumaya, Bailus Walker, and
Martin Wasserman.

I have been fortunate to work with many of the major public health
organizations in the United States and globally. These organizations, and
the people with whom I have worked, have contributed a great deal to
my development as a public health law scholar. In the United States, I
have been associated with the following agencies, boards, and commit-
tees: the Office of the General Counsel, Department of Health and
Human Services (e.g., Eugene W. Matthews and Verla S. Neslund); the
Centers for Disease Control and Prevention (e.g., Edward L. Baker,
Kevin DeCock, Helene Gayle, Richard A. Goodman, Robert Janssen,
Martha Katz, Patricia Fleming, Anthony Moulton, Dixie Snyder, Ronald
Valdisseri, and John Ward); Institute of Medicine, National Academy of
Sciences, Board on Health Promotion and Disease Prevention (e.g.,
Robert E. Fullilove, Rose Martinez, Donald R. Mattison, Hugh H.
Tilson, Kathleen Stratton, Kathleen E. Toomey, and Kenneth E. Warner),
Institutional Review Board (e.g., Robert Cook-Deegan and Roger
Herdman), and several committees (e.g., Edward Brandt, Chair,
Committee on Health and Behavior, and colleagues to whom I am grate-
ful for their inspiration for chapter 6); the Council of State and
Territorial Epidemiologists (e.g., Guthrie Birkhead, David Fleming,
Willis Forrester, Donna Knutson, Kristine Moore, John Middaugh, and
Michael Osterholm); the Turning Point Project, Robert Wood Johnson
Foundation (e.g., Bobbie Berkowitz, Deborah Erickson, Peter
Nakamura, and Jack Thompson); the Hastings Center (e.g., Daniel
Callahan, Bruce Jennings, and Bette-Jane Crigger); and the National
Conference of State Legislatures (e.g., Tracey A. Hooker, Richard
Merritt, and Lisa Speissegger).

Internationally, I have served on the following boards and committees:
Joint United Nations Programme on AIDS (previously WHO's pro-
gramme on AIDS) (e.g., the late Jonathan Mann, Daniel Tarantola, Peter
Piot, Susan Timberlake, and Helen Wachirs); World Health Organization
(e.g., Sev Fluss); and the Council of International Organizations of
Medical Sciences (e.g., Zbigniew Bankowski and Jack Bryant).

The book contains a series of images from the history of public
health. Visual expressions of the relationship between public health and

the law are difficult to find, organize, and explain. I received considerable assistance from one of the most important national figures in this area—the U.S. Public Health Service historian John Parascandola.

I thank, most of all, the people who mean the most to me and to whom this book is dedicated: my family, Jean, Bryn, and Kieran. In addition to providing the kind of support that only a lifetime of love can assure, my wife Jean worked on the graphics that are so helpful in clarifying and visualizing the intellectual ideas presented in this book.

COPYRIGHT NOTE

Lawrence O. Gostin
Washington, D.C.
December 1999

PART ONE

Conceptual Foundations of Public Health Law

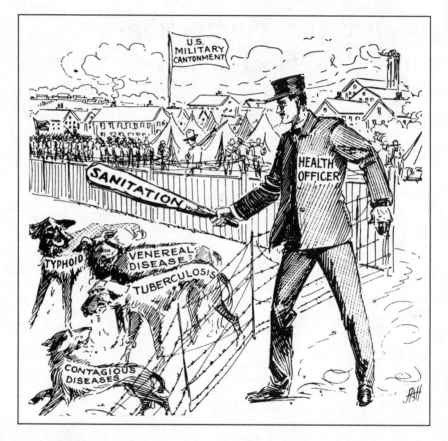

During the First World War, the U.S. Public Health Service cooperated with local health departments to contain infectious diseases, which were assumed to be the principal threats to public health, in the areas around the military training camps. Sanitation and public health regulation were health officers' principal weapons against these diseases.

1 A Theory and Definition of Public Health Law

> [Public health law] should not be confused with medical jurisprudence, which is concerned only in legal aspects of the application of medical and surgical knowledge to individuals. . . . [P]ublic health is not a branch of medicine, but a science in itself, to which, however, preventive medicine is an important contributor. Public health law is that branch of jurisprudence which treats of the application of common and statutory law to the principles of hygiene and sanitary science.
>
> *James A. Tobey (1926)*

The literature, both academic and judicial, on the intersection of law and health is pervasive. The subject of law and health is widely taught (in schools of law, medicine, public health, and health administration), practiced (by "health lawyers"), and analyzed (by scholars in the related fields of health law, bioethics, and health policy). Organized groups of teachers, scholars, and practitioners in law and health are active and visible, including the American Society of Law, Medicine & Ethics; the American Health Lawyers Association; and the American College of Legal Medicine.

The fields that characterize these branches of study are variously called health law, health care law, law and medicine, forensic medicine, and public health law. Do these names imply different disciplines, each with a coherent theory, structure, and method that sets it apart? Notably absent from the extant literature is a theory of the discipline of public health law, an exploration of its doctrinal boundaries, and an assessment of its analytical methodology.

Public health law shares conceptual terrain with the field of law and medicine, or health care law, but is a distinct discipline. My claim is not that public health law is contained within a tidy doctrinal package; its boundaries are blurred and overlap other paths of study in law and health. Nor is public health law easy to define and operationalize; the field is as complex and confused as public health itself. Rather, I posit that public health law is susceptible to theoretical and practical differentiation from other disciplines at the nexus of law and health.

Public health law can be defined, its boundaries circumscribed, and its analytical methods detailed in ways that distinguish it as a discrete discipline—just as the disciplines of medicine and public health can be demarcated. With this book I hope to provide a fuller understanding of the varied roles of law in advancing the public's health. The core idea that I propose is that law can be an essential tool for creating the conditions that enable people to lead healthier and safer lives.

In this chapter, I construct a definition of public health law, borrowing from ideas in constitutional law, theories of democracy and community, and public health history and practice. My definition of public health law follows, and the remainder of this chapter offers a justification for each component of the definition.

Public health law is the study of the legal powers and duties of the state to assure the conditions for people to be healthy (e.g., to identify, prevent, and ameliorate risks to health in the population) and the limitations on the power of the state to constrain the autonomy, privacy, liberty, proprietary, or other legally protected interests of individuals for the protection or promotion of community health.

Through this definition, I suggest five essential characteristics of public health law (see Figure 2):

Government: Public health activities are a special responsibility of the government.

Populations: Public health focuses on the health of populations.

Relationships: Public health addresses the relationship between the state and the population (or between the state and individuals who place themselves or the community at risk).

Services: Public health deals with the provision of population-based services grounded on the scientific methodologies of public health (e.g., biostatistics and epidemiology).

Coercion: Public health authorities possess the power to coerce individuals and businesses for the protection of the community, rather than relying on a near universal ethic of voluntarism.

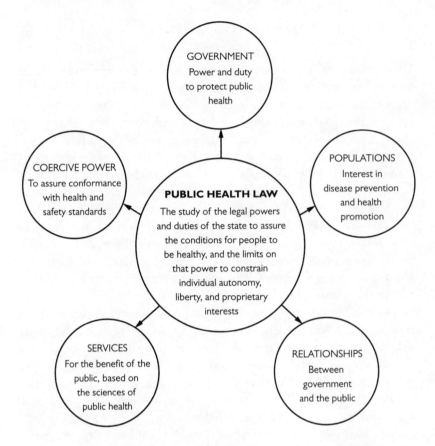

Figure 2.   Public health law: a definition and essential characteristics.

GOVERNMENT POWER AND DUTY IN PUBLIC HEALTH: WHAT IS "PUBLIC" IN PUBLIC HEALTH LAW

A systematic understanding of public health law requires a careful examination of what is "public." A public entity acts on behalf of the people and gains its legitimacy through a political process. A characteristic form of "public" or state action occurs when a democratically elected government exercises powers or duties to protect or promote the population's health. What follows is a systematic justification of government's special responsibility in matters of public health. I base my argument on the primacy of government in the constitutional design, the obligations of government in a democracy, and governmental health regulation in history and practice. I do not mean to suggest, however, that government is exclusively engaged in the work of public health. The private and charitable sectors have played, and continue to play, a vital role in improving the health of the populace.[1]

THE ROLE OF GOVERNMENT
IN THE CONSTITUTIONAL DESIGN

The Constitution, it is widely assumed, is conceived in negative terms to restrain government from invading a sphere of individual liberty and property interests. According to this settled view, the Constitution does not oblige the government to act for the common good. I will return to the idea of a negative constitution in the next chapter. For the present, it is important to understand that the constitutional design shows that the government is empowered to, and actually does, defend the common welfare.

The Preamble to the Constitution reveals the influence of republican ideals of government as the wellspring of communal life and mutual security:[2] "We the People of the United States, in Order to form a more perfect Union, establish Justice, insure domestic Tranquility, provide for the common defence, promote the general Welfare, and secure the Blessings of Liberty to ourselves and our Posterity, do ordain and establish this Constitution. . . ."

The common defense and the general welfare could not have been conceived as relating solely to physical security, for perhaps the principal threat to civil society during the generation in which the Constitution was ratified (the "framing era") was epidemic disease and other forms of ill health. After examining public and private roles during the framing era, Wendy Parmet concludes, "Despite the disagreement and uncertainty over the actual meaning of 'the common good,' it seems likely that the preservation of public health . . . was one meaning that all would share. Tradition and practice pointed to it. Theorists such as Montesquieu supported it. So did popular political discourse."[3]

The constitutional design reveals a plain intent to vest power in government, at every level, to protect community health and safety. In its very first sentence, the Constitution provides sole legislative, or policy-making, authority to the Congress,[4] and the first enumerated legislative power is expressly to provide for the "common Defence" and "general Welfare" of the United States.[5] The legislative role is to enact laws necessary to safeguard the population from harms, including harms relating to health and safety risks. The executive branch, pursuant to its constitutional obligation to "take Care that the Laws be faithfully executed," enforces and amplifies legislative health and safety standards.[6] Executive agencies have developed special expertise in matters of health and have long promulgated regulations to safeguard public health and safety.[7] The judicial role is to construe the law and to ensure that legislative and executive actions are congruent with the Constitution.[8] Since the earliest times, the courts have authorized compulsion—notably through common law nuisance abatement—to protect the public health.[9]

From a constitutional perspective, only government—whether federal, state, or local—can collect taxes and expend public resources, and only government can require members of the community to submit to inspection and regulation. The Constitution grants no residual power to the private sector to tax, spend, or regulate—all necessary for the preservation of the public's health. To the extent that the private sector uses public funds or demands compliance with health and safety standards, it does so principally through delegated governmental authority. The private sector's role in public health is simply not found in the constitutional design.

THE RESPONSIBILITIES OF GOVERNMENT IN DEMOCRACIES

Why is it that a political, or governmental, entity possesses principal, if not sole, responsibility to protect and promote public health? Theories of democracy and political communities help to explain the primacy of government in matters of public health. Michael Walzer has articulated an essential truth about the nature and purposes of political communities: "Membership is important because of what the members of a political community owe to one another . . . and the first thing they owe is the communal provision of security and welfare."[10] Public health, according to Walzer, is the "easy" case of a general communal provision because public funds are expended to benefit all or most of the population without any specific distribution to individuals. To contrast public health with medicine, the former is most often a general communal provision, while the latter is most often particular.[11]

A political community stresses a shared bond among members: organized society safeguards the common goods of health, welfare, and security, while members subordinate themselves to the welfare of the community as a whole.[12] Public health can be achieved only through collective action, not through individual endeavor. Acting alone, individuals cannot assure even minimum levels of health. Individuals may procure personal medical services and many of the necessities of living; any person of means can purchase a home, clothing, food, and the services of a physician or hospital. Yet no single individual, or group of individuals, can assure his or her health. Meaningful protection and assurance of the population's health require communal effort. The community as a whole has a stake in environmental protection, hygiene and sanitation, clean air and surface water, uncontaminated food and drinking water, safe roads and products, and control of infectious disease. These collective goods, and many more, are essential conditions for health. Yet these goods can be secured only through organized action on behalf of the population.

Moreover, the population, or electorate, legitimizes systematic community activity for the public health. Public health activities in a democracy cannot be organized, funded, or implemented without the assent of the people. It is government that possesses the sole authority to empower, regulate, or carry out activities designed to protect or promote the general health, safety, and welfare of the population. It is the public that bands together to achieve social goods that could not be secured absent collective action. And it is the public, or electorate, that legitimizes or authorizes government to act for the common welfare. Walzer argues that every set of political officials is at least putatively committed to securing health for the population, and every set of members of a political community is committed to bear the necessary burdens (and does so). "The first commitment has to do with the duties of office; the second, with the duties of membership."[13] Consequently, the communal efforts of the body politic to protect and promote the population's health represent a central theoretical tenet of what we call public health law.

Political philosophers, such as Norm Daniels and Dan Brock, show that health takes on a special meaning and importance in political communities.[14] Public health is indispensable not only to individuals, but to the community as a whole. The benefits of health to each individual are indisputable. Health is necessary for much of the joy, creativity, and productivity that a person derives from life. Perhaps not as obvious, however, health is also essential for political communities. Without minimum levels of health, populations cannot fully engage in the social interactions of a community, participate in the political process, generate wealth and assure economic prosperity, and provide for common defense and security. Public health, then, becomes a transcendent value because a fundamental level of human functioning is a prerequisite for engaging in activities that are critical to communities—social, political, and economic.

I do not mean to suggest that the political commitment to public health must be absolute. What constitutes "enough" public health? How much? What kinds of services? How will they be paid for and distributed? These remain political questions.[15] Democratic government will never devote unlimited resources to public health; core public health functions compete for scarce resources with other demands for services, and resources are allocated through a prescribed political process. In this sense, Dan Beauchamp is instructive in suggesting that a healthy republic is not achieved solely through a strong sense of communal welfare, but is also the result of a vigorous and expanded democratic discussion about the population's health.[16]

GOVERNMENTAL HEALTH REGULATION
IN HISTORY AND PRACTICE

Constitutional law and democratic theory support the basic power or obligation of organized society (principally through government) to protect and preserve the health of populations. But in a very real sense, governmental health activities form part of the fabric and experience of public health in America. Throughout the history of public health, the line between public and private action has never been hard and fast. Moreover, private, charitable, and religious influences have been manifest.[17] Still, from the colonial and framing periods to the Progressive Era and the New Deal—and continuing to modern times—government in all its various forms has assumed responsibility for public health.

The early history of public health in America has been widely chronicled and need not be reiterated here.[18] Public health regulation had become a common feature by the colonial and federalist periods.[19] Health regulation, which reaches at least as far back as the seventeenth century, included conditions of travel at sea; isolation and quarantine; inoculation with smallpox pus; sanitary controls on dead fish, animals, and garbage; and quality controls on bread, meat, and drinking water (see chapters 7, 8, and 9).[20] From the earliest times of the republic, public bodies acted in cases of necessity and were prepared to subordinate the freedoms of individuals for the sake of the common welfare.[21]

During the early nineteenth century, the sanitary movement emerged in response to epidemic diseases (e.g., cholera, smallpox, yellow fever, and tuberculosis).[22] Local sanitary surveys, notably the Shattuck report in Massachusetts,[23] assessed the health effects of decaying waste, foul air, and an immoral lifestyle.[24] During this period, local government began to expand sanitary regulation to improve sewage, drinking water, and garbage disposal.[25] As the Institute of Medicine observed, "Sanitation changed the way society thought about health. Illness came to be seen as an indicator of poor social and environmental conditions, as well as poor moral and spiritual conditions. . . . Sanitation also changed the way society thought about public responsibility for citizen's health. Protecting health became a social responsibility."[26]

The Progressive Era of the early twentieth century is often regarded as a high-water mark of local government regulation, principally regarding sanitary controls introduced by city and, later, state boards of health.[27] This was a complex period during which public health activities were influenced by many factors. Remarkable successes of bacteriology inspired by the pioneering work of Koch and Pasteur foreshadowed the discoveries of Dubos, Fleming, and Waksman. W.T. Sedgwick, a familiar name in sanitary and bacteriologic research in Massachusetts, remarked, "[B]efore 1880 we knew nothing; after 1890 we knew it all."[28] Public health began to embrace medicine and science, so the identification and treatment of persons with infectious disease took on a new importance. Legislatures enacted disease reporting requirements, while public health agencies traced sexual contacts and established clinics for treating tuberculosis. It was clear even then, however, that efforts to identify and treat persons with infectious disease were insufficient. Sanitary and hygienic conditions aggravated by industrialization and immigration were regarded as potent causes of ill health.[29] The health risks associated with urban growth were thought to demand a collective, governmental response in the form of expanded sewer systems, creative drain designs, improved garbage collection, and other hygienic measures.[30] "Public health once again became a task of promoting a healthy society."[31] During the Progressive Era, this goal was pursued through scientific analysis of disease and epidemics, medical treatment of individuals, education, and advancements in social conditions.

Although the American Public Health Association (APHA) was formed in 1879 and the United States Public Health Service emerged from the Marine Hospital Service in 1912,[32] most public health initiatives of the early twentieth century concentrated on local activity.[33] Many observers saw the New Deal in Franklin Delano Roosevelt's administration (and, to a lesser extent, the Great Society in Lyndon Johnson's administration) as an important juncture in developing an active federal role in public health.[34] During this period, the federal government asserted regulatory jurisdiction over adulterated or otherwise harmful food, drugs, and cosmetics;[35] established national standards for drinking water;[36] enacted a venereal disease control program in response to a reemergent sexually transmitted infection epidemic;[37] and formed a federal grant-in-aid program requiring the states to establish and maintain public health services and training for public health professionals.[38] Also during this period, the National Hygienic Laboratory moved to Bethesda, Maryland, and was renamed the National Institutes of Health. Meanwhile, the states expanded their capacity to engage in classic public health activities, including the collection of vital statistics, communicable disease reporting, venereal disease investigation, milk pasteurization, and institution of school hygiene standards.[39]

Public health activities, both federal and state, are omnipresent in the late twentieth century. Government assesses population health status, investigates health threats, sets policies and standards, regulates the private sector, funds research, finances and delivers personal health services, and performs other health-related functions. Federal regulation now reaches broad aspects of public health, such as air and water quality, food and drug safety, tobacco advertising, pesticide production and sales, consumer product protection, and occupational health and safety. States exercise jurisdiction in virtually all areas of public health—ranging from surveillance, disease reporting, and control of injury and disease to regulating sanitation and hygienic conditions in schools, child care facilities, and restaurants.

This brief historical overview is not intended to provide a systematic account of American public health practice. Rather, it demonstrates the ubiquity of health regulation and underscores the historic governmental authority in public health. From the founding of the republic to the present day, government has assumed a significant level of responsibility for community well-being. Earlier this century, Tobey noted this central role of government within the discipline of public health law: "The protection and promotion of the public health has long been recognized as the responsibility of the sovereign power. Government is, in fact, organized for the express purpose, among others, of conserving the public health and cannot divest itself of this important duty."[40]

THE POPULATION-BASED PERSPECTIVE OF PUBLIC HEALTH

The crux of public health, as I have sought to demonstrate, is a public, or governmental, entity that harbors the power and responsibility to assure community well-being. Public health, however, also focuses on persons or groups that stake a claim to health protection or promotion. Most scholars who have compared public health with medicine have noted that, generally, public health focuses on the health of populations, while medicine focuses on the health of individuals.[41] Elizabeth Fee observes that medicine and public health have contradictory interests. "Public health is oriented to-

ward the analysis of the determinants of health and disease on a population basis, while medicine is oriented toward individual patients."[42]

Public health is organized to provide an aggregate benefit to the mental and physical health of all the people in a given community. Classic definitions of public health emphasize this population-based perspective:
"As one of the objects of the police power of the state, the 'public health'
means the prevailingly healthful or sanitary condition of the general body
of people or the community in mass, and the absence of any general or
widespread disease or cause of mortality. The wholesome sanitary condition of the community at large."[43] Consequently, while the art or science
of medicine seeks to identify and ameliorate ill health in the individual
patient, public health seeks to improve the health of the population.

Admittedly, it is not easy to separate individual and population-based
health interventions. A direct relationship exists between the health of
each individual and the health of the community at large. After all, the
well-being of the whole may be accomplished by little more than assuring the health of each individual. This is not to suggest, however, that the
public health system is, or should be, solely responsible for population-
level approaches and the health care system responsible for individual-
level approaches. Sometimes the dividing line between health care and
public health is exceedingly difficult to draw. The medical treatment of an
infectious disease, for example, benefits both the individual and the wider
population. The boundaries between medicine and public health become
obfuscated in such cases, and it is not unusual to see both the health care
and public health systems accept responsibility for patient care, health education, and follow-up for infectious diseases.

Despite the lack of clarity, strong arguments exist—based on theory
and practice—that the quintessential feature of public health is its concentration on communal well-being, and that this feature separates
public health from medicine. The organized community activity known
as public health is conceptually designed to benefit the collective population. If political communities form for the communal provision of security and welfare, it is the community—not individuals—that stakes a
claim to disease prevention and health promotion. Public health services are those shared by all members of the community, organized and
supported by, and for the benefit of, the people as a whole.

The focus on populations rather than individual patients is grounded
not only in theory, but in the methods of scientific inquiry and the services offered by public health. The analytical methods and objectives of
the primary sciences of public health—epidemiology and biostatistics—

are directed toward understanding risk, injury, and disease within populations. Epidemiology, literally translated from the Greek, is the study (*logos*) of what is among (*epi*) the people (*demos*). Roger Detels notes that "[a]ll epidemiologists will agree that epidemiology concerns itself with populations rather than individuals, thereby separating itself from the rest of medicine and constituting the basic science of public health."[44] Epidemiology examines the frequencies and distributions of disease in the population.[45] The population strategy "is the attempt to control the determinants of incidents, to lower the mean level of risk factors, [and] to shift the whole distribution of exposure in a favourable direction."[46] The advantage of a population strategy is that it seeks to reduce underlying causes that make diseases common in populations.

In his authoritative article "Sick Individuals and Sick Populations," Geoffrey Rose compares the scientific methods and objectives of medicine with those of public health. "Why did *this* patient get *this* disease at this time?" is a prevailing question in medicine, and it underscores a physician's central concern for sick individuals.[47] Other accounts of the medical profession emphasize its reductionist tendencies, even while recognizing its cyclical interest in broader issues, such as the ecological and social meanings of disease. "It follows from disease theory," writes Eric Cassell, "that the purpose of the clinician is to discover in the sick patient that unique phenomenon with its unique cause that is the disease (and thus the source of the sickness), and to base diagnostic and therapeutic actions accordingly."[48]

The concentration on aggregate health effects in populations helps construct a thoughtful definition of public health that I incorporate into my broader definition of public health law. Definitions of public health vary widely, ranging from the utopian conception of the World Health Organization of an ideal state of physical and mental health[49] to a more concrete listing of public health practices.[50] The Institute of Medicine has proposed one of the most influential contemporary definitions of public health:[51]

> Public health is what we, as a society, do collectively to assure the conditions for people to be healthy. This requires that continuing and emerging threats to the health of the public be successfully countered. These threats include immediate crises, such as the AIDS epidemic; enduring problems, such as injuries and chronic illness; and growing challenges, such as the aging of our population and the toxic by-products of a modern economy, transmitted through air, water, soil, or food. These and many other problems raise in common the need to protect the nation's health through effective, organized, and sustained efforts led by the public sector.

This definition can be appreciated by examining its constituent parts. The emphasis on cooperative and mutually shared responsibility ("we, as a society") reinforces that people form political communities precisely because the collective entity can best protect and promote the population's health. What do communities do to preserve health? Notably, communal responsibilities are intended to "assure the conditions for people to be healthy." These conditions of health include a variety of behavioral, economic, and environmental interventions to reduce the burden of injury and disease in populations. Finally, the definition emphasizes the "public sector" responsibility to engage in "effective, organized, and sustained efforts" to safeguard communal health.

The foundational article by Michael McGinnis and William Foege examines the leading causes of death in the United States, revealing different forms of thinking in medicine and public health. Medical explanations of death point to discrete pathophysiological conditions, such as cancer, heart disease, cerebrovascular disease, and pulmonary disease. Public health explanations, on the other hand, examine the root causes of disease. From this perspective, the leading causes of death are environmental, social, and behavioral factors, such as smoking, alcohol and drug use, diet and activity patterns, sexual behavior, toxic agents, firearms, and motor vehicles. McGinnis and Foege observe that the vast preponderance of government expenditures is devoted to medical treatment of diseases ultimately recorded on death certificates as the nation's leading killers. Only a small fraction is directed to control the root determinants of death and disability.[52]

THE RELATIONSHIP BETWEEN THE PEOPLE AND THE STATE

Public health law studies the relationship between the state and the community at large (or between the state and individuals who place themselves or the community at risk) rather than the relationship between health care providers and patients. Public health is interested in organized community efforts to improve the health of populations. Accordingly, public health law observes collective action—principally by government through federal, state, and local health agencies—and its effects on various populations.

Public health law similarly examines the benefits and burdens placed by government on legally protected interests. As government acts to promote or protect public health, it may enhance or diminish individual interests in autonomy, liberty, privacy, or property. The powers and obligations of government itself, as well as the limitations on state action, capture the attention of students of public health. Thus, public health law considers how government acts, or fails to act, to address the major health problems facing large populations (e.g., tobacco use, drug or alcohol dependency, communicable diseases, injuries, violence, and occupational or environmental risks). And when government acts, or fails to act, public health law studies the effects on personal and organizational interests (e.g., restraints on commercial speech, free association, liberty, and control of property).

In contrast, health care law has an abiding and material interest in the microrelationships between health care providers and patients. The duties of physicians and the "rights" claims of individual patients in the course of the therapeutic relationship are central to the discipline of health care law. Consequently, issues regarding informed consent and confidentiality shape the discourse of health care law. The doctor has certain obligations to the patient to provide information concerning treatment alternatives and to respect confidences divulged during the therapeutic exchange. Similarly, malpractice law involves the study of duties of care owed by physicians to patients and, more recently, the duties—if any—owed by systems of care to patients.[53]

Health care law, moreover, studies the organization, financing, and provision of personal medical services. It focuses on the relationships among health care providers (e.g., managed care organizations and integrated delivery systems), third-party payers (e.g., state or employer-sponsored health care benefits and private insurers), and regulators (e.g., government oversight of access, quality, and costs of personal medical services). Scholars in the field of health care law scrutinize each of the major components of a well-functioning system in providing personal medical services. Who has *access* to the health care system? Is the system *fair* for various economic, racial, and social groups? Does the system provide adequate *choice* of physicians and providers? Are the services provided of high *quality*? Is the health care system *cost-effective*? Thus, the field of health care law is concerned with relationships between physicians and patients and with indicators of access, equity, choice, quality, and cost of personal medical services.

Seldom do students of health care law focus on the questions that dominate thinking in public health: What is the health status of the population, and what broad societal measures can reduce the overall level of injury and disease?

THE MISSION, FUNCTIONS, AND SERVICES OF THE PUBLIC HEALTH SYSTEM

Public Health is purchasable. Within natural limitations every community can determine its own death rate.

Hermann Biggs (1894)

It has been shown that external agents have as great an influence on the frequency of sickness as on its fatality; the obvious corollary is, that man has as much power to prevent as to cure disease. . . . Yet, medical men, the guardians of public health, never have their attention called to the prevention of sickness; it forms no part of their education. . . . The public do not seek the shield of medical art . . . till the arrows of death already rankle in the veins. . . . Public health may be promoted by placing the medical institutions of the country on a liberal scientific basis; by medical societies co-operating to collect statistical observations; and by medical writers renouncing the notion that a science can be founded upon the limited experience of an individual.

William Farr (1837)

If government has the primary responsibility to assure the conditions of health for populations, then what public health activities best assure health, and what organizational arrangements are necessary to provide these services? The answers to these questions inform not only traditional methods for population-based health improvement but, more important, the critical differences between medical and public health services.

The literature is replete with attempts to identify the mission of public health, classify "core" functions, and set national and international[54] standards for "essential" services.[55] The mission of public health is broad, encompassing systematic efforts to promote physical and mental health and to prevent disease, injury, and disability.[56] The core functions of public health agencies are to prevent epidemics, protect against environmental hazards, promote healthy behaviors, respond to disasters and assist communities in recovery, and assure the quality and accessibility of health services.[57]

The "essential services" of public health are to monitor community health status; diagnose and investigate health problems; inform and educate people about health; mobilize community partnerships; develop and enforce health and safety protection; link people to needed personal health services; assure a competent health workforce; foster health-enhancing public policies; evaluate the quality and effectiveness of services; and research for new insights and innovations.[58]

Public health professionals have devised a set of "leading health indicators" to help measure the health of communities. Modeled on economic indicators, these criteria evaluate whether communities are becoming healthier or sicker. The leading health indicators measure the most important attributes of health in populations: physical activity, overweight and obesity, tobacco use, substance abuse, responsible sexual behavior, mental health, injury and violence, environmental quality, immunization, and access to health care.[59]

This description of the mission, functions, services, and leading indicators shows the breadth of public health activities. Public health addresses the root causes of disease and disability; agencies identify these causes and intervene at various levels. Notably, public health subsumes personal medical services as one of many conditions necessary to preserve the population's health. Contrary to popular belief, the public sector assumes considerable responsibility for health care. Taking into consideration public insurance programs, such as Medicare and Medicaid, and forgone revenue as a result of tax exclusion of employee health benefits, the public sector accounts for roughly 58 percent of total health care spending.[60] Additionally, the public health system traditionally provides direct medical services for pregnant women, persons with contagious diseases (e.g., TB, STDs, and HIV/AIDS), and other discrete populations.

The dividing line between medicine and public health is not always clear. Both fields are concerned with prevention. Clinical prevention services, such as immunizations, mammograms, Pap smears, PPD skin tests and chest X-rays, HIV antibody tests, and colorectal screening, are central to the mission of both the health care and public health systems. So, too, are both systems concerned with counseling and health education to change individual behavior.

Despite the absence of a clear boundary, major differences exist between the services performed in the health care and public health systems. At its core, health care is devoted to personal medical diagnosis, clinical prevention, and treatment, while public health is devoted to strategies to identify health risks and improve behavioral, environmental, social, and economic conditions that affect the health of wider populations. The dividing line is not neat, but the methodologies, practices, and services in these respective disciplines are distinct.

THE ROLE OF COERCION AND INDIVIDUAL RIGHTS IN PUBLIC HEALTH LAW

I have suggested that public health law is concerned with governmental responsibilities to the community; the well-being of the population; the relationship between the state and the community at large; and a broad range of services designed to identify, prevent, and ameliorate health threats within society. These ideas encompass what can be regarded as "public" and what constitutes "health" within a political community. Although it may not be obvious, I am also suggesting that the use of coercion must be part of an informed understanding of public health law.

Government can do many things to promote public health and safety that do not require the exercise of compulsory powers. Yet government alone is authorized to require conformance with publicly established standards of conduct. Governments are formed not only to attend to the general needs of their constituents, but to insist, through force of law if necessary, that individuals and businesses act in ways that do not place others at unreasonable risk of harm. To defend the common welfare, political communities assert their collective power to tax, inspect, regulate, and coerce. Of course, different ideas exist about what compulsory measures are necessary to safeguard the public health. Reconciling divergent interests about the desirability of coercion in a given situation (should government resort to force, what kind, and under what circumstances?) is an issue for political resolution. I propose standards for evaluating public health regulation in chapter 4.

Protecting and preserving community health is not possible without the constraint of a wide range of private activities. Private actors—whether individuals, groups, or corporate entities—have incentives to engage in behaviors that are personally profitable or pleasurable but may threaten other individuals or groups.[61] Individuals with sexually transmitted infections derive satisfaction from intimate relationships; industry finds it profitable to produce goods without considering broader social or environmental costs; and manufacturers find it economical to offer products without the highest available safety or hygiene standards. In each instance, individuals or organizations act rationally for their own interests, but their actions may adversely affect communal health and safety. Absent a governmental authority, and willingness, to coerce, these threats to public health and safety could not easily be reduced.

Although regulation in the name of public health is theoretically intended to safeguard the health and safety of whole populations, it often benefits those most at risk of injury and disease. Everyone gains value from public health regulations, such as food and water standards, but some regulation protects the most vulnerable. For instance, the elimination of a toxic waste site, a building code in a crowded tenement, and the closure of an unhygienic restaurant hold particular significance for those at immediate risk.

Perhaps because engaging in risk behavior may promote personal or economic interests, individuals and businesses frequently oppose government regulation. Resistance is sometimes based on philosophical grounds of autonomy or freedom from government interference. Citizens, and the groups that represent them, claim that self-regarding behaviors, such as the use of seatbelts or motorcycle helmets, are not the business of government. Sometimes these arguments are extended to behavior that threatens others, such as sex or needle sharing by persons with bloodborne infections.

Industry often asserts that economic principles militate against government control. Entrepreneurs tend to accept as a matter of faith that governmental health and safety standards often retard economic development and should be avoided. In political arenas, they contest these standards in the name of economic liberty, holding out government taxation and regulation as inefficient.

Debates such as these should take place within a democratic society. My intention is not to say whether, in any particular case, government control is desirable. Governments of all description have historically used force to benefit communal health; compulsion is sometimes necessary to avert obvious social risks. The study of the coercive powers of the state is a staple of what we call public health law. Charles V. Chapin, a pioneering city health officer from the Progressive Era, reached one of the core understandings of public health law—that the state, in the exercise of its police powers, sets boundaries on the behavior of individuals that poses risks to the public:[62]

[It is well to cite] the oft quoted aphorism of the Earl of Derby that "sanitary instruction is even more important than sanitary legislation." Sanitarians work toward the ideal that all people will in time know what healthful living is, and that they will in time reach that moral plane when they will practice what they know. While hopeful for the millennium we must work. Law is still necessary. People still incline to acts which are not for their neighbors' good. In our complicated civilization, many restrictions must be placed on individual conduct in order that we may live happily and healthfully one with another.

Public health, then, historically has constrained the rights of individuals and organizations to protect community interests in health.[63] Whether through the use of reporting requirements that affect privacy, mandatory testing or screening that affects autonomy, environmental standards that affect property, industrial regulation that affects economic freedom, or isolation and quarantine that affect liberty, public health has not shied from controlling individuals and organizations for the aggregate good.

Assuredly, public health is empowered to restrict human freedoms and rights to achieve a collective good, but it must do so consistent with constitutional constraints on state action. The inherent prerogative of the state to protect and promote the public health, safety, and welfare (known as the police powers) is limited by individual rights to liberty, autonomy, property, and other constitutionally protected interests (see chapter 3). Achieving a just balance between the powers and duties of the state to defend and advance the public health and constitutionally protected rights poses an enduring problem for public health law.

Any theory of public health law presents a paradox. Government, on the one hand, is compelled by its role as the elected representative of the community to act affirmatively to promote the health of the people. To many, this role requires vigorous measures to control obvious health risks. On the other hand, government cannot unduly invade individuals' rights in the name of the communal good. Health regulation that overreaches, in that it achieves a minimal health benefit with disproportionate human burdens, is not tolerated in a society based on the rule of law. Consequently, scholars and practitioners often perceive an irreconcilable conflict between the claim of the community to reduce obvious health risks and the claim of individuals to be free from government interference. This perceived conflict may be agonizing in some cases and absent in others. Thus, public health law must always pose the questions, Does a coercive intervention truly reduce aggregate health risks, and what, if any, less intrusive interventions might reduce those risks as well or better?

It has become fashionable to claim that no real conflict exists between the protection of individual rights and the promotion of public health.[64] According to this view, safeguarding rights is always (or virtually always) consistent with preserving communal health.[65] Indeed, according to this perspective, individual rights and public health are synergistic—the defense of one enhances the value of the other, and vice versa. This rhetorical position serves a purpose but is simplistic. It suggests that a decision to avert a discrete health risk actually may result in an aggregate increase in injury or disease in the population as a whole. The exercise of compulsory powers (e.g., isolation or quarantine) may prevent individuals from, say, transmitting a communicable infection. But the social decision to coerce affects group behavior and, ultimately, the population's health. By provoking distrust in, or alienation toward, medical and public health authorities, coercion may shift behaviors to avoidance of testing, counseling, or treatment.

Public health decision-making involves complex trade-offs. Will coercive measures to avert a known individual risk be the correct course of action (e.g., isolating a person with tuberculosis who refuses to take the full course of medication), even if doing so may produce a greater aggregate risk? The social calculation is hardly scientific or precise regarding whether compulsion will alter behavior and, if so, in what direction.[66]

Distinct tensions exist in public health law between voluntarism and coercion; civil liberties and public health; and discrete (or individual) threats and aggregate health outcomes. These competing interests, together with the substantive standards and procedural safeguards that circumscribe the lawful exercise of state powers, form the corpus of public health law.

CONCLUSION

The definition of public health law I have proposed and defended does not depict the field of public health law narrowly as a complex set of technical rules buried within state health codes. Rather, public health law should be seen broadly as the authority and responsibility of government to assure the conditions for the population's health. The study of the field requires a detailed understanding of the various legal tools available to prevent injury and disease and to promote the health of the populace.

Several important characteristics of the field help to separate public health law from other disciplines at the intersection of law and health. First, even though the private and voluntary sectors make important contributions, the *government* retains a special responsibility for ensuring the health of the people. Second, government carries out its public health duties to benefit *populations*. Third, public health law scholars study the *relationships* between the state and the public (or between the state and individuals who place themselves or the community at risk). Fourth, public health authorities deliver *services* to the public based on the sciences of public health. Finally, public health authorities possess the power to *coerce* individuals and businesses for the protection of the community. These characteristics—government, populations, relationships, services, and coercion—form the basis of public health law, a field that poses enticing intellectual challenges, both theoretical and essential to the body politic.

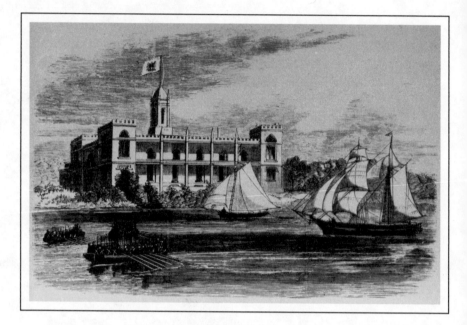

A 1798 law for the relief of sick and disabled seamen created a major role for the federal government in the public health arena by establishing the Marine Hospital Service (forerunner of the Public Health Service). Marine hospitals such as this one in New Orleans were built in many American port cities.

2   Public Health in the Constitutional Design

No inquiry is more important to public health law than understanding the role of government in the constitutional design. If, as I argue in chapter 1, public health law principally addresses government's assurance of the conditions for the population's health, then what activities must government undertake? The question is complex, requiring an assessment of duty (what government must do), authority (what government is empowered, but not obligated, to do), and limits (what government is prohibited from doing). In addition, this query raises a corollary question: Which government is to act? Some of the most divisive disputes in public health are among the federal government, the states, and the localities about which government has the power to intervene.[1]

Legal reasoning in public health embraces constitutional doctrine, legislation, regulation, and common law. This chapter and the next view public health through the lens of constitutional law by exploring government duty and authority, the division of powers under our federal system, and the limits on government power. I begin with a general discussion of constitutional functions and their application to public health.

CONSTITUTIONAL FUNCTIONS AND THEIR APPLICATION TO PUBLIC HEALTH

The Constitution serves three primary functions: to allocate power between the federal government and the states (federalism), to divide power among the three branches of government (separation of powers), and to limit government power (protection of individual liberties).[2] These functions are critical to public health. The Constitution enables government to act to prevent violence, injury, and disease, and to take measures to promote health. At the same time, the Constitution limits government's power to interfere with a personal sphere of liberty and autonomy. In the realm of public health, then, the Constitution acts as both a fountain and a levee: it originates the flow of power (to preserve the public health) and curbs that power (to protect individual freedoms).[3]

AMERICAN FEDERALISM

If the Constitution is a fountain from which governmental powers flow, federalism is its foundation, or structure.[4] Federalism separates the pool of legislative authority into two tiers of government, federal and state. American federalism, as a precept of constitutional design, preserves the balance of power among national and state authorities (see Figure 3).

Theoretically, American federalism grants the national government only limited powers, while the states possess plenary powers. Under the doctrine of enumerated powers, the United States Congress is granted certain specific powers. For public health purposes, the chief powers are the power to tax, to spend, and to regulate interstate commerce. These powers provide Congress with independent authority to raise revenue for public health services and to regulate, both directly and indirectly, private activities that endanger public health. The Necessary and Proper Clause in Article I, Section 8 of the Constitution permits Congress to employ all means reasonably appropriate to achieve the objectives of the enumerated national powers.[5] This "implied powers" doctrine has enabled the federal government to expand greatly the network of public health regulation.

The federal government is a government of limited power whose acts must be authorized in the Constitution to be valid. The states, in contrast, retain the power they possessed as sovereign governments before the Constitution was ratified.[6] The Tenth Amendment enunciates the plenary power retained by the states: "The powers not delegated to the United States by the Constitution, nor prohibited by it to the States, are reserved to the States respectively, or to the people."

The "reserved powers" doctrine holds that states may exercise all the powers inherent in government—that is, all the authority necessary

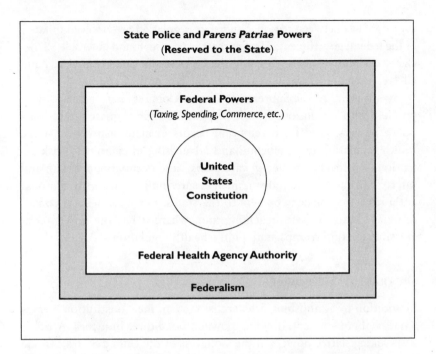

Figure 3.   Public health and federalism in the constitutional design.

Diagram explanation: This figure represents an overhead view of the principle of federalism. The U.S. Constitution is a fountain that provides the source of federal public health powers. Limited federal powers are circumscribed by the source of the constitutional fountain (e.g., power to tax, spend, and regulate inter-state commerce). State governmental powers exist outside the federal sphere (i.e., state police and parens patriae powers). Federalism is represented by the boundary dividing the pool of governmental powers. This line represents a permeable boundary between federal and state governmental powers. In theory, neither federal nor state powers may intrude on one another, but the judiciary has often permitted federal public health activities to invade traditional state territory.

to govern that is neither granted to the federal government nor prohibited to the states. Two specific powers—the police power (protecting the health, safety, and morals of the community) and the *parens patriae* power (protecting the interests of minors and incompetent persons)—express the state's inherent sovereignty to safeguard the community's welfare.

Federalism functions as a sorting device for determining which government, federal or state, may legitimately respond to a public health threat. Often, the national and state governments exercise public health powers concurrently. A national, state, and local presence exists in most spheres of public health (e.g., injury prevention, clean air and water, and infectious disease surveillance and control). Pursuant to the Supremacy Clause, however, conflicts between national and state regulation are resolved in favor of the federal government. The Supremacy Clause, found in Article VI, declares that the "Constitution, and the Laws of the United States . . . and all Treaties made . . . shall be the supreme law of the Land."

By authority of the Supremacy Clause, Congress may preempt state public health regulation, even if the state is acting squarely within its police powers.[7] Federal preemption occurs in many aspects of public health regulation (e.g., labeling and advertising of cigarettes,[8] risk retention (self-insurance) health care plans,[9] and occupational health and safety[10]). American federalism, then, ensures limited powers to national authorities and plenary powers to the states. However, federal constitutional authority is far-reaching, and, where it has the power, congressional action trumps state public health regulation.[11]

SEPARATION OF POWERS

In addition to establishing a federalist system, the Constitution creates a national government, dividing power among three branches. Article I vests all legislative powers in the Congress of the United States; Article II vests executive power in the president of the United States; and Article III vests judicial power in one supreme court and in such inferior courts as the Congress may establish. The states, pursuant to their own constitutions, have adopted similar schemes of governance. This separation of power provides a system of checks and balances, where no single branch of government can act without some degree of oversight and control by another, to reduce the possibility of government oppression (see Figure 4).

The separation of powers doctrine is essential to public health, for each branch of government possesses a unique constitutional authority to create, enforce, or interpret health policy. The legislature creates health policy and allocates the necessary resources to effect it. Some commentators contend that legislators are ill equipped to make complex public health decisions: legislators often fail to dwell sufficiently or carefully on any single issue to gather the facts and consider the implications; they characteristically lack expertise in the health sciences; and they are influenced by popular beliefs that may be uninformed, prejudicial, or both. Yet the legislature, as the only "purely" elected branch of government, is politically accountable to the people. If the legislature enacts an ineffective or overly intrusive policy, the electorate has a remedy at the ballot box. Legislatures, in addition, are re-

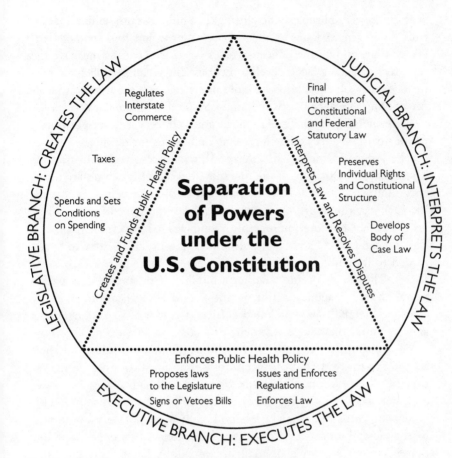

Figure 4.   Public health law functions: "checks and balances."

sponsible for balancing public health services with competing claims, say, for tax relief, national defense, transportation, and education.

The executive branch enforces health policy, but it has come to occupy a far greater role in modern America (see chapter 9). Most of the influential public health agencies reside in the executive branch—for example, the Department of Health and Human Services at the federal level and public health departments at the state and local level. Executive agencies are charged not only with implementing legislation, but with establishing complex health regulation. Although the legislature establishes general policy goals, agencies frequently devise a network of rules and conduct detailed oversight and enforcement. The executive branch possesses many attributes for effectively governing public health: agencies are created for the very purpose of advancing the public's health within their jurisdiction; agencies focus on the same set of problems for extended periods of time; and agency officials possess specific expertise and have the resources to gather facts, develop theories, and generate policy alternatives. Agency officials, however, are not elected, and the duration in office of nonpolitical civil servants can result in stale thinking and complicity with the subjects of regulation. In addition, they are not positioned politically to balance competing values and claims for resources.

The judiciary's task is to interpret law and resolve legal disputes. These may appear to be sterile pursuits, devoid of much policy influence, but the courts' role in public health is deceptively broad. Increasingly, the courts have exerted substantial control over public health policy by determining the boundaries of government power. The judiciary erects a zone of autonomy, privacy, and liberty to be afforded to individuals and economic freedoms to be afforded to businesses. The courts decide whether a public health statute is constitutional, whether agency action is authorized by legislation, whether agency officials have marshaled sufficient evidence to support their actions, and whether government officials and private parties have acted negligently. The judicial branch has the independence and legal training to make thoughtful decisions about constitutional claims regarding, for example, federalism or individual rights. Courts, however, may be less equipped to review critically the substance of health policy choices: judges may be less politically accountable,[12] are bound by the facts of a particular case, may be influenced by expert opinion that is unrepresentative of mainstream public health thought, and may focus too intently on individual rights at the expense of communal claims to public health protection.[13]

Is it possible to conclude from this discussion which particular branch of government, if any, is best suited for formulating and executing public health policy?[14] Public health practitioners, from time to time, lament the influence wielded by legislators and judges in matters of public health. They claim that legislation and adjudication are time-consuming and costly endeavors, that legislators and judges are not trained or experienced in the sciences of public health, and that legislatures devote insufficient resources to the public health infrastructure.[15] Yet the separation of powers doctrine does not aspire to achieve maximum efficiency or even the best result in public health governance. Rather, the constitutional design appears to value restraint in policymaking: Elected officials reconcile demands for public health funding with competing claims for societal resources, the executive branch straddles the line between congressional authorization and judicial restrictions on that authority, and the judiciary tempers public health measures with compassion for individuals. As a society, we forgo the possibility of bold public health governance by any given branch in exchange for constitutional checks and balances that prevent overreaching and assure political accountability.

LIMITED POWERS

A third constitutional function is to limit government power for the purpose of protecting individual liberties. When government acts to promote the communal good, it frequently infringes upon the rights and freedoms of individuals and businesses. For example, isolation and quarantine restrict liberty; cigarette advertising restrictions limit free expression; bathhouse closures constrain free association; and product regulation impedes economic freedom. Consequently, public health and individual rights, at least to some extent, conflict; efforts to promote the common welfare may compel a trade-off with personal and proprietary interests.

Protection of "rights" is commonly regarded as the Constitution's most important function. The Constitution grants extensive government power, but curtails it as well. The Bill of Rights (the first ten amendments to the Constitution), together with other constitutional provisions, creates a zone of individual liberty, autonomy, privacy, and economic freedom that exists beyond the reach of the government.[16] The Framers, moreover, believed that people retain rights not specified in the Constitution. The Ninth Amendment states, "The enumeration in the Constitution, of certain rights, shall not be construed to deny or disparage others retained by the people."

The constitutional design, then, is one where government is afforded ample power to safeguard the common weal but is prohibited from wielding it to trample individual rights. The constant quest of students of public health law is to determine the point at which government authority to promote the population's health should yield to individual rights claims. Put another way, to what degree should individuals forgo freedom to achieve improved health, a higher quality of life, and enhanced safety for the community? Much of the remainder of this book strives to answer that question.

THE NEGATIVE CONSTITUTION:
THE ABSENCE OF GOVERNMENT DUTY

[Nothing] in the language of the Due Process Clause
itself requires the State to protect the life, liberty, and
property of its citizens against invasion by private
actors. The Clause is phrased as a limitation on the
State's power to act, not as a guarantee of certain minimal levels of safety and security. It forbids the State
itself to deprive individuals of life, liberty, or property
without "due process of law," but its language cannot
fairly be extended to impose an affirmative obligation
on the State to ensure that those interests do not come
to harm through other means. Nor does history support such an expansive reading of the constitutional
text. . . . Its purpose was to protect the people from
the State, not to ensure that the State protected them
from each other. The Framers were content to leave
the extent of governmental obligation in the latter area
to the democratic political processes.

William Rehnquist (1989)

Individuals rely on government to organize social and economic life to
promote healthy populations. Given the importance of government in
maintaining public health (and many other communal benefits), one
might expect the Constitution to create affirmative obligations for government to act. Yet, by standard accounts, the Constitution is cast
purely in negative terms.[17]

The Constitution, it is often said, imposes no affirmative obligation
on the government to act, to provide services, or to protect. For the
most part, the Bill of Rights is classically defensive, or negative, in character (e.g., the First Amendment declares that government may not
abridge free speech).

The Supreme Court remains faithful to this negative conception of
the Constitution, even in the face of dire personal consequences. In
DeShaney v. Winnebago County Department of Social Services
(1989),[18] a Wyoming court granted a divorce and awarded custody of
a one-year-old child, Joshua DeShaney, to his father. Two years later,
county social workers began receiving reports that Joshua's father was
physically abusing him. The suspicious injuries were carefully noted,
but the department of social services took no action. Eventually, at four
years of age, Joshua was beaten so badly that he suffered permanent

brain injuries. He was left profoundly retarded and institutionalized. The *DeShaney* Court found no government obligation to protect children from harm of which the state is acutely aware. The Court held that, since no affirmative government duty to protect exists, citizens have no constitutional remedy.[19]

The Supreme Court has applied this line of reasoning in cases that bitterly divided the Court and the nation. In *Webster v. Reproductive Health Services* (1989),[20] the majority saw no government obligation to provide services—in this case, medical services—for the poor[21] when a Missouri statute barred state employees from performing abortions and banned the use of public facilities for such procedures. Referring to *DeShaney,* the Court rejected a positive claim for basic procedures government services: "[O]ur cases have recognized that the Due Process Clause generally confers no affirmative right to governmental aid, even where such aid may be necessary to secure life, liberty, or property interests of which the government itself may not deprive the individual."[22] According to the Court, if "no state subsidy, direct or indirect, is available, it is difficult to see how any procreational choice is burdened by the State's ban on the use of its facilities or employees for performing abortions."[23] The majority found irrelevant the fact that, if a woman is poor, her only realistic access to medical services may be through government assistance. In *DeShaney, Webster,* and other cases,[24] the judiciary has disavowed the idea of positive social rights by finding that the Constitution affords no affirmative obligations, but only negative liberties; government inaction is constitutionally immaterial, and government's failure to act brings no constitutional remedy. This negative theory of constitutional design, though well accepted, is oversimplified and, in the words of Justice Blackmun, represents "a sad commentary upon American life and constitutional principles."[25]

A weakness of the negative theory of constitutional law is that its distinctions, as between action and inaction, are difficult to sustain. The Supreme Court has repeatedly held that government has no obligation to prevent harms to health or to provide services to ameliorate ill health; that is, a government act that causes harm is actionable, while government passivity in an existing state of affairs is not. Although the Court appears to know instinctively what constitutes a governmental act, the difference between an act and an omission is often difficult to determine.[26] Any government failure to act is usually embedded in a series of affirmative policy choices (e.g., which agency will be established; the agency's objectives and how its staff will be trained; what resources, if any, will be devoted to certain problems). When government deliberately chooses to intervene (or to allocate scarce resources) in one sphere and conspicuously fails to perform in another, can that fairly be characterized as "inaction"?

Another problem with the negative constitution is that citizens rely on the protective umbrella of the state. When the state establishes an agency to detect and prevent child abuse (or to prevent any other cause of injury or disease), it promises, at least implicitly, that it will respond in cases of obvious threats to health. If an agency represents itself to the public as a defender of health, and citizens justifiably rely on that protection, is government "responsible" when it knows that a substantial risk exists, fails to inform citizens so they might initiate action, and passively avoids a state response to that risk?

Finally, judicial refusal to examine government's failure to act, irrespective of the circumstances, leaves the state free to abuse its power and cause harm to citizens. Government more often exerts its power, and its potential to harm, by withholding services in the face of obvious threats to health.[27] The state's neglect of the poor and vulnerable, its calculated failure to respond to obvious risk, or its arbitrary or discriminatory enforcement of public health law is a certain, and direct, cause of harm. Seidman and Tushnet suggest that the Fourteenth Amendment's historical purpose was to expand government's power to contend with private acts of violence. This history is consistent with the view that "the state *is* inflicting . . . deprivation [of life, liberty, or property] when officials organize their activities so that people fall prey to private violence."[28] A constitutional rule, moreover, that punishes government misfeasance (when the state intentionally or negligently causes harm) but not nonfeasance (when the state simply does not act) provides an incentive to withhold services and interventions.[29] The rule requiring state action as a prior condition for judicial review, therefore, provides a limited and uninspired vision of the Constitution.

FEDERAL POWER TO ASSURE THE CONDITIONS FOR PUBLIC HEALTH

Article I, Section 1 of the Constitution endows Congress with the "legislative Powers herein granted," not with plenary legislative authority. The federal government must draw its authority to act from specific, enumerated powers. Thus, before an act of Congress is deemed constitutional, two questions must be asked: Does the

Constitution affirmatively authorize Congress to act, and does the exercise of that power improperly interfere with any constitutionally protected interest?

In theory, the United States is a government of limited powers, but the reality is quite different. The federal government possesses considerable authority to act and exerts extensive control in the realm of public health and safety. The Supreme Court, through an expansive interpretation of Congress's enumerated powers, has enabled the federal government to maintain a vast presence in public health in matters ranging from biomedical research and the provision of health care to the control of infectious diseases, occupational health and safety, and environmental protection.

Congress derives its sweeping powers, in part, from Article I, Section 8 of the Constitution: Congress may "make all Laws which shall be necessary and proper for carrying into Execution" all powers vested by the Constitution in the government of the United States. The Necessary and Proper Clause, the subject of many great debates in American history, incorporates within the Constitution the doctrine of implied powers. Thus, the federal government may employ all means reasonably appropriate to achieve the objectives of constitutionally enumerated national powers. Chief Justice Marshall's authoritative construction of the Necessary and Proper Clause in *McCulloch v. Maryland* suggests that Congress may use any reasonable means not prohibited by the Constitution to carry out its express powers: "Let the end be legitimate, let it be within the scope of the constitution, and all means which are appropriate, which are plainly adapted to that end, which are not prohibited, but consistent with the letter and spirit of the constitution, are constitutional."[30] The Constitution delegates diverse authority to the United States.[31] The foremost powers for public health purposes are the power to tax, spend, and regulate interstate commerce.

THE POWER TO TAX IS THE POWER TO RAISE REVENUE, REGULATE RISK BEHAVIOR, AND INDUCE HEALTH-PROMOTING BEHAVIORS

No attribute of sovereignty is more pervading [than taxation], and at no point does the power of government affect more constantly and intimately the relations of life than through the exactions made under it.
                        Thomas M. Cooley (1890)

Article I, Section 8 states that "[t]he Congress shall have Power To lay and collect Taxes, Duties, Imposts and Excises." On its face, the power to tax has a single, overriding purpose—to raise revenue to provide for the good of the community. Absent the ability to generate sufficient revenue, the legislature could not provide services such as transportation, education, medical services to the poor, sanitation, and environmental protection. Historically, constitutional constraints have been imposed on Congress's revenue-raising capacity. Drawing a distinction between direct taxes (imposed upon property) and indirect taxes (imposed on the performance of an act),[32] the Supreme Court, at the turn of the century, declared a federal income tax unconstitutional.[33] The Sixteenth Amendment, ratified in 1913, restored the federal income tax and made possible an almost limitless revenue-raising potential within the federal government.

The power to tax is closely aligned with the power to spend.[34] Economists regard congressional decisions to provide tax relief for certain activities as indirect expenditures because government is, in fact, subsidizing the activity from the national treasury. Economists project, for example, that favorable tax treatment afforded to employer-sponsored health care plans will cost the federal government $438 billion between the years 1999 and 2003.[35]

The taxing power, while affording government the financial resources to provide public health services, has another, equally important purpose. The power to tax is also the power to regulate risk behavior and influence health-promoting activities.[36] Virtually all taxes achieve ancillary regulatory effects by imposing an economic burden on the taxed activity or providing economic relief for certain kinds of private spending. Consequently, the tax code provides incentives and disincentives to perform, or to refrain from performing, certain acts. The more onerous the tax (in terms of the economic and administrative costs) or the more generous the tax relief, the more powerful the ancillary regulatory effects.

The taxing power is a primary means for achieving public health objectives. As Daniel Fox and Daniel Schaffer observe, "tax law and health policy come together" to affect fundamentally the health of the community.[37] Broadly speaking, the tax code influences health-related behavior through tax relief and tax burdens: tax relief encourages private, health-promoting activity and tax burdens discourage risk behavior.

Through various forms of tax relief (e.g., excluding benefits from taxable income, deducting spending from gross income, and providing credits against tax owed), government provides incentives for private activities that it views as advantageous to community health. Employer-sponsored health plans, for example, receive generous tax incentives. By excluding employer contributions for health benefits from federal and state taxable income,[38] the Internal Revenue Code "deeply affects how health care is provided in the United States, to whom it is provided, and who provides it."[39] Similarly, federal and state income and property tax exemptions afforded to the nonprofit sector demonstrate a distinct government preference for nonprofit over investor-owned health care institutions. Government preferences for nonprofit entities have significant effects on hospital care in America.[40] The tax code influences private health-related spending in many other ways: encouraging child care to enable parents to enter the work force;[41] inducing investment in low-income housing;[42] promoting clinical testing of pharmaceuticals for rare diseases;[43] and stimulating charitable spending for research and care in areas such as heart disease, cancer, and mental retardation.[44]

Public health taxation also regulates private behavior by economically penalizing risk-taking activities. Tax policy discourages a number of activities that government regards as unhealthy or dangerous.[45] Consider excise or manufacturing taxes on tobacco,[46] alcoholic beverages,[47] or firearms.[48] Tax policy also penalizes certain behavior regarded as "immoral," such as gambling.[49] Finally, tax policy influences individual and business decisions that adversely affect health or the environment; examples are taxes on gasoline[50] or on ozone-depleting chemicals[51] that contribute to environmental degradation. It is difficult to imagine a public health threat caused by human behavior or business activity that cannot be influenced by the taxing power.

The taxing power provides an independent source of federal legislative authority. Congress may regulate through the tax system for purposes that may not be authorized under its enumerated powers. The Supreme Court, in its early jurisprudence, was concerned about federal taxes that were designed to punish or regulate rather than to raise revenue. Thus, the Court distinguished between revenue-raising taxes, which it upheld, and purely regulatory taxes, which it found constitutionally troubling.[52] This distinction, however, has all but disappeared. For example, the Court has upheld federal taxes on firearms capable of being concealed and on persons who "deal in" or prescribe marijuana, stating that a "tax does not cease to be valid because it regulates, discourages, or even definitely deters the activities taxed."[53] Today, a federal tax is likely to be constitutional unless it requires behavior conformance extraneous to any tax need.[54]

The power to tax, then, is the power to govern. Taxes amass the resources necessary for public health services and provide an effective
regulatory mechanism for controlling individual and corporate behavior. Tax incentives and disincentives are powerful tools for promoting
or discouraging anything legislators deem important for the health and
well-being of the population.

THE POWER TO SPEND IS THE POWER TO ALLOCATE
RESOURCES AND TO INDUCE CONFORMANCE WITH
PUBLIC HEALTH STANDARDS

The powers to tax and spend both are found in the same constitutional
phrase of Article I, Section 8: "Congress shall have Power To lay and
collect Taxes . . . and provide for the common Defence and general
Welfare of the United States." The spending power provides Congress
with independent authority to allocate resources for the public good;
Congress need not justify its spending by reference to a specific enumerated power.[55] Closely connected to the power to tax, the spending
power has two purposes. First, it authorizes expenditures expressly for
the public's health, safety, and well-being. Secondly, it effectively induces state conformance with federal regulatory standards.

The power to spend is expressly to promote "general welfare," that
is, all reasonable public health purposes. Theoretically, the spending
power may be exercised only to pursue a common benefit, as distinguished from a local purpose, but Congress determines whether expenditures are for the common benefit, and the Supreme Court has historically concurred: "Nor is the concept of the general welfare static.
Needs that were narrow or parochial a century ago may be interwoven
in our day with the well-being of the Nation."[56] Laurence Tribe believes that such judicial deference is understandable "in an era lacking
any coherent theory of the public good as more than an aggregate of
private needs and wants."[57] Nonetheless, the Court is not well placed
to adopt any particular theory of governmental appropriation, or any
other inherently political function.

The spending power does not simply grant Congress the authority to
allocate resources; it is also an indirect regulatory device. Congress may
prescribe the terms upon which it disburses federal money to the states.
The conditional spending power is akin to a contract: In return for federal funds, the states agree to comply with federally imposed conditions.[58] The Supreme Court permits conditional appropriations, pro-

vided the conditions are clearly expressed in the statute[59] and a reasonable relationship exists between the condition imposed and the program's purposes.[60] If Congress wants states to conform to federally imposed standards to receive federal funds, it must say so clearly enough to permit the states to make an informed choice. Moreover, states must be cognizant of the consequences in advance of their participation in a federal grant program.[61]

The strings attached to federal resources must also bear some reasonable relationship to the purposes of the grant. The conditional spending cannot be so coercive as to pass the point at which "pressure turns into compulsion."[62] Despite these theoretical limits, the Supreme Court grants Congress substantial leeway and appears to search for permissible relationships between the appropriation and the conditions. For example, the Court saw a direct relationship between the appropriation of highway funds and the states' acceptance of a 21-year-old drinking age. Since a major purpose of highway funds is traffic safety, the drinking age limits were deemed constitutionally acceptable.[63]

Congress's power to set the terms upon which state appropriations shall be distributed is an effective regulatory device. States and localities can seldom afford to decline federal public health grants.[64] Congress and the federal agencies use conditional appropriations to induce states to conform to federal standards in numerous public health contexts. Federal funding programs for HIV/AIDS, for example, require involuntary postconviction testing of sex offenders,[65] adoption of CDC guidelines (or their "equivalent") for preventing transmission of infection during invasive medical procedures,[66] acceptance of CDC guidelines for counseling and testing of pregnant women,[67] and compliance with specific community planning and program priorities.[68] Conditional spending induces states to conform to federal regulatory requirements in other areas as well: eligibility and quality standards relating to Medicare and Medicaid;[69] prohibition on family-planning fund recipients from engaging in abortion counseling, referral, and activities advocating abortion as a method of family planning;[70] and state and local planning for land use and solid waste management.[71]

It is obvious from this discussion that the power to tax and spend is not value neutral, but rather is laden with political overtones. Collection of revenues and allocation of resources go to the very heart of the political process. Legislators, as influenced by the public and interest groups, purport to promote public health, safety, and security. Many of their economic decisions do promote the common good, such as taxes on cigarettes and expenditures for antismoking campaigns. But their vision is also influenced by moral, cultural, and social values so that government's economic power may be used to discourage abortions, fetal research, sex education, or needle exchange.

THE POWER TO CONTROL COMMERCE IS
THE POWER TO BROADLY REGULATE

The Commerce Clause, more than any other enumerated power, affords Congress potent regulatory authority. Article I, Section 8 states that "[t]he Congress shall have the power . . . to regulate Commerce with foreign Nations, and among the several states, and with the Indian Tribes." The Supreme Court's expansive construction of the Commerce Clause since Franklin Delano Roosevelt's New Deal has facilitated a marked increase in federal regulatory authority in public health matters.

On its face, the Commerce Clause is limited to controlling the flow of goods and services across state lines. Yet, as interstate commerce has become ubiquitous, activities once considered purely local have come to have national effects, and have, accordingly, come within Congress's commerce power.[72] The Court's post-1937 construction of "commerce among the states" has been broad—the commerce power has been described by the judiciary as "plenary" or all-embracing,[73] and has been exerted to affect virtually every aspect of social life.[74]

The broad interpretation of the Commerce Clause has enabled national authorities to reach deeply into traditional realms of state public health power, and has significantly diminished the force of the Tenth Amendment. The courts have upheld exercises of the Commerce Clause in the fields of environmental protection,[75] food and drug safety,[76] and other public health matters.[77] In Hodel v. Virginia Surface Mining & Reclamation Association (1981), for example, the Supreme Court sustained federal regulation of surface mining, even though regulation of land use is a traditional state function. Congress's intent was to prevent "hazards dangerous to life," such as soil erosion and water pollution, and to "conserve soil, water, and other natural resources."[78]

The Rehnquist Court has begun to rethink the Commerce Clause as part of its agenda of gradually returning power from the federal government to the states. In the process, the Court has held that Congress lacks the power to engage in social and public health regulation primarily affecting intrastate activities (see "New Federalism" below).

COOPERATIVE FEDERALISM

Where it has authority under the Commerce Clause, Congress may offer states the choice of either establishing regulatory schemes that reflect federal standards or having federal regulation preempt state law. This model, known as "cooperative federalism," is found in federal public health statutes concerning water quality,[79] occupational health and safety,[80] and conservation.[81] It is the predominant approach to federal-state relations in environmental law. Under this model, federal agencies (e.g., the EPA) establish minimum national standards, and states retain the choice to administer the federal standards themselves or have federal authorities implement national standards.[82]

THE DORMANT COMMERCE CLAUSE

The Commerce Clause, in addition to affording Congress considerable police power authority, implicitly limits the states' public health power. The Dormant Commerce Clause limits state authority to regulate in ways that place an undue burden on interstate commerce. Thus, even if Congress has not entered a field of public health, states may not regulate if doing so obstructs commerce among the states. The Supreme Court has a history of invalidating state public health legislation on Dormant Commerce Clause grounds. Thus, the Court has struck down state or local police power regulation involving milk sales;[83] liquor taxes;[84] groundwater use;[85] and solid,[86] liquid,[87] or hazardous[88] waste disposal and processing. The Constitution, therefore, does not simply empower Congress to control "commerce among the states" but implicitly limits state public health authority that unduly burdens interstate commerce.

THE FEDERAL PRESENCE IN PUBLIC HEALTH

Historically, public health functions have been the responsibility of the states. From modest beginnings, the federal presence in public health has grown steadily. In 1798 President John Adams signed a law creating the first Marine Hospital as part of the United States Marine Hospital Services (USMHS) with a mandate to care for ailing seamen.[89] Three-quarters of a century later, in 1862, a Bureau of Chemistry was founded; it eventually led to the creation of the Food and Drug

TABLE I
THE FEDERAL AGENCY ROLE IN PUBLIC HEALTH

U.S. Department	Agency/Administration	Date/Authority		Public Health Function
HHS	Health and Human Services (www.hhs.gov)	1953 1980	HEW est. HHS est.	Principal agency for protecting the health of all Americans and providing essential human services
	Public Health Service (phs.os.dhhs.gov/phs/phs.html)	1798 1902 1912 1995	Marine Hospital Service est. Public Health and Marine Hospital Service est. Public Health Service est. Reorganized (Fed. Reg. 60, No. 217)	Public Health Service agencies comprise many of the operating divisions of DHHS, and the PHS Commissioned Corps assigns health officers to other agencies
	Administration on Aging (www.aoa.gov)	1961 1965	First White House Conference on Aging Admin. on Aging est. under the Older Americans Act (amended in 42 USC 3001 et seq.)	Provides policy and program leadership on aging to the federal government; develops programs for the aging; and collects, analyzes, and disseminates information on aging
	Administration for Children and Families (www.acf.gov)	1991	Est. under § 6 of Reorganization Plan No. 1 of 1953	Provides executive direction and guidance relating to issues surrounding children and families
	Agency for Health Research and Quality (www.ahrq.gov)	1989	Est., reorganized Oct. 31, 1995 (42 USC 299)	Provides resources for research designed to improve the quality of health care

Agency for Toxic Substances and Disease Registry (www.atsdr.cdc.gov)	1980	Est.	Aims to prevent exposure and subsequent harmful effects from hazardous substances in the environment
	1986	Received additional responsibilities with passage of Superfund Amendments and Reauthorization Act, reorganized Oct. 31, 1995	
Centers for Disease Control and Prevention (www.cdc.gov)	1942	Office of National Defense Malaria Control Activities est.	Provides leadership and coordination in efforts to prevent and control diseases and unhealthy conditions, and responds to health emergencies
	1942	Office of Typhus Fever health Control est.	
	1946	Communicable Disease Center est.	
	1970	Centers for Disease Control est.	
	1973	Est., reorganized Oct. 31, 1995	
Food and Drug Administration (www.fda.gov)	1862	Bureau of Chemistry est.	Ensures that food, drugs, cosmetics, and medical devices are safe and effective
	1907	Food and Drug Act passed	
	1931	FDA est. under the Agriculture Appropriation Act (46 Stat. 392), reorganized Oct. 31, 1995	
Health Care Financing Administration (www.hcfa.hha.gov)	1977	Est.	Serves the elderly, disabled, and poor Americans through the administration and oversight of the Medicare and Medicaid programs
Health Resources and Services Administration (www.hrsa.gov)	1995	Est. as an operating division within HHS	Makes essential primary care services available to underserved populations

(continued)

TABLE 1 *(continued)*

U.S. Department	Agency/Administration	Date/Authority		Public Health Function
Health Resources and Services Administration (www.hrsa.gov)	Indian Health Service (www.ihs.gov)	1787	Federal govt. to Indian tribal govt. relationship est. to provide health services to federally recognized tribes	Provides health services to American Indians and Native Alaskans, while including tribal involvement in managing health needs
		1995	Est. as an operating division within HHS	
	National Institutes of Health (www.nih.gov)	1887	Est. one-room laboratory for disease research	Serves as the principal biomedical research agency, supporting research and development
	Substance Abuse and Mental Health Services Administration (www.samhsa.gov)	1992	Est.	Works to improve access to programs and services for individuals, families, and communities who are at risk or suffer from mental disorders
USDA	Food Safety and Inspection Service (www.fsis.usda.gov)	1981	Est. (5 USC 301)	Regulates the meat and poultry industry to ensure safety and accurate labeling
	Food, Nutrition and Consumer Services (www.fns.usda.gov/fns)	1969	Est. (5 USC 301)	Ensures access to nutritious, healthy diets, and nutrition education
DOL	Occupational Safety and Health Administration (www.osha.gov)	1970	Est. under the Occupational Safety and Health Act (29 USC 651 et seq.)	Develops and enforces safety and health standards and regulations in the workplace

	Mine Safety and Health Administration (www.msha.gov)	1969	Est. under the Federal Coal Mine Health and Safety Act (30 USC 801 et seq.)	Develops safety and health standards, promotes research, and aims to prevent mine accidents and occupational diseases in the mining industry
EPA	Environmental Protection Agency (www.epa.gov)	1970	Est. under the reorganization plan No. 3 (5 USC app)	Created to coordinate and provide effective governmental action on behalf of the environment
SSA	Social Security Administration (www.ssa.gov)	1935	Social Security Act passed	Manages the nation's social insurance program; administers the Supplemental Security Income program for the aged, blind, and disabled; and recommends methods for solving the problem of poverty
		1946	SSA est. under the reorganization plan no. 2 (5 USC app)	
		1994	Became an independent agency (42 USC 901)	
FEMA	Federal Emergency Management Agency (www.fema.gov)	1979	Est.	Coordinates activities to ensure a broad-based effort to protect life and property and provide assistance after a disaster

Administration.[90] In 1887 the USMHS established a one-room labora-tory on Staten Island that would later become the National Institutes of Health.[91] In 1912 the USMHS was reorganized into the United States Public Health Service (USPHS). Among its other responsibilities in the nineteenth century, the USPHS performed public health functions, such as imposing and enforcing quarantine regulations in immigration.[92] In the years following the New Deal, Congress greatly expanded the fed-eral presence in public health. The Social Security Act of 1935 began to address problems of poverty and its harmful health effects, and the Federal Security Agency was established in 1939 to deal with health, education, social insurance, and human services.[93] In 1946, the Communicable Disease Center was founded, which later became the Centers for Disease Control and Prevention (CDC).[94]

The Department of Health, Education, and Welfare (HEW), created in 1953, incorporated the USPHS. Since then, advancements in public health have continued. The 1960s saw the creation of Medicare and Medicaid, the Head Start program, and the Administration on Aging. In 1970 the National Health Service Corps was established, and by 1977 the Health Care Financing Administration (part of HEW) as-sumed the administration of the Medicare and Medicaid programs from the Social Security Administration. In 1979 a reorganization split HEW into the Department of Education and the future Department of Health and Human Services. What began in the eighteenth century as a Marine hospital has grown into a massive federal presence in the area of health.

The modern role of the federal government in public health is broad and complex. Public health functions, which include public funding for health care, safe food, effective drugs, clean water, a beneficial envi-ronment, and prevention services, can be found in an array of agencies. The bulk of all health responsibilities lies with the Department of Health and Human Services and its many subparts. However, the Department of Agriculture, the Department of Labor, and the Envi-ronmental Protection Agency, to name a few, also have important pub-lic health functions (for an overview, see Table 1). As the United States has garnered more resources (principally through a national income tax) and as the Supreme Court has permitted direct and indirect regu-lation (under the powers to tax, spend, and control commerce), the fed-eral presence in public health has grown. Today, it is nearly impossible to find a field of public health that is not heavily influenced by United States government policy.

STATE AND LOCAL POWER TO ASSURE
THE CONDITIONS FOR PUBLIC HEALTH

salus populi est suprema lex

Despite a contemporary federal presence, the states and localities have had the predominant public responsibility for population-based health services since the founding of the republic. Even today, the states account for the majority of traditional public health spending, including the kinds of population-based services discussed in chapter 1, but excluding funding for personal medical services and for the environment. Early public health law employed a legal maxim that embodied the intrinsic purposes of a sovereign government: *Salus populi est suprema lex*—the welfare of the people is the supreme law.[95] *Salus populi* demonstrates the close connection between state power and historic understandings of the public's well-being. From a constitutional perspective, there exist historic wellsprings of state authority to protect the common good—the police power to protect the public's health, safety, and morals and the *parens patriae* power to defend the interests of persons unable to secure their own interests.

POLICE POWERS: REGULATION FOR
HEALTH, SAFETY, AND MORALS

sic utere tuo ut alienum non laedas

OF OFFENCES AGAINST THE PUBLIC HEALTH, AND
THE PUBLIC POLICE OR ŒCONOMY. [A] species of
offences, more especially affecting the commonwealth,
are such as are against the public health of the nation;
a concern of the highest importance. . . . By public
police and œconomy I mean the due regulation and
domestic order of the kingdom: whereby individuals of
the state, like members of a well-governed family, are
bound to conform their general behaviour to the rules
of propriety, good neighbourhood, and good manners;
and to be decent, industrious, and inoffensive in their
respective stations.

William Blackstone (1769)

The "police power" is the most famous expression of the natural authority of sovereign governments to regulate private interests for the public good. I define police power as

The inherent authority of the state (and, through delegation, local government) to enact laws and promulgate regulations to protect, preserve, and promote the health, safety, morals, and general welfare of the people. To achieve these communal benefits, the state retains the power to restrict, within federal and state constitutional limits, private interests—personal interests in autonomy, privacy, association, and liberty as well as economic interests in freedom to contract and uses of property (see Figure 5).

The linguistic and historical origins of the concept of "police" demonstrate a close association between government and civilization: *politia* (the state), *polis* (city), and *politeia* (citizenship).[96] "Police" traditionally connoted social organization, civil authority, or formation of a political community—the control and regulation of affairs affecting the general order and welfare of society.[97] Such was the context in which Hamilton used the term in the *Federalist Papers,* to suggest civil peace and public law.[98] "Police" was meant to describe those powers that permitted sovereign government to control its citizens, particularly for the purpose of promoting the general comfort, health, morals, safety, or prosperity of the public.[99] The word had a secondary usage as well: cleansing or keeping clean. This use resonates with early twentieth-century public health connotations of hygiene and sanitation.

The police power represents the state's authority to further the goal of all government, to promote the general welfare of society.[100] States possess the police power as an innate attribute of sovereignty. As sovereign governments before the formation of the United States, the states still retain sovereignty except as surrendered under the Constitution.[101] Part of the constitutional compact of our Union was that states would remain free to govern within the traditional sphere of health, safety, and morals. All states, to a greater or lesser degree, delegate police powers to local government: counties, parishes, cities, towns, or villages.[102]

The definition of "police power" encompasses three principles: The governmental purpose is to promote the public good; the state authority to act permits the restriction of private interests; and the scope of state powers is pervasive. States exercise police powers to ensure that communities live in safety and security, in conditions conducive to good health, with moral standards, and, generally speaking, without unreasonable interference in human well-being. Police powers legitimize state action to protect and promote broadly defined social goods.

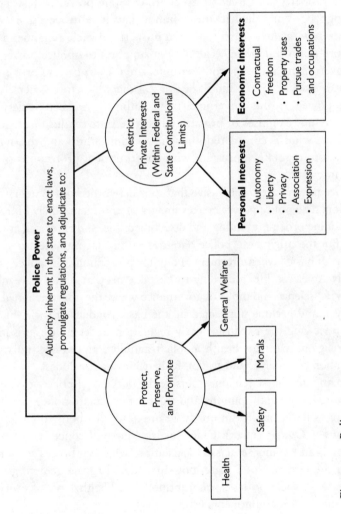

Figure 5. Police power.

Government, in order to achieve common goods, is empowered to enact legislation, regulate, and adjudicate in ways that necessarily limit, or even eliminate, private interests. Thus, government has inherent power to interfere with personal interests in autonomy, privacy, association, and liberty as well as economic interests in ownership, uses of private property, and freedom to contract. State power to restrict private rights is embodied in the common law maxim *sic utere tuo ut alienum non laedas*—"use your own property in such a manner as not to injure that of another." The maxim supports the police power, giving government authority to determine safe uses of private property to diminish risks of injury and ill health to others.[103] More generally, the police power affords government the authority to keep society free from noxious exercises of private rights. The state retains discretion to determine what is considered injurious or unhealthful and the manner in which to regulate, consistent with constitutional protections of personal interests.

Police powers are so pervasive that they defy orderly or systematic description. The police power evokes images of an organized civil force for maintaining order, preventing and detecting crime, and enforcing criminal laws. But the origins of "police" are deeper and far more textured than notions of basic law enforcement and crime prevention. The police power in early American life, according to Novak, was part of a well-regulated society, a "science and mode of governance where the polity assumed control over, and became implicated in, the basic conduct of social life."[104] After reviewing the expansive early regulation under police jurisdiction (e.g., religion, manners, health, public tranquility and safety, transportation, labor, commerce, and trade), Robert Novak concludes, "No aspect of human intercourse remained outside the purview of police science."[105]

Countless judicial opinions and treatises articulate police powers as a deep well of public authority granted to the body politic.[106] In *Gibbons v. Ogden* (1824), Chief Justice Marshall conceived of police powers as an "immense mass of legislation, which embraces every thing within the territory of a state, not surrendered to the general government. . . . Inspection laws, quarantine laws, health laws of every description . . . are components of this mass."[107]

Police powers in the context of public health include all law and regulation directly or indirectly intended to improve morbidity and mortality in the population. Police powers have enabled states and their subsidiary municipal corporations to promote and preserve public health in areas ranging from injury and disease prevention [108] to sanitation, waste disposal, and clean water and air.[109] Police powers exercised by the states include vaccination,[110] isolation and quarantine,[111] inspection of commercial and residential premises,[112] abatement of unsanitary conditions or other health nuisances,[113] regulation of air and surface water contaminants as well as restriction of public access to polluted areas,[114] standards for pure food and drinking water,[115] extermination of vermin,[116] fluoridization of municipal water supplies,[117] and licensure of physicians and other health care professionals.[118]

The courts have often used the police power as a rough sorting device to separate authority rightfully retained by the states from that appropriately exercised by the federal government. If the authority exercised was traditionally part of the corpus of police powers, states, at least presumptively, were thought to have a valid claim of jurisdiction. Although the extent of permissible state public health regulation has not been easy to measure, a state's power is "never greater than in matters traditionally of local concern" to the health and safety of its population.[119] Courts in many contexts, such as the quality standards for meat,[120] fruits, and vegetables,[121] have emphasized the legitimacy of state authority. Even in assessing express federal preemption, courts acknowledge that police powers are "primarily, and historically, . . . matters of local concern."[122] Thus, the judiciary adopts a presumption that "the historic police powers of the States [are] not to be superseded by the Federal Act unless that was the clear and manifest purpose of Congress."[123]

PARENS PATRIAE POWERS: STATE POWER TO PROTECT CHILDREN AND INCOMPETENT PERSONS

This prerogative of *parens patriae* is inherent in the
Supreme power of every state, whether that power is
lodged in a royal person, or in the legislature . . . [and] is
a most beneficent function . . . often necessary to be exercised in the interests of humanity, and for the prevention
of injury to those who cannot protect themselves.
                              Joseph P. Bradley (1890)

Parens patriae—literally, parent of the country—refers to the state's role as sovereign and as the guardian of persons under legal disability (principally minors and incompetent persons).[124] *Parens patriae* powers derive from the Royal Prerogative in England, which arose in the early years of Edward I (1275–1306).[125] The *Statute de Prerogativa Regis*[126] recognized the existence of the Prerogative and imposed limits on its operation: "The King shall have the custody of the lands of natural fools, taking the profits of them without waste or destruction, and shall find them their necessaries." It was the job of the crown "to take care of people legally unable, on account of mental incapacity, whether it proceed[ed] from 1. nonage 2. idiocy or 3. lunacy: to take proper care of themselves and their property."[127]

In America, the *parens patriae* function belongs to the states, which have the power to protect and care for those who cannot care for themselves. The *parens patriae* power is traditionally invoked in two contexts: to make decisions on behalf of individuals who are incapable of doing so for themselves,[128] and to assert the state's general interest and standing in communal health, comfort, and welfare (see Figure 6).[129]

The state, as *parens patriae*, has the authority to protect the welfare of persons who are unable to understand the nature and consequences of their decisions and who require protection in their own interests (e.g., minors, comatose or incompetent patients, the mentally ill, and the mentally retarded). The *parens patriae* power is used in diverse contexts, including custody and other decisions relating to children;[130] guardianship over money, property, and personal affairs;[131] treatment decisions for incompetent, terminally ill patients; and civil commitment of persons with mental illness.[132]

The exercise of *parens patriae* powers in this individualized context can deprive individuals of autonomy, privacy, and liberty: "[A]n inevitable consequence of exercising the *parens patriae* power is that the ward's personal freedom will be substantially restrained, whether a guardian is appointed to control his property, he is placed in the custody of a private third party, or committed to an institution."[133] Consequently, courts adopt legal standards and processes for decision-making to safeguard individuals' interests,[134] and require fair and nondiscriminatory treatment.[135] Depending upon the circumstance, the legal standards adopted may be either the person's best interests (the decision that would best secure the individual's welfare) or substituted judgment (the decision the person would have made were she competent to decide for herself).[136] Courts also require procedural due process, depending upon the context and the potential burden on individual interests.[137] Because of the potential for diminution of individual rights, then, courts adopt standards and procedures to ensure that the state's *parens patriae* powers, intended to be wielded beneficently, do not inflict harm.

The *parens patriae* function is asserted not only to protect incompetent individuals, but also to safeguard the general community interest in health,

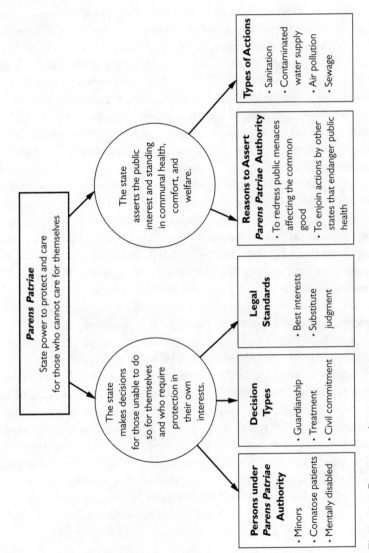

Figure 6. *Parens patriae* power.

welfare, and economic benefit. This meaning of *parens patriae* is quite different from the first; it is a concept used to describe a state's standing or right to sue in court, to promote the communal interest. The legal theory is that the state litigates to defend the well-being of its citizens, not to defend the economic interests of the state. A state's ability to bring an action under the doctrine of *parens patriae* is not conditioned upon whether private individuals in that state would have standing to bring suit.[138] As a result, a state can redress public menaces in situations where private individuals would be unable to sue because of a lack of specific injury. Likewise, in situations where a state cannot legislate or institute a regulatory scheme to protect its citizens, it can sue in federal court under the *parens patriae* doctrine to enjoin another state from actions that pose a threat to health or welfare (e.g., where polluted water from another state threatens the health of its citizens).[139] At the turn of the century, the Supreme Court accepted this understanding of the *parens patriae* power in a quarantine case,[140] setting in motion a chain of litigation dealing with matters of public health: sanitation,[141] water supply,[142] air pollution,[143] and sewage.[144]

For a state to maintain a *parens patriae* action, it must have an interest separate from that of private parties;[145] that is, a state cannot enter a controversy as a nominal party to forward claims of individual citizens.[146] However, if a state is pursuing its own interests and, in the process, advances the interests of others, it can sue in *parens patriae*. The state's interests are expressed as "quasi-sovereign," which are those interests that a state has in the well-being of its populace; the state's interests must be sufficiently concrete to engender a conflict between the state and a defendant. A state's "quasi-sovereign" interests have two general characteristics: (1) they must affect the economic or physical health and well-being of its residents, and (2) a state has an interest in not being discriminated against and denied its rightful status in the federal system. Although the courts have not delineated a quantifiable formula for determining what part of a state's population must be affected to reach a substantial segment and, therefore, trigger *parens patriae*, a state in making its claim is allowed to consider, in addition to direct harm, the indirect effects on its population.[147]

The state's ultimate goal in utilizing *parens patriae* is to protect individuals who are unable to protect themselves. An example of a *parens patriae* action in the area of public health was an action brought by the state of New York to redress the denial of a zoning approval for a residence for homeless persons living with HIV/AIDS.[148] The "quasi-sovereign" interest alleged by the state was the damage to its population's health and welfare by the denial of benefits that a residential care facility would provide. The population affected appeared to be the small number of people who would reside in the facility. However, the court felt that these kinds of policies would indirectly affect an ever-larger population of HIV-infected individuals who would be denied care. Thus, the court agreed that New York State had *parens patriae* standing to litigate on behalf of the health and welfare of its HIV-infected population. Although holdings of this sort may infringe on the liberty of some, the result of the *parens patriae* doctrine is to create a safer environment for those citizens who cannot provide for themselves, as well as for the society at large.

NEW FEDERALISM: PUBLIC HEALTH IN THE AMERICAN FEDERALIST SYSTEM

This nation has long struggled with the problem of attaining the proper balance of powers between the federal government and the states. This problem is particularly acute in matters of public health because both levels of government want to be seen as responding to the electorate's concerns about health and safety. States and localities are closer to the people and understand better threats to their health. Because they are closer to the community, they can adapt prevention strategies to meet the needs of localities. States also are better placed to experiment with solutions to complex health problems. By permitting states to act as laboratories for innovative health policies, the federalist system can, in theory, sort out effective from less effective interventions. The federal government, on the other hand, has greater resources and scientific expertise with which to tackle complicated health policy problems. Many public health problems, moreover, transcend state borders, such as pollution, infectious disease, and traffic hazards. Other public health problems are so worrying or pervasive that they demand a national response (e.g., mass firearm fatalities in schools).

It would be comforting to think that the struggles between federal and state public health authorities have been resolved by force of logic (i.e., by systematically determining which level of government is likely to be more effective in reducing health threats). The reality, however, is that this struggle has been fought more on political than policy grounds. The Supreme Court, moreover, has dramatically shifted its stance as the ideological composition of the Court has changed.

In the early twentieth century (the so-called *Lochner* era; see chapter 3), the Court carved out a zone of state power that could not be infringed by national authorities. During this era, a politically conservative Court found the freedom of contract to be a fundamental "economic" right under the Due Process Clause, and struck down a great deal of social and economic regulation.[149] Franklin Delano Roosevelt's New Deal ushered in a period in which the Court granted Congress expansive powers. Indeed, from 1937 to 1995, the Supreme Court did not find a single piece of social or economic legislation unconstitutional on the basis that Congress had exceeded its Commerce Clause authority.[150]

In the most recent manifestation of the federalism debate, the Rehnquist Court has explored the contours of a "new federalism" where states retain a sphere of autonomy in matters of public health.[151] A reenergized majority on the Supreme Court, led by Justices Rehnquist and Scalia, has been actively recentering the balance between national and state power.[152] The Rehnquist Court has implemented its interpretation of a states-rights agenda in three ways: limiting federal commerce powers, expanding state reserved powers, and undertaking a sustained defense of state sovereign immunity.

THE COMMERCE POWER REVISITED

The Supreme Court's 1995 decision in *United States v. Lopez*[153] signaled a change in the Court's view about the balance of federal and state powers in the constitutional design.[154] In *Lopez*, the Court held that Congress exceeded its Commerce Clause authority by making gun possession within a school zone a federal offense. Concluding that possessing a gun within a school zone did not "substantially affect" interstate commerce, the Court declared the statute unconstitutional. Here is a case where the nation's highest court invalidated a politically popular measure thought to be important to the public's safety. The Court did not invalidate this legislation on grounds that regulating guns in school zones was an unimportant aim of government, but only that it was outside the reach of the federal government. States would still be free to legislate in traditional realms of public health, but *Lopez* left little doubt that the Rehnquist Court would henceforth examine the exercise of federal police power authority.

Lopez probably does not indicate a wholesale retreat from the liberal interpretation of the Commerce Clause. Certainly, Congress will continue to have wide power to regulate businesses and individuals when they engage in explicitly economic or commercial activity. Courts in the post-*Lopez* era have found social and public health activities to "substantially affect" interstate commerce in fields ranging from access to abortion clinics[155] and firearm control[156] to environmental cleanups[157] and protection of endangered species.[158] For example, in 2000 the Supreme Court upheld, on

Commerce Clause grounds, the Drivers Privacy Protection Act, which restricts the state's ability to disclose personal information in drivers' licenses. Because driver information is an article of commerce, the Court found that its sale or release into the interstate stream of business is sufficient to support congressional regulation.[159]

The important question *Lopez* leaves open is the constitutionality of social and public health regulation of intrastate activity. A wide range of public health regulation remains vulnerable to Commerce Clause attacks. For example, in 2000 the Supreme Court invalidated the private civil remedy provision of the Violence Against Women Act as an unconstitutional exercise of the commerce power. The act created a civil rights remedy, permitting survivors to bring federal lawsuits against perpetrators of sexually motivated crimes of violence. Congress proclaimed that violence impairs women's abilities to work, harms businesses, and increases national health care costs. However, the Court found that the gender-motivated crimes of violence are primarily state and local concerns.[160] Additionally, Commerce Clause challenges threaten important environmental regulations.[161] For example, the Court accepted a new and potentially far-reaching case about federal authority in its 2001 term. The new case, *Solid Waste Agency v. U.S. Army Corps of Engineers,* is a challenge to federal juristiction under the Clean Water Act over isolated wetlands.

RESERVED POWERS REVISITED

In *New York v. United States* (1992), the Supreme Court, for only the second time in more than half a century,[162] struck down a federal statute as violating the Tenth Amendment.[163] Congress had enacted monetary and other incentives to induce states to provide for disposal of radioactive waste generated within their borders. To ensure effective action, if a state was unable to dispose of its own waste, it was required under the statute to "take title" and possession of the waste. The Court invalidated the "take title" provision because the Constitution does not confer upon Congress the ability to "commandeer the legislative processes of the States by directly compelling them to enact and enforce a federal regulatory program." According to the Court, although Congress may exercise its legislative authority directly over private persons or businesses, it lacks the power to compel states to regulate according to the federal standards. Congress, of course, may offer incentives to the states to influence their policy choices, through, for instance, conditional spending or cooperative federalism. In both of these two methods, however, the electorate retains the ultimate authority to decide whether the state will comply. By contrast, where national authorities direct the state to regulate, state officials "bear the brunt of public disapproval, while the federal officials who devised the regulatory program may remain insulated from the electoral ramifications of their decision."[164]

In 1997 the Supreme Court used its reasoning in *New York v. United States* to overturn provisions in the Brady Handgun Violence Prevention Act, which directed state and local law enforcement officers to conduct background checks on prospective handgun purchasers.[165] The *New York* Court held that state legislatures are not subject to federal direction. In the Brady handgun case, the Court held that federal authorities may not supplant the state executive branch. In this instance, Congress did not require the state to make policy, but only to assist in implementing the federal law. The Court rejected the distinction between "making" law or policy on the one hand and merely enforcing or implementing it on the other hand.

As a result of the *New York* and Brady handgun cases, the Tenth Amendment has become a vehicle for challenging federal statutes that compel state legislative or administrative action. In an era of "new federalism," a body of public health law may be vulnerable to challenges on Tenth Amendment grounds—for example, environmental regulations that direct states to adopt or enforce a federal regulatory scheme.

STATE SOVEREIGN IMMUNITY REVISITED

The Eleventh Amendment grants states immunity from certain law suits in federal court without the state's consent.[166] Known as "sovereign immunity," this doctrine is highly important to states' autonomy because it limits Congress's power to authorize private law suits against states.[167] In *Seminole Tribe of Florida v. Florida*[168] (a case of great importance in American federalism decided in 1996), the Supreme Court held that Congress lacks the power, when acting under the Commerce Clause, to abrogate the states' sovereign immunity in federal court. This means that the federal government may not authorize private individuals to sue states.

The Rehnquist Court perceives the states' immunity from suit to be a fundamental precept of sovereignty: "Federalism requires that Congress accord States the respect and dignity due them as residuary sovereigns and joint participants in the Nation's governance."[169] The Court finished its 1998/99 term with three decisions that demonstrate its profound commitment to state sovereignty in the national constitutional system. The most far-reaching of the three cases declared for the first time that states cannot be sued, without their consent, by private parties in the state's own courts for violations of federal law.[170] The other two cases nullified congressional abrogations of state Eleventh Amendment immunity from suits in federal courts for patent infringement[171] and for product misrepresentation.[172]

In 2000 the Court continued to limit federal powers under the sovereign immunity doctrine. Notably, the Court decided that the federal government may not authorize suits against the states under the Age Discrimination in Employment Act (ADEA).[173] The federal courts are also struggling with important public health cases, such as whether persons with disabilities may sue states for violation of the Americans with Disabilities Act (ADA)[174] or the Individuals with Disabilities Education Act (IDEA).[175]

With these decisions on national commerce powers, state reserved powers, and state sovereign immunity, the Rehnquist Court has been defending traditional states' rights against federal political domination.[176] Beyond the jurisprudential debate about the most appropriate level of government in a federal system lies an important question about the population's health and safety. If the states do not act effectively or uniformly to reduce health threats such as firearms, cigarettes, or pollution, will the judiciary permit national authorities to exercise a police function? The current political thrust evident in the judiciary may impede the federal government's power to act for the health of the population.[177] At the same time, an activist court is invalidating social legislation enacted through the democratic process, not to safeguard individual liberty, but to pursue an ideal of governance that is much disputed within the nation.

CONCLUSION

The constitutional design is complex, seeking a balance between federal and state power (federalism); legislative, executive, and judicial power (separation of powers); and government authority and individual liberties (limited government). In this chapter, I have explored federalism and separation of powers, both of which pose intriguing problems in the context of public health. Much of the history of public health, however, involves earnest debate over the relationship between the power of government and the freedom of individuals. How much power should we afford government to act for the collective good? How important are individual values in liberty, privacy, association, and expression, or economic values in control of property and freedom of contract? How shall we balance personal liberty and business interests against communal goods of health, safety, and wellbeing? These are the tasks that I turn to in the next chapter.

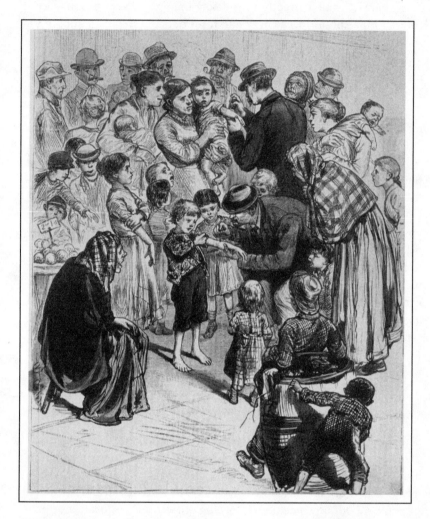

An 1800s engraving depicting smallpox vaccination in Jersey City, New Jersey: a street scene during the smallpox scare. By 1905, in *Jacobson v. Massachusetts*, the Supreme Court would find compulsory smallpox vaccination constitutional.

3 Constitutional Limits on the Exercise of Public Health Powers

Safeguarding Individual Rights and Freedoms

[T]he very existence of government presupposes the right of the sovereign power to prescribe regulations demanded by the general welfare for the common protection of all. This principle inheres in the very nature of the social compact. . . . This power of government, the power, as expressed by Taney, C.J., "inherent in every sovereignty, the power to govern men and things," is not, however, uncontrollable or despotic authority, subject to no limitation, exercisable with or without reason in the discretion or at the whim or caprice of the legislative body. . . . [The constitutional guaranty] was designed for the protection of personal and private rights against encroachments by the legislative body . . . as held and understood when the Constitution was adopted.

John A. Andrews (1889)

Personal coercion and economic regulation remain staples of public health practice in America.[1] Throughout most of the major infectious disease epidemics—smallpox, tuberculosis, and sexually transmitted diseases (STDs)—health officials have resorted to compulsory programs of testing, vaccination, physical examination, treatment, isolation, and quarantine. Government agencies license health care providers, inspect food establishments, regulate food and drugs, set standards for occupational health and safety, control pollutants, and abate nuisances. Even the most cursory examination of public health practice reveals the extensive forms of personal coercion and economic regulation that pervade society. I am not suggesting that coercion and regulation are the preferred strategies for ameliorating health threats. Nevertheless, any careful discussion of public health law must confront the inevitability of governmental exercise of power, as well as the potential trade-offs between personal freedom and the common good.

What limits exist on government powers to restrict personal and economic interests in the search for a healthy society? Chapter 2 examined the powers of the federal government (through the authority to tax, spend, and control commerce) and the states and localities (through the police and *parens patriae* powers) to protect the public's health. This chapter, and much of the remainder of this book, examine the *limitations* on government power to protect public health. That is, under what circumstances may the government interfere with a person's autonomy, privacy, liberty, or property to achieve health benefits for the population as a whole?

PUBLIC HEALTH AND THE BILL OF RIGHTS

The Bill of Rights, the first ten amendments to the Constitution, was ratified by the states in 1791. The first eight amendments guarantee certain fundamental rights and freedoms.[2] Table 2 describes each amendment in the Bill of Rights, presents selected public health issues relating to those amendments, and gives the holdings of one or more public health cases. Although constitutional provisions apart from the Bill of Rights safeguard personal liberties,[3] they are not highly relevant to public health. The Bill of Rights is directed to the federal government, but the Supreme Court has found that most of the Bill of Rights applies to the states as well by virtue of the Fourteenth Amendment.[4] Some constitutional rights, such as the Second Amendment's right to bear arms,[5] apply only to the federal government and not to the states.[6]

THE PUBLIC/PRIVATE DISTINCTION IN PUBLIC HEALTH: PROBLEMS AND ILLUSTRATIONS

The Constitution prohibits government, at every level, from invading certain fundamental rights and freedoms. However, the Constitution does not constrain merely private conduct, however discriminatory or wrongful.[7] The public/private distinction in constitutional law may, at first, appear straightforward. However, the activities of governmental, private ("for profit" and charitable), and community actors are frequently intertwined in public health; it is quite difficult in some cases to separate public from purely private behavior.

Any affirmative measure taken by a branch of government constitutes "state action" (e.g., public health laws enacted by the legislature, regulations

TABLE 2
PUBLIC HEALTH AND THE BILL OF RIGHTS

Selected Public Health Issues	Selected Public Health Cases*
First Amendment: Freedom of religion, speech, press, assembly, petition	
Religious exemption to vaccination	*Mason*[1]—upholding religious exemption to mandatory vaccination
Advertising restrictions (e.g., cigarettes, alcoholic beverages)	*44 Liquormart*[2]—ban on advertising the price of alcoholic beverages held unconstitutional
Closure of bath houses	*St. Marks*[3]—upholding closure of private bath houses as a public health nuisance
Second Amendment: Right to keep and bear arms	
Gun control legislation	*Fresno Rifle & Pistol Club*[4]—upholding regulation of gun manufacture and sale
Third Amendment: Right to refuse to quarter soldiers in home	
Not directly applicable to public health	
Fourth Amendment: Freedom from unreasonable search and seizure	
Compulsory testing and screening (e.g., drug, alcohol, HIV testing)	*Skinner*[5]—upholding drug tests following train accidents
Inspection of premises/administrative searches	*Camara*[6]—routine housing and building code inspections require search warrants
Fifth Amendment: Due process, equal protection of the law, and "just compensation" for private property taken for public use	
Public health regulation that deprives a person of liberty or property must provide procedural due process	*Greene*[7]—fair procedures for quarantine *Addington*[8]—fair procedures for civil commitment of the mentally ill *Goldberg*[9]—fair procedures for denial of welfare benefits
Public health regulation must not be arbitrary or discriminatory	*Jacobson*[10]—compulsory vaccination is a legitimate use of state's police power
Just compensation for land use restrictions for environmental and other public health purposes	*Lucas*[11]—landowner entitled to "just compensation" for environmental land use restrictions that deprived land of all value

(continued)

TABLE 2 *(continued)*

Sixth Amendment: Right to speedy and public trial by an impartial jury in criminal prosecution

Not directly applicable to public health

Seventh Amendment: Trial by jury in civil cases

Not directly applicable to public health

Eighth Amendment: Prohibition against excessive bail or fines, or cruel and unusual punishment

Not directly applicable to public health

*Some of the cases listed were decided under the Fourteenth Amendment, which incorporates many provisions in the Bill of Rights to the states.

1. Mason v. General Brown Cent. Sch. Dist., 851 F.2d 47 (2d Cir. 1988). See chapter 7.
2. 44 Liquormart, Inc. v. Rhode Island, 517 U.S. 484 (1996). See chapter 6.
3. City of New York v. New St. Mark's Baths, 562 N.Y.S.2d 642 (N.Y.A.D. 1 Dept., 1990). See chapter 9.
4. Fresno Rifle & Pistol Club, Inc. v. Van de Kamp, 965 F.2d 723 (9th Cir. 1992). See chapter 3.
5. Skinner v. Railway Labor Executives' Ass'n, 489 U.S. 602 (1989). See chapter 7.
6. Camara v. Municipal Court of the City & County of San Francisco, 387 U.S. 523 (1967). See chapter 9.
7. Greene v. Edwards, 263 S.E. 2d 662 (W. Va. 1980). See chapter 8.
8. Addington v. Texas, 441 U.S. 418 (1979). See chapter 8.
9. Goldberg v. Kelly, 397 U.S. 254 (1970). See chapter 3.
10. Jacobson v. Massachusetts, 197 U.S. 11 (1905). See chapter 3.
11. Lucas v. South Carolina Coastal Council, 505 U.S. 1003 (1992). See chapter 9.

and orders issued by the health department, and nuisance abatements adjudicated through the courts). Individuals who are adversely affected by these governmental acts are entitled to the full protection of the Constitution. Additionally, if the state mandates a private breach of constitutional norms, there is state action[8] (e.g., an environmental agency that requires a private contractor to discriminate in access to public lands). Beyond these obvious forms of governmental activity exist numerous ambiguities. This section discusses four interesting public health law problems.[9]

Official State Acts by Health Care Professionals.   Health care professionals who are employed by the government and act in an official capacity are "state actors."[10] Consequently, professionals who work in prisons, state mental hospitals, or municipal STD clinics may be acting in an official capacity and thereby are bound by the Constitution.

Licensed, Inspected, or Regulated Private Entities.   Private individuals and businesses that are subject to government licensing, inspection, or regulation are not "state actors."[11] A regulatory scheme, "however detailed it may be in some particulars," does not, by itself, invoke the state action doctrine.[12] There may be no state action, for example, if a licensed, inspected, or regulated entity discriminates on grounds of race or sex,[13] censors certain sexually explicit or politically sensitive material,[14] or fails to provide fair procedures.[15] The government, through its regulatory network, must be "entangled" with the private entity to establish state action; a "close nexus" must exist between the state and the regulatory entity.[16]

Organizations in Receipt of Government Funding.   The Supreme Court rarely finds state action based solely on government funding, even if subsidies are substantial: "Acts of . . . private contractors do not become acts of the government by reason of their significant or even total engagement in performing public contracts."[17] Thus, private health care providers, businesses, researchers, and community organizations that are funded by public health agencies are not bound to conform with constitutional norms.

Privatization of Public Health Functions.   Government may not privatize the exercise of powers traditionally associated with sovereignty.[18] Consequently, delegation of legislative, regulatory, or judicial powers to the private sector is impermissible (e.g., granting private entities police power authority to quarantine, compel medical treatment, or regulate businesses).[19] Although government may not delegate police powers, there is ample scope for delegation of a broad range of public health services to the private sector.[20]

Private entities that exercise "public functions" are bound by the Constitution, but the definition of "public functions" is so narrow that it is unlikely to include the private exercise of many public health services. Public functions are "traditionally exclusively reserved to the State,"[21] but many public health services (e.g., vaccination, testing and counseling, treatment for infectious diseases, and surveillance) are also undertaken by private health care and community-based organizations. The Supreme Court, for example, has held that education[22] (and other important public services)[23] are not public functions.

CONSTITUTIONAL LIMITATIONS ON THE POLICE POWER IN THE EARLY TWENTIETH CENTURY

When government acts, even for the well-being of the community, it must abide by constitutional constraints. What exactly are the constitutional limits placed on public health activities? This apparently simple question requires a complex response. The beginning point, as in all discourse on public health law, is the Due Process Clause in the Fifth (applying to the federal government) and Fourteenth (applying to the states) Amendments, and, in particular, the foundational Supreme Court case of *Jacobson v. Massachusetts* (1905).[24]

In early American jurisprudence, before *Jacobson*, the judiciary periodically suggested that public health regulation was immune from constitutional review,[25] expressing the notion that "where the police power is set in motion in its proper sphere, the courts have no jurisdiction to stay the arm of the legislative branch."[26] The core issue, of course, was to understand what was meant by the "proper legislative sphere," for it was never supposed in American constitutional history that government could act in an arbitrary manner free from judicial control.[27]

JACOBSON V. MASSACHUSETTS: PERSONAL FREEDOM

Massachusetts enacted a law at the turn of the century empowering municipal boards of health, if necessary for public health or safety, to require the vaccination of inhabitants. The Cambridge Board of Health, under authority of this statute, adopted the following regulation: "Whereas, smallpox has been prevalent . . . in the city of Cambridge and still continues to increase; and whereas, it is necessary for the speedy extermination of the disease . . . ; be it ordered, that all inhabitants of the city be vaccinated." Henning Jacobson, who refused the vaccination, was convicted by the trial court and sentenced to pay a fine of five dollars. The Massachusetts Supreme Judicial Court upheld the conviction, and the case was decided by the U.S. Supreme Court in 1905. Jacobson's legal brief asserted that "a compulsory vaccination law is unreasonable, arbitrary and oppressive, and, therefore, hostile to the inherent right of every freeman to care for his own body and health in such way as to him seems best."[28] His was a classic claim in favor of a laissez-faire society and the natural rights of persons to bodily integrity and decisional privacy.

The Supreme Court preferred a more community-oriented philosophy where citizens have duties to one another and to the society as a whole. Justice Harlan, writing for the Court, states

> [T]he liberty secured by the Constitution of the United States . . . does not import an absolute right in each person to be, at all times and in all circumstances, wholly freed from restraint. There are manifest restraints to

which every person is necessarily subject for the common good. On any other basis organized society could not exist with safety to its members. Society based on the rule that each one is a law unto himself would soon be confronted with disorder and anarchy. Real liberty for all could not exist under the operation of a principle which recognizes the right of each individual person to use his own, whether in respect of his person or his property, regardless of the injury that may be done to others. . . . In the constitution of Massachusetts adopted in 1780 it was laid down as a fundamental principle of the social compact that the whole people covenants with each citizen, and each citizen with the whole people, that all shall be governed by certain laws for the "common good," and that government is instituted "for the common good, for the protection, safety, prosperity and happiness of the people, and not for the profit, honor or private interests of any one man, family or class of men."[29]

Under a social compact theory, then, "a community has the right to protect itself against an epidemic of disease which threatens the safety of its members."[30] The Court's opinion is filled with examples ranging from sanitary laws and animal control to quarantine, demonstrating the breadth of valid police powers. The legacy of *Jacobson* surely is its defense of social welfare philosophy and unstinting support of police power regulation.[31]

Jacobson is a classic case about separation of powers and federalism, and these doctrines were used to support deference to the legislative branch and to the states. The Court's political theory about separation of powers led to an almost unquestioning acceptance of legislative findings of scientific fact. Quoting the New York Court of Appeals (which had recently upheld compulsory vaccination as a condition of school entry),[32] Justice Harlan argued that[33]

the legislature has the right to pass laws which, according to the common belief of the people, are adapted to prevent the spread of contagious diseases. In a free country, where the government is by the people, through their chosen representatives, practical legislation admits of no other standard of action; for what the people believe is for the common welfare must be accepted as tending to promote the common welfare, whether it does in fact or not. Any other basis would conflict with the spirit of the Constitution, and would sanction measures opposed to a republican form of government.

Under a theory of democracy, Justice Harlan would grant considerable leeway to the elected branch of government to formulate public health policy. The Supreme Court, relying on principles of federalism, also asserted the primacy of state authority over federal in the realm of public health. "[I]t is of last importance," wrote Justice Harlan, that the judiciary "should not invade the domain of local authority except when it is plainly necessary. . . . The safety and the health of the people of Massachusetts are, in the first instance, for that Commonwealth to guard and protect. They are matters that do not ordinarily concern the National Government."

The *Jacobson* standard, assuredly, is deferential to public health authorities. The Supreme Court during the *Jacobson* era upheld numerous public health activities including the regulation of food,[34] milk,[35] and garbage disposal.[36] Beyond its passive acceptance of state legislative discretion in matters of public health, however, was the Court's first systematic statement of the constitutional limitations imposed on government. The *Jacobson* Court established a floor of constitutional protection. Public health powers are constitutionally permissible only if they are exercised in conformity with four standards that I shall call public health necessity, reasonable means, proportionality, and harm avoidance. These standards, while permissive of public health intervention, nevertheless require a deliberative governmental process to safeguard autonomy.

Public Health Necessity.   Public health powers are exercised under the theory that they are necessary to prevent an avoidable harm. Justice Harlan, in *Jacobson*, insisted that police powers must be based on the "necessity of the case" and could not be exercised in "an arbitrary, unreasonable manner" or go "beyond what was reasonably required for the safety of the public."[37] Early meanings of the term "necessity" are consistent with the exercise of police powers: to necessitate was to "force" or "compel" a person to do that which he would prefer not to do, and the "necessaries" were those things without which life could not be maintained.[38] Government, in order to justify the use of compulsion, therefore, must act only in the face of a demonstrable health threat.[39]

The standard of public health necessity requires, at a minimum, that the subject of the compulsory intervention must actually pose a threat to the community. In the context of infectious diseases, for example, public health authorities could not impose personal control measures (e.g., mandatory physical examination, treatment, or isolation) unless the person was actually contagious or, at least, there was reasonable suspicion of contagion (see chapter 8.)

Reasonable Means.   Under the public health necessity standard, government may act only in response to a demonstrable threat to the community. The methods used, moreover, must be designed to prevent or ameliorate that threat. The *Jacobson* Court adopted a means/ends test that required a reasonable relationship between the public health intervention and the achievement of a legitimate public health objective. Even though the objective of the legislature may be valid and beneficent, the methods adopted must have a "real or substantial relation" to protection of the public health, and cannot be "a plain, palpable invasion of rights."[40]

Proportionality.   The public health objective may be valid in the sense that a risk to the public exists, and the means may be reasonably likely to achieve that goal—yet a public health regulation is unconstitutional if the human burden imposed is wholly disproportionate to the expected benefit. "[T]he police power of a State," said Justice Harlan, "may be exerted in such circumstances or by regulations so arbitrary and oppressive in particular cases as to justify the interference of the courts to prevent wrong, . . . and oppression."[41]

Public health authorities have a constitutional responsibility not to overreach in ways that unnecessarily invade personal spheres of autonomy. This suggests a requirement for a reasonable balance between the public good to be achieved and the degree of personal invasion. If the intervention is gratuitously onerous or unfair it may overstep constitutional boundaries.

Harm Avoidance.   Those who pose a risk to the community can be required to submit to compulsory measures for the common good. The control measure itself, however, should not pose a health risk to its subject. Justice Harlan emphasized that Henning Jacobson was a "fit person" for smallpox vaccination, but asserted that requiring a person to be immunized who would be harmed is "cruel and inhuman in the last degree."[42] If there had been evidence that the vaccination would seriously impair Jacobson's health, he may have prevailed in this historic case.[43]

Jacobson-era cases reiterate the theme that public health actions must not harm subjects. For example, a quarantine of a district in San Francisco was held unconstitutional, in part, because it created conditions likely to spread bubonic plague.[44] Similarly, courts required safe and habitable environments for persons subject to isolation on the theory that public health powers are designed to promote well-being, and not to punish the individual (see chapter 8).

LOCHNER V. NEW YORK: ECONOMIC FREEDOM

Jacobson v. Massachusetts was decided in the same term as *Lochner v. New York*,[45] the beginning of the so-called *Lochner* era in constitutional law—from 1905 to 1937.[46] During the *Lochner* era, the Supreme Court afforded individuals greater protection in the realm of economic affairs than in personal affairs.[47] The exercise of public health powers, of course, can substantially affect economic freedoms. Public health regulation, for example, requires landlords to maintain sanitary premises, employers to provide safe workplaces, restaurant workers to take precautions in food preparation, businesses to avoid pollution, and health care professionals to adhere to minimum standards of practice—all of which fetter economic freedom.

In *Lochner*, the Supreme Court held that a limitation on the hours that bakers could work violated the Due Process Clause of the Fourteenth Amendment. Justice Peckham, writing for the Court, perceived a limitation on bakers' hours as an interference with the freedom of contract, rather than as a legitimate police power regulation.[48] Yet, Justice Harlan, in dissent, professed that the New York statute was expressly for the public health: "labor in excess of sixty hours during a week . . . may endanger the health of those who thus labor."[49] Quoting standard public health treatises, Justice Harlan observed that "[d]uring periods of epidemic diseases the bakers are generally the first to succumb to disease, and the number swept away during such periods far exceeds the number of other crafts."[50]

Under the reasoning in *Lochner*, public health authorities could enact reasonable rules "to the full extent of providing for the cleanliness and the healthfulness" of the premises (inspection, wash rooms, drainage, and plumbing).[51] However, the legislature could not interfere with economic freedoms unless its purposes were indisputably for the public health. This was a basic economic substantive due process message. The Due Process Clause requires that government objectives be permissible and the means adopted be reasonably likely to achieve those objectives.

The *Lochner* era posed deep concerns for those who realized that much of what public health does interferes with economic freedoms involving contracts, business relationships, the use of property, and the practice of trades and professions. *Lochner*, in the words of Justice Harlan, in dissent, "would seriously cripple the inherent power of the states to care for the lives, health, and well-being of their citizens."[52] So it was. For in the next three decades, the Supreme Court struck down important health and social legislation protecting trades unions,[53] setting minimum wages for women,[54] protecting consumers from products that posed health risks,[55] and licensing or regulating businesses.[56]

By the time of the New Deal, the laissez-faire philosophy that undergirded Lochnerism was challenged by those who believed that all people did not have unfettered contractual freedom, and that economic transactions were naturally constrained by unequal wealth and power relationships. This was also a time when people looked toward government to pursue actively the values of welfare, health, and greater social and economic equity. It was within this political context that the Supreme Court repudiated the principles of *Lochner:* "What is this freedom? The Constitution does not speak of freedom of contract. It speaks of liberty and prohibits the deprivation of liberty without due process of law."[57] The post–New Deal period led to a resurgence of a permissive judicial approach to public health regulation, irrespective of . its effects on commercial and business affairs (see further chapter 9).[58]

PUBLIC HEALTH POWERS IN THE MODERN CONSTITUTIONAL ERA

Jacobson, as explained earlier, established a floor of constitutional protection for individual rights, including four standards of judicial review: necessity, reasonable methods, proportionality, and harm avoidance. Arguably, these standards remain in the modern constitutional era, but the Supreme Court has developed a far more elaborate system of constitutional adjudication. Modern constitutional law is complicated and the analysis of public health measures affecting personal autonomy, liberty, privacy, and property will unfold in subsequent chapters. For now, I will review "first principles": due process of law (both substantive and procedural), equal protection of the laws, and levels of scrutiny used by the Court to balance public goods and individual rights.

It will be obvious from the discussion of federalism in the last chapter and the *Jacobson* and *Lochner* era in this chapter that the march toward more rigorous constitutional scrutiny of governmental action has been slow, cyclical, and politically charged. During the two decades beginning in the 1960s, constitutional doctrine changed markedly. It is important to remember that constitutional law reflects culture, society, and politics. Many cultural developments brought about this revolutionary shift: the civil rights movement for African-Americans, protests against the

Vietnam War, and the reemergence of feminism.[59] Responding to these and other social movements, the Supreme Court, principally under Chief Justice Earl Warren, revitalized and strengthened the Court's position on issues of equality and civil liberties. The Warren Court set a liberal agenda that prized personal freedom and nondiscrimination, and exhibited a healthy suspicion of government. The modern courts, however, are in the process of halting, and even reversing, this liberal doctrine.

PROCEDURAL DUE PROCESS

The Fifth and Fourteenth Amendments prohibit government from depriving individuals of "life, liberty, or property, without due process of law." The Due Process Clause imposes two separate obligations: a "substantive" element that requires government to provide sound reasons for invading personal freedoms, and a procedural element that requires government to provide a fair process for individuals subject to state regulation or coercion.[60] Consider a state requirement for the licensing of physicians or the inspection of food establishments. These governmentally imposed conditions on the ability to practice a profession or to run a business meet the substantive part of the test if the state has a legitimate public health rationale (e.g., to assure the competent practice of medicine or the safe preparation of food). Actual decisions to deny or withdraw the license meet the procedural part of the test if the state affords professionals or businesses a reasonable opportunity to be heard.[61]

The procedural element of due process requires government to provide a fair process—principally notice, a hearing, and an impartial decision-maker—before depriving life, liberty, or property. Affording individuals an opportunity to present their case is so essential to basic fairness that Europeans refer to procedural due process as "natural justice." Procedural due process is important in many different public health contexts ranging from licenses and inspections of businesses to isolation of persons with infectious disease. This section explains "property" and "liberty" interests in the context of public health, and briefly discusses the kinds of procedures that are required in particular cases.

Property Interests.   Government must provide a fair process before depriving individuals of property. The Supreme Court defines a "property interest" as more than an abstract need, desire, or unilateral expectation. The person must "have a legitimate claim of entitlement."[62] Certainly, an individual has an "entitlement" to the legitimate ownership of real or personal property. However, does a person have an entitlement to a benefit, a job, a professional license, or a business permit?

The Supreme Court, until the 1970s, limited "property interests" to cases where the person had a legal right, and not a simple privilege. However, in *Goldberg v. Kelly,* the Supreme Court abandoned the "rights/privilege" distinction, holding that individuals have a property interest in the continued receipt of welfare benefits.[63] While the Court has officially rejected the distinction between rights and privileges, demonstrating an "entitlement" can be difficult. Under the reasoning of *Goldberg,* an entitlement is measured by the importance of the interest to the person's life; without welfare, for example, a person may not obtain the necessities of life. The modern Court's preferred approach is to examine whether the person has a reasonable expectation to the property interest based on an independent source such as state law.[64]

Health departments possess the statutory authority to take, destroy, or restrict property uses to prevent risks to the health or safety of the community.[65] Except in urgent cases,[66] due process generally requires notice and an opportunity to be heard before the deprivation of a property interest.[67] Deprivations of property interests, which trigger procedural due process safeguards, occur in a variety of public health contexts: inspections of goods and buildings;[68] licenses of health care professionals,[69] hospitals,[70] nursing homes,[71] or restaurants;[72] and staff privileges in public hospitals.[73]

Liberty Interests.   Government must provide procedural due process before depriving individuals of liberty. The Supreme Court broadly defines a "liberty interest" as "not merely freedom from bodily restraint, but also the right to contract, to engage in any of the common occupations of life, to acquire useful knowledge, to marry, establish a home and bring up children, to worship God . . . , and generally to enjoy those privileges long recognized . . . as essential to the orderly pursuit of happiness by free men."[74]

Procedural due process classically is required in any case where public health authorities interfere with freedom of movement (e.g., isolation and quarantine) or bodily integrity (e.g., compulsory physical examination and medical treatment). See chapter 8 for a discussion of procedural due process for civil confinement of persons with infectious disease.

The Elements of Procedural Due Process.   Fair procedures are constitutionally required if an individual or business suffers a deprivation of property or liberty.[75] However, this does not decide the question of exactly what kinds of procedures the government must provide. Due process is a flexible concept that varies with the particular situation. The Supreme Court has said that, in deciding which procedures are required, courts should balance several factors.[76] First, the courts consider the nature of the private interests affected. The more intrusive or coercive the state intervention, the more rigorous the procedural safeguards. In cases of plenary deprivation of liberty,[77] such as civil commitment of a person with mental illness[78] or tuberculosis,[79] the state must provide the full panoply of procedures—notice, counsel, presentation of evidence at a hearing, cross-examination, a written decision, and an appeal. The justification for rigorous procedural protections is found in the fundamental invasion of liberty occasioned by long-term detention.[80]

Second, the courts consider the risk of an erroneous deprivation and the probable value, if any, of additional or substitute procedural safeguards. Here, the courts are concerned with the value of procedures as a method of protecting against erroneous decision-making. If the court feels that an informal process is likely to lead to a "correct" result, it will not require procedural formalities that it regards as unnecessary. In *Parham v. J.R.*, "mature minors" were "voluntarily" admitted to a mental hospital by their parents, although the minors opposed the admission. The Supreme Court ruled that the hearing did not have to be formal or conducted by a court. Since juvenile admission was "essentially medical in character," an independent review by hospital physicians was sufficient for due process purposes.[81]

Third, the courts consider the fiscal and administrative burdens in providing additional procedures and the extent to which the government's interests would be undermined. Most mental health or public health statutes permit an expedited form of due process in cases of emergency. Reduced due process is justified by the fact that the state's interests in rapid confinement of immediately dangerous persons would be undermined by elaborate, time-consuming procedures.

In sum, in ascertaining the procedures that are constitutionally required, the courts weigh three factors—the extent of the deprivation of liberty or property, the risk of an erroneous decision, and the burdens that additional procedures will entail. Thus, the procedures in any given circumstance depend on the public health context and vary from case to case.

SUBSTANTIVE DUE PROCESS

Substantive due process is a legal theory that requires government to justify deprivations of life, liberty, or property. Under this theory, government must have adequate reasons for its interventions. The police power represents a classically adequate justification under substantive due process. Thus, government may act for the purposes of protecting the health, safety, or morals of the community. Depending on the level of judicial scrutiny applied, government action must be justified by a legitimate, a substantial, or even a compelling public interest.

Another way of thinking about substantive due process is its proscription against arbitrary and capricious government activity. Since government must produce adequate reasons, it cannot intervene in ways that are indiscriminate, haphazard, or purposeless. If public health authorities coerce without a comprehensible rationale, they violate substantive due process. So, too, must the state avoid regulation influenced by animosity toward a politically unpopular constituency. If government's principal purpose is to disadvantage a person or population, the "enactment [is] divorced from any factual context from which [the Court] could discern a relationship to legitimate state interests."[82]

Substantive due process is controversial because it permits the judiciary to find constitutional rights where none are expressed in the Constitution. The Rehnquist Court has repeatedly declared its reluctance to expand substantive due process "because guideposts for responsible decision-making in this unchartered area are scarce and open-ended."[83] The Court sees substantive due process as being in conflict with democratic values by placing policy questions outside the "arena of public debate and legislative action."[84] The Court's concern is that, absent objective criteria, substantive due process would permit members of the Court to inject their policy preferences. The Supreme Court's substantive due process analysis has two features designed to facilitate objective reasoning. The Court requires, first, a "careful description" of the asserted liberty interest and, second, that the interest is "deeply rooted in the Nation's history and traditions."[85]

The ongoing debate between those with an expansive, and those with a restrictive, view of due process is highly important in public health. Few public health measures directly infringe on a right or freedom declared in the Bill of Rights. The Constitution, for example, does not explicitly mention bodily integrity, which is implicated in mandatory testing and treatment, or privacy, which is implicated in mandatory reporting and partner notification. Moreover, since groups at risk of certain diseases have never gained protection within our constitutional history (e.g., gays and prostitutes), the Court might not see their freedoms as "deeply rooted in the Nation's history."

EQUAL PROTECTION OF THE LAWS

The Fourteenth Amendment commands that no state shall "deny to any person within its jurisdiction the equal protection of the laws." The Supreme Court, in a 1954 school segregation case, held that the federal government must also afford persons equal protection of the laws.[86]

The law usually classifies for one purpose or another, with resulting disadvantage to various persons or groups.[87] The law can discriminate among people in two ways. First, the law can expressly make distinctions among persons or groups. This kind of discrimination is called a facial classification because the distinction among people is "on the face" of the statute. A statute that requires homeless people with tuberculosis to undergo directly observed therapy facially discriminates between people with residences and those without. Second, the law can be "facially neutral" in that it applies a general standard to all people. Statutes of general applicability, nonetheless, often disproportionately affect particular persons or groups. For instance, a law that requires prenatal screening in all communities with a specified high prevalence of HIV infection will have a disparate impact on women of color and low income. The Supreme Court will not necessarily find that a law of general applicability violates equal protection even if a demonstrably inequitable effect on vulnerable groups exists. If a law is facially neutral, the disproportionately burdened class must demonstrate that the government's actual purpose was to discriminate against that group.[88] For example, if a health department applies an inspection law disproportionately against landlords of a certain ethnic origin or social class, an intent to discriminate may be apparent.

If a law expressly discriminates or if a facially neutral law adversely affects persons or groups and the government intends to discriminate, an equal protection problem exists. Contrary to popular belief, however, government is not obliged to treat all people identically. Instead, the Equal Protection Clause requires that government treat like cases alike, but permits government to treat unlike cases dissimilarly.[89] Virtually any public health policy establishes a class of people that receives a benefit or burden and a class that does not. The critical inquiry is whether a sufficient justification exists for the distinction among classes. Put another way, do public health authorities have a valid reason for distinguishing among people and, if so, how substantial is that reason? Medicare eligibility, for example, is based on a person's age, but the government has a plausible reason for offering the benefit to the elderly and excluding others. On the other hand, quarantining Asian-

Americans but not Caucasians in an area where disease is endemic appears to have no justification.[90]

If the government engages in particularly pernicious forms of discrimination or infringes on particularly important rights, then it must provide a more cogent justification for the unequal treatment. Equal protection analysis, therefore, requires an examination of the class created by the statute and the right that is denied to that class. The Court strictly scrutinizes laws that create "suspect classifications" (e.g., race, national origin, or alienage) or burden "fundamental rights" (e.g., procreation, marriage, interstate travel, and voting) (see "Levels of Constitutional Review" below). For example, the courts would closely examine a policy that required all African-Americans to be tested for sickle cell. Similarly, the courts would carefully examine a quarantine placed at the border of New York and New Jersey that inhibited movement across state lines.

LEVELS OF CONSTITUTIONAL REVIEW
OF PUBLIC HEALTH ACTIVITIES

As this brief discussion of substantive due process and equal protection suggests, the Supreme Court adopts different levels of constitutional review, depending on the form of discrimination or the nature of the civil liberty in question. The level of review signals how the courts will balance the various interests in a particular case—the government's interest in preventing injury or disease and the individual's interest in avoiding infringement of autonomy, privacy, or liberty. The level of review also signals how carefully the Court will examine the public health policy or, to put it another way, how much deference the courts will give to public health regulation. The lower the level of scrutiny, the more the Court will grant a presumption of constitutionality. The three formal levels of constitutional review, ranging from the most to the least deferential, are rational basis (minimum rationality), intermediate review, and strict scrutiny.

Rational Basis Review.   The Court's lowest, and most commonly used, standard of constitutional review is the rational basis test. All public health regulation must, at least, comply with this minimum rationality standard.[91] Rational basis review requires both a legitimate government objective and means that are reasonably related to attaining that objective. Police power regulation is a classically valid objective: "Public safety, public health, morality, peace, law and order—these are some of the more conspicuous examples of [legitimate governmental interests]."[92] The Court has expressly upheld numerous public health objectives, including traffic safety,[93] detection of underdiagnosed disease,[94] and disease prevention.[95] Not only must the government's purpose be valid, the means adopted must be reasonably directed toward achieving the public health objective.[96] For example, an ordinance requiring owners of vacant lots to clear-cut all vegetation was invalidated because the town's claim that noxious vines could grow was implausible.[97]

Rationality review is highly permissive of public health regulation, with the Court granting a strong presumption of constitutionality.[98] Constitutional review "is not a license for courts to judge the wisdom, fairness, or logic of legislative choices."[99] The judiciary leaves the desirability of public health regulation to the legislature. Further, the legislature need not "actually articulate at any time the purpose or rationale" for its public health policy.[100] Rather, public health regulation is upheld if there is "any reasonably conceivable state of facts that could provide a rational basis for the classification."[101]

Scientific evidence of risk is the raison d'être of public health action. Yet, under rational basis review, the state is not obliged to produce scientific evidence.[102] "A legislative choice is not subject to courtroom fact finding and may be based on rational speculation unsupported by evidence or empirical data."[103] Indeed, the courts often defer to expert agencies on matters of public health policy because agencies are faced with complex practical problems that require "rough accommodations—illogical, it may be, and unscientific."[104] The courts, under rationality review, have upheld a wide spectrum of public health regulations ranging from infectious disease screening[105] and mandatory treatment[106] to regulation of landfills[107] and licensing of fishermen.[108]

Rationality review almost always results in a finding that police power regulation is constitutional. However, several Supreme Court decisions suggest that rational basis review may be more rigorous when the government engages in invidious discrimination. Earlier this century, in a famous footnote in the Carolene Products case, the Court hinted that it might engage in a more searching judicial inquiry when legislation discriminates against "discrete and insular minorities" who could not easily redress their injuries through democratic processes.[109] While the modern Court seldom applies the Carolene Products standard, it has on several occasions engaged in more exacting scrutiny of discriminatory government action, while purporting to apply the rational basis test—so-called "rational basis with a bite."

In *City of Cleburne v. Cleburne Living Center, Inc.*,[110] the Supreme Court, using rational basis review, declared unconstitutional a zoning ordinance that effectively prevented the operation of a group home for persons with mental retardation. Under conventional rationality review, the judiciary would be deferential, but the Court felt that the legislature was motivated by animosity against a traditionally disenfranchised group. Similarly, in *Romer v. Evans*,[111] the Supreme Court saw prejudice against homosexuals, another group that is disadvantaged in the political process. Colorado had amended its state constitution to prohibit all legislative, executive, or judicial action designed to protect lesbians or gay men from discrimination. The Court held that the state constitutional amendment "fails, even defies," the rational basis test.[112] The State's reason, said the Court, "seems inexplicable by anything but animus toward the class that it affects; it lacks a rational relationship to legitimate state interests."[113] Both *Cleburne* and *Romer* suggest that there may be areas where legislatures act against politically disfavored groups with such hostility that the Court will be prepared to examine legislative motives more carefully than in conventional applications of rationality review. In the Court's words, "a bare congressional desire to harm a politically unpopular group cannot constitute a legitimate government purpose."[114]

Rationality review is extraordinarily important in public health because most prevention strategies will be measured against this standard. Since risk assessment and scientific evidence are so important in evaluating public health measures (see chapter 4), rationality review hardly seems sufficient.[115] This lowest standard of review does not force public health authorities to justify their actions by demonstrating a significant risk and that the intervention is likely to ameliorate that risk; nor does it usually require authorities to explain why they chose to target particularly vulnerable or unpopular groups such as gays, prostitutes, homeless persons, or drug users. Discrimination on the basis of sexual orientation, disability, and socioeconomic class has played an important role in the history of public health. The future of rationality review in light of cases such as *Cleburne* and *Romer* may well demonstrate whether the Court is prepared to look more carefully at disfavored treatment of politically unpopular groups.

Intermediate Review.   The Supreme Court adopts an intermediate level of review where government discriminates on the basis of sex[116]

or against "illegitimate" children.[117] Gender discrimination triggers
this intermediate scrutiny whether discrimination is against women or
men.[118] Under this middle level of constitutional review, the state must
establish that its classification serves important governmental objectives
and must be substantially related to those objectives.[119] Thus, the government's interest must be "important," not simply legitimate, and the
relationship between means and ends must be "substantial," not merely
reasonable. The Court exercises great care in examining government
policy under this middle tier of review. In invalidating gender discrimination at the Virginia Military Institute (VMI), Justice Ginsberg emphasized that the state must demonstrate "an exceedingly persuasive
justification. . . . The burden of justification is demanding and rests entirely on the State."[120]

Public health actions that classify on the basis of sex, therefore, are
subject to a rigorous form of judicial review. Consider, for example,
mandatory syphilis testing of female, but not male, applicants for a
marriage license. This sexual classification probably would be unconstitutional because it does not serve a substantial public health purpose.[121] The prenatal HIV testing of women, however, might withstand
constitutional scrutiny, because the state could demonstrate a substantial reason for focusing the intervention on women.[122]

Strict Scrutiny.   As explained earlier, the Supreme Court strictly reviews laws that create "suspect" classifications or which burden "fundamental" rights and liberty interests. The Court has emphasized several reasons why it might find a suspect classification: (1) *immutable
characteristics*—personal statuses acquired at birth that individuals do
not choose and cannot change; (2) *political powerlessness*—discrete minorities who have ineffective access to the political process to safeguard
their own rights; (3) *history of discrimination*—groups that have suffered from long periods of prejudice and unfavorable treatment;
(4) *stereotypes*—classifications that are rarely justified by rational public policy choices. The Court has decided that race,[123] national origin,[124] and, with some exceptions, alienage[125] are suspect classes.[126]

The Court also strictly reviews government actions that burden fundamental rights and liberty interests including procreation,[127] marriage,[128] interstate travel,[129] and bodily integrity.[130] Fundamental
rights and interests receive heightened protection because of their
value in our constitutional system. The Supreme Court, during its
modern history, has used different forms of reasoning to determine if

a right is "fundamental." Liberties that are explicitly protected within the text of the Constitution, such as the freedoms of expression, religion, and the right to vote, are always regarded as fundamental. Other liberties, such as the right to procreate, are deemed fundamental because they involve "the most intimate and personal choices a person may make in a lifetime, choices central to personal dignity and autonomy."[131] Finally (as explained earlier), rights are deemed fundamental if they "are deeply rooted in this Nation's history and tradition."

Under strict scrutiny, the government must demonstrate a "compelling interest," a tight relationship between means and ends, and that its objectives could not be achieved by less restrictive or discriminatory purposes. First, the government must demonstrate an interest that is "compelling" or truly vital to community well-being. Public health and safety are quintessentially regarded as compelling interests.

Second, the government must demonstrate that the methods chosen are strictly necessary to achieve its objectives. Thus, legislation must avoid underinclusiveness and, particularly, overinclusiveness (see further chapter 4). Policies that are underinclusive apply only to certain individuals or groups, but not to others who are in a similar position— for example, the policy uses compulsion against one group, but not against another group that poses the same risk to the public. By itself, underinclusiveness is not necessarily fatal from a constitutional position. Government may use its limited resources "one step at a time" to address part of a public health problem without having to address the entire problem.

Overinclusiveness, or overbreadth, occurs when a policy extends to more people than it needs to in order to achieve the public health objective. An overinclusive exercise of a compulsory power is frequently unacceptable because it subjects individuals who pose no health risk to loss of liberty. For example, isolation of all persons with *Mycobacterium* tuberculosis infection who are not contagious could be fatally overinclusive because most people in this population do not pose a risk.[132]

Finally, strict scrutiny requires the adoption of the "least restrictive alternative." Thus, the government must demonstrate that its public purpose could not be achieved as well, or better, through less restrictive or less discriminatory policies. The principle of the least restrictive alternative does not require public health authorities to adopt policies that are ineffective, or even less effective, than the proposed policy. It simply requires government to utilize the policy that achieves the public health objective with the least intrusion on personal rights and freedoms.

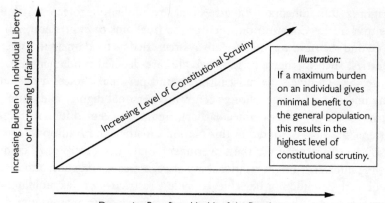

Figure 7.   Evaluating the constitutionality of public health policies: a proposal for a graduated approach.

BEYOND LEVELS OF CONSTITUTIONAL SCRUTINY

Constitutional scholars, and members of the Court itself, often criticize the levels of review because they are inflexible and outcome determinative.[133] Where the Court sees certain touchstones of constitutional concern such as a suspect classification or the violation of a fundamental right, the government almost invariably loses—strict scrutiny is "strict in theory, but fatal in fact."[134] In the absence of these specific gauges of constitutional concern, the Court uses the rational basis test and the government almost invariably wins. Certainly, different standards ought to apply depending on the class affected or the right infringed; yet it is far from clear why such sharply different constitutional standards, and outcomes, should result. Strict scrutiny is invoked for classifications based on race, national origin, and alienage, but not sexual orientation,[135] disability,[136] or socioeconomic status.[137] Yet each of these groups has experienced discrimination based on irrational fears and prejudices. Similarly, strict scrutiny is invoked for invasions of fundamental interests such as contraception, abortion, and interstate travel, but not for breaches of confidentiality[138] or interference with the doctor-patient relationship.[139] Yet each of these liberty interests has importance to human dignity and individual freedom. Whatever differences exist between various status classifications and liberty interests, they are differences of degree, not of kind.

At the same time, when the Court applies rationality review, it fails to ask public health authorities to justify their actions in the most elemental ways: What are the specific public health goods sought by the intervention? What scientific evidence exists demonstrating a significant health risk? Are the interventions proposed likely to be effective?

Two problems, then, are evident in constitutional analysis. First, the standards provide a rigid "all-or-nothing" assessment, rather than a graduated examination based on the burdens posed by discriminatory classifications or infringements on autonomy, privacy, and liberty. Second, rationality review, by far the most common form of scrutiny, places few demands on public health authorities to justify their actions based on scientific evidence of risk reduction.

For a different way of thinking about levels of constitutional review, think of a sliding scale that subjects public health policies to increasingly demanding levels of constitutional review. As the intrusiveness and un-fairness of the public health policy grows, so would the level of scrutiny. As a policy moves across the continuum because of its restrictive or dis-criminatory quality, public health would gradually give way to individual liberty (see Figure 7). In the next chapter, I propose a more systematic method of assessing the appropriateness of public health interventions.

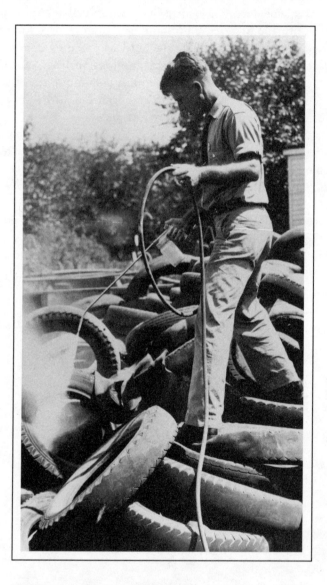

A Public Health Service officer sprays water-filled tires with insecticide to eliminate mosquitoes, 1939.

4 Public Health Regulation

A Systematic Evaluation

> One very simple principle [justifies state coercion]. That principle
> is, that the sole end for which mankind are warranted, individually
> or collectively, in interference with the liberty of action of any of
> their number, is self-protection. That the only purpose for which
> power can be rightfully exercised over any member of a civilized
> community, against his will, is to prevent harm to others. . . . His
> own good, either physical or moral is not a sufficient warrant. He
> cannot be rightfully compelled to do or forbear because it will be
> better for him to do so, because it will make him happier, because,
> in the opinion of others, to do so would be wise, or even right.
>
> *John Stuart Mill (1856)*

Public health regulation entails potential trade-offs between public
goods and private interests. When public health authorities act, they
face troubling conflicts between the collective benefits of population
health on the one hand, and personal and business interests on the
other. Table 3 summarizes the major trade-offs in public health regulation. For each public health activity, one side of the table explains the
probable public benefits of the policy and the other side explains the
probable burdens on private rights and interests.

These trade-offs between the collective benefits of public health and
personal interests in liberty and property are much discussed within the
public health literature. But how do we know when the public good to
be achieved is worth the infringement of individual rights? In this chapter, I propose a systematic evaluation of public health regulation that
analyzes regulatory justifications, public risks, the intervention's effectiveness, economic costs, personal burdens, and the policy's fairness.

This chapter, unlike the previous two, is more prescriptive than descriptive. Thus, I suggest criteria for courts and policymakers to adopt

TABLE 3
PUBLIC HEALTH REGULATION:
TRADE-OFFS BETWEEN PUBLIC BENEFITS AND
PRIVATE INTERESTS AND RIGHTS

Public Health Activity	Public Benefits	Private Interests/Rights
Surveillance, monitoring, and epidemiologic investigations Reporting Outbreak investigations Case control studies	Identify injuries and diseases, understand prevalence and incidence in the population, understand causes of disease	Physician-patient confidentiality and health information privacy
Case finding Testing Screening Partner notification	Identify injuries and diseases as a prerequisite to counseling, education, treatment, and support services	Personal autonomy, bodily integrity, and health information privacy
Medical interventions Physical examination Compulsory treatment Immunization Directly observed therapy	Prevent and diagnose disease, clinical benefits, reduce infectiousness, reduce drug-resistant strains of pathogens	Personal autonomy, bodily integrity, religious freedom
Personal control measures Cease-and-desist orders Isolation Quarantine Compulsory hospitalization	Prevent spread of infectious diseases by requiring behavior change or separating infectious persons from the public	Personal autonomy, liberty, and travel
Prohibition of behavior Illicit drug use Driving while intoxicated Smoking in public places	Protect health and safety of person or others by restricting risk behaviors	Personal autonomy and freedom of action
Required behavior Seatbelt use Motorcycle helmet use	Prevent personal injury, reduce health care and related costs by requiring safer behaviors	Personal autonomy and freedom of action
Product design Passive restraints in cars Locks on firearms Negligence under tort law Product liability under tort law	Prevent injuries by regulation or incentives for safer product design, and compensate injured persons	Freedom of contract (manufacturer-consumer), business interests, property uses, consumer costs

TABLE 3 *(continued)*

Public Health Activity	Public Benefits	Private Interests/Rights
Informational constraints and required disclosures Advertising restrictions Labeling requirements Mandated warnings	Restrict content of commercial messages that encourage harmful behavior, provide consumer information to avoid hazards	Freedom of speech, freedom of press, business and property interests
Youth access restrictions Cigarettes Alcoholic beverages Firearms Automobiles	Reduce health and safety risks among children and adolescents	Autonomy of youth, spill-over effects in denying access to adults
Nuisance abatement Closure/regulation of: Bath houses Adult theaters Food establishments Unsafe premises	Reduce health or safety risks in businesses, recreational facilities, homes, and other places	Property and business interests, consumer costs, free association
Regulation of businesses, professionals, food, drugs, and medical devices Inspection of premises Business permits Professional licenses Approval of pharmaceuticals	Reduce health and safety risks in the conduct of businesses, the provision of health care services, and the sale of drugs and medical devices	Property and business interests, freedom of contract, consumer costs, freedom to engage in occupations
Environmental regulation Emission controls of pollutants Toxic waste cleanup Drinking water standards	Prevent acute and long-term risks to health, beautify the environment, preserve habitat and animal life	Business and property interests, consumer costs
Occupational health and safety Infection control Health and safety standards Maximum work hours	Reduce health and safety hazards in the workplace, such as exposure to toxic materials, dangerous workplace environments, and stressful conditions	Freedom of contract (employer-employee), business and property interests, consumer costs
Taxation Taxes on cigarettes Taxes on alcoholic beverages	Reduce demand for hazardous products by price increases, create disincentives or incentives to promote healthier behavior	Consumer costs, business and property interests, and possible fairness problem with regressive taxation

in reviewing public health regulation. However, I do not mean to suggest that these standards are already a part of existing legal doctrine; nor do I mean to suggest that these standards, if conscientiously applied, will lead to the "correct" public health policy. Public health problems and interventions are too diverse and complicated to meet a single, ordered test of any kind. My claim, therefore, is that the following standards are important, but not determinative, in analyzing complex public health policy problems.

GENERAL JUSTIFICATIONS FOR PUBLIC HEALTH REGULATION

Convention holds that government intervention designed to promote population health and well-being is an unmitigated good. Why wouldn't society want to organize itself in ways that maximize the health of populations? To fulfill many of the aspirations of human life requires a healthy mind and body.[1] Because health is so highly valued, sometimes American society assumes that government need not justify public health interventions. But government should justify interventions because, almost invariably, they intrude on individual rights and interests and incur economic costs. Before proposing a systematic evaluation of public health regulation, it will be helpful to think about the three general justifications commonly asserted: risk to others, protection of incompetent persons, and risk to self.

RISK TO OTHERS: THE "HARM PRINCIPLE"

The risk of serious harm to other persons is the most commonly asserted justification for public health regulation. The so-called harm principle holds that competent adults should have freedom of action unless they pose a risk to the community.[2] The reason for permitting such a wide range of freedom is that people have a strong interest in autonomy.

Autonomy, literally, "self-governance," has acquired meanings as diverse as liberty, privacy, individual choice, and even economic freedom.[3] The legal community uses autonomy to support rules such as informed consent and confidentiality. At its core, autonomy is the personal governance of the self that is free from controlling interferences.[4] Autonomous persons are free to hold views, to make choices, and to take actions based on personal values and beliefs.[5] Respect for autonomy, according to Immanuel Kant, demands respect for a person's unconditional worth and freedom of will; persons should be treated as an end and never as a means only.[6] Thus, an individual should not be treated in a fashion exclusively for the objectives of others without regard to his own goals.

Theories of autonomy hold that government, or others, should not restrain competent adults in the absence of some overriding justification. Avoidance of serious harm to others is often thought to be an adequate justification for constraining autonomy. John Stuart Mill argued that persons should be free to think, speak, and behave as they wish, provided they do not interfere with a like expression of freedom by others.[7] This is a classic argument that personal freedoms extend only so far as they do not intrude on the health, safety, and other legitimate interests of other individuals. Under this view, public health regulation is justified by the competing, and overriding, obligation not to harm or interfere with the rights of the community. If autonomy extended so far as to permit the invasion of others' spheres of liberty, there would be an overall diminution of autonomy in the population. Seen in this way, genuine autonomy requires a certain amount of security, so that persons are free to live without risks of serious injury or disease. For a constitutional explanation, see the police powers discussion in chapters 2 and 3.

PROTECTION OF INCOMPETENT PERSONS: "BEST INTERESTS"

Autonomous persons should not only be free from controlling interferences by others, but also from internal limitations that impede meaningful choice. Persons who have insufficient understanding to make informed choices, to deliberate, and to act according to their desires or plans have diminished autonomy. Thus, two conditions are essential for autonomy: freedom from external control and internal capacity for deliberative action. Children and persons with mental illness or mental retardation may, to a greater or lesser degree, have diminished capacity. In these circumstances, government may step in to ensure their health or safety such as by civilly committing a person with mental illness or controlling the financial affairs of a person with mental retardation.

A justification for personal regulation based on incapacity does not give the state license to restrict freedoms without purpose. Rather, the state should further justify its intervention in two ways. First, the government should demonstrate that the individual is not capable of making the particular decision. Since a finding of incompetency seriously undermines a person's right of self-determination, there should be just cause for believing that he cannot understand the risks and benefits entailed in the decision to be taken. Second, the substitute decision should be either consistent with the person's known wishes (if he was once competent) or in the person's best interests. Since the rationale for interference with autonomy is to make those decisions a person would have made if he were competent, the government should act beneficently in the interests of the individual. For a constitutional explanation, see the *parens patriae* powers discussion in chapter 2.

RISK TO SELF: SELF-REGARDING BEHAVIOR

Of the three traditional justifications for public health regulation, risk to self is, by far, the most controversial. Risk to self is highly controversial because the behavior is "self-regarding"—that is, the conduct appears to affect only the person concerned and not others. Classical regulation of self-regarding behavior includes mandatory motorcycle helmet[8] and seat belt use,[9] gambling prohibitions,[10] and fluoridation of drinking water.[11] In addition to direct control over personal activity, government heavily taxes, and restricts advertising of, cigarettes and alcoholic beverages. One can also imagine taxation or other regulation of high-calorie and high-fat foods.[12]

Regulation of self-regarding behavior is justified, if at all, by *paternalism:* Interference with a person's liberty of action is justified exclusively by the need to protect the health, safety, welfare, and happiness, or other interests or values, of the person subject to coercion.[13] The case against paternalism rests on the assumption that individuals are most informed about their own needs and value systems, and most self-interested.[14] After all, a person declines to wear a motorcycle helmet not because he is oblivious to the risk, but presumably because he places one value (freedom) above another (physical security). Anti-paternalists are not simply saying that persons make wiser decisions by taking into account their own value systems; rather, they find intrinsic value in permitting the individual to decide for himself even if, objectively, he makes the "wrong" choice. In short, allowing individuals to make decisions respects the person as an autonomous agent, while coercion undermines dignity.

A defense of paternalism usually relies on the fact that people face constraints (both internal and external) on the capacity to pursue their own interests.[15] Because personal behavior is heavily influenced, government regulation is sometimes necessary to protect the individual's health. First, individuals have cognitive limits—either inadequate information or the inability to process complex scientific information. People frequently make choices without full information about the risks. Everyone does not know that children are at risk of severe injury from front-seat air bags or that radon is prevalent, and dangerous, in homes. Even when information is available, consumers may misapprehend the risks. Media discussions of a "good diet" or the health effects of vigorous exercise are, at best, contradictory and confusing.

Second, individuals have limited willpower. They may know, objectively, what is in their best interests, but find it difficult to behave accordingly. This point is obvious in the case of physical and psychological dependencies on illicit drugs, alcoholic beverages, tranquilizers, diet medication, or nicotine. But individuals may have difficulty controlling many behaviors that are not conventionally regarded as addictive: A person understands that high-fat foods will cause adverse health effects or that excessive spending or gambling will cause financial hardship, but it is not always easy to refrain.

Finally, individuals face social, economic, and environmental constraints on their behavior. Human behavior is influenced by many external factors including parents and family, peers and community, media, and commercial advertising. An adolescent's decision about whether to use a condom is affected not only by what he knows about sexually transmissible infections, but also by the social meaning associated with condoms among his peers and particularly his sexual partners.[16] Similarly, a person's decision about what to eat and whether to smoke cigarettes or drink alcoholic beverages (and what brand) is influenced by commercial messages (see chapter 6). Social, structural, and physical factors in the environment also influence behavioral decisions. Consider a poor inner-city neighborhood where most food shopping is fast food, and where there are no supermarkets to purchase fresh fruits and vegetables at reasonable prices.[17] Or think about the same neighborhood where there are no parks or recreational areas and people fear violence if they travel in the streets. In such an environment, voluntary choice is constrained even if public health messages about a healthy diet and exercise are being heard and understood.

The courts routinely uphold regulation of classically self-regarding behaviors, emphasizing the aggregate consequences for society's health and economic resources—the risk to safety (e.g., an unprotected motorcyclist

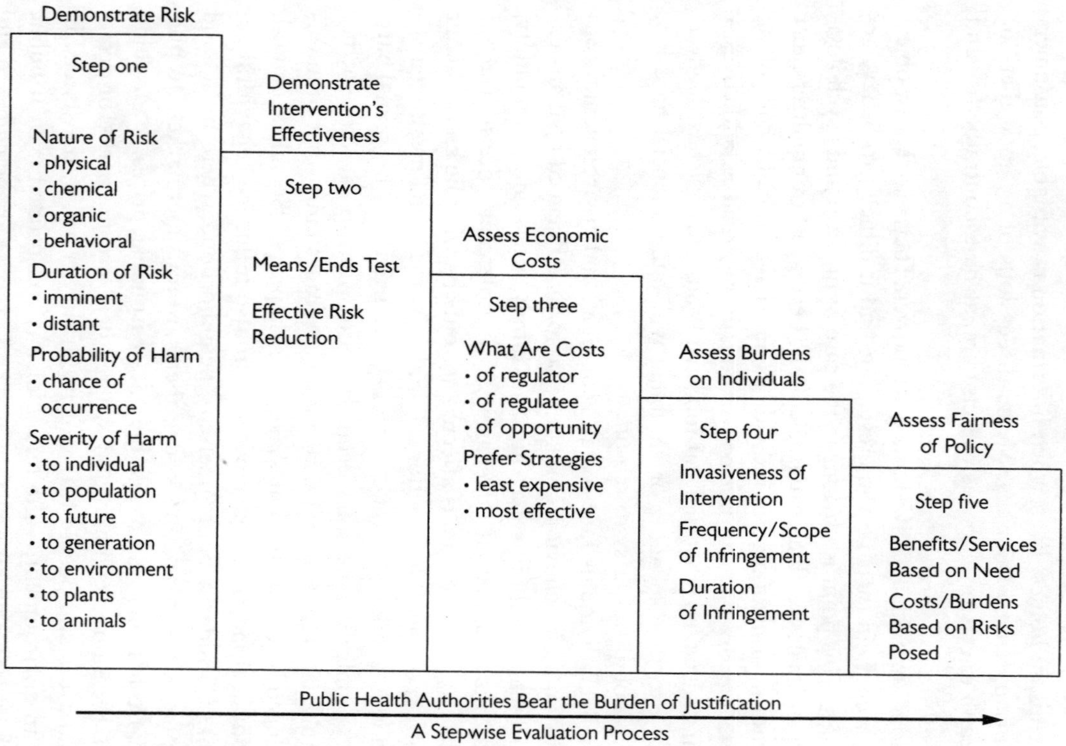

Demonstrate Risk

Step one

Nature of Risk
- physical
- chemical
- organic
- behavioral

Duration of Risk
- imminent
- distant

Probability of Harm
- chance of occurrence

Severity of Harm
- to individual
- to population
- to future
- to generation
- to environment
- to plants
- to animals

Demonstrate Intervention's Effectiveness

Step two

Means/Ends Test

Effective Risk Reduction

Assess Economic Costs

Step three

What Are Costs
- of regulator
- of regulatee
- of opportunity

Prefer Strategies
- least expensive
- most effective

Assess Burdens on Individuals

Step four

Invasiveness of Intervention
Frequency/Scope of Infringement
Duration of Infringement

Assess Fairness of Policy

Step five

Benefits/Services Based on Need
Costs/Burdens Based on Risks Posed

Public Health Authorities Bear the Burden of Justification

A Stepwise Evaluation Process

Figure 8.   Public health regulation: a stepwise evaluation.

presenting a traffic hazard),[18] health (e.g., sidestream tobacco smoke),[19] or the economy (e.g., urgent care costs and burdens on government benefits such as Medicaid):[20]

> From the moment of the [motorcycle] injury, society picks the person up off the highway; delivers him to a municipal hospital and municipal doctors; provides him with unemployment compensation if, after recovery, he cannot replace his lost job, and, if the injury causes permanent disability, may assume the responsibility for his and his family's continued subsistence. We do not understand a state of mind that permits plaintiff to think that only he himself is concerned.[21]

These kinds of judicial decisions, however, fail to confront the real issue of paternalism. After all, the principal reason that society requires citizens to wear motorcycle helmets or seat belts is to protect the person himself. These court decisions reduce the justification for regulation of self-regarding behavior to a strained conception of social harms rather than recognizing certain public health interventions as justified paternalism.

Having considered the general justifications for public health regulation,[22] it is important to systematically evaluate whether particular interventions are warranted. Next, I propose that public health authorities should bear the burden of justification and, therefore, should demonstrate

Significant risk (based on scientific methods)

The intervention's effectiveness (by showing a close fit between means and ends)

Reasonableness of economic costs (compared with the probable benefits)

Fair distribution of benefits, costs, and burdens so that services are provided only where needed and that regulatory burdens are imposed only where a risk to the community exists

These four factors are summarized in Figure 8.

UNDERSTANDING RISK

Risk. A concept used to give meaning to things, forces, or circumstances that pose danger to people or to what they value. Descriptions of risk are typically stated in terms of the likelihood of harm or loss from

a hazard and usually include: an identification of what
is "at risk" and may be harmed or lost (e.g., health of
human beings or an ecosystem, personal property,
quality of life, ability to carry on an economic activity); the hazard that may occasion this loss; and a
judgment about the likelihood that harm will occur.

National Research Council (1996)

The mission of public health is to identify risks and prevent and/or ameliorate harms or other undesirable consequences to humans and what
they value. Populations face hazards from many different sources: from
physical forces (e.g., radioactivity, sound waves, and magnetic fields),
chemicals (e.g., ozone, mercury, dioxins, and drugs), organisms (e.g.,
viruses and bacteria), and human behavior (e.g., sex, smoking, drunk
driving, and firearm use).[23] People also face social consequences from
the unauthorized disclosure of health information such as embarrassment, stigma, and discrimination in employment, insurance, and housing.[24] Risk is a highly complex concept, and a vast literature exists about
the analysis,[25] perception,[26] characterization,[27] communication,[28] and
management[29] of risk. I will not attempt to synthesize systematically the
extant literature regarding risk. However, I will propose a framework
for risk analysis, discuss value choices in risk regulation, and explain the
difficult trade-offs among competing risks to health.

RISK ANALYSIS IN PUBLIC HEALTH REGULATION

Public health regulation is an attempt to control risk. However, we need
to know more about the evidence needed to assess the risk and the
level, or seriousness, of the risk that warrants regulation.[30] Risk assessments are almost always made in circumstances of uncertainty, so an
accurate calculation is usually difficult. Nevertheless, to the extent possible, risk assessments should be based on objective and reliable scientific evidence provided by the multiple disciplines of public health, including medicine, virology, bacteriology, and epidemiology.[31]
Science-based risk assessments provide a surer grounding for decision-
making and avoid reflexive actions based upon irrational fears, speculation, stereotypes, or pernicious mythologies.[32]

Risk assessments should also be made on a case-by-case basis.
Individualized risk assessments avoid decisions made under a blanket
rule or generalization about a class of persons. A fact-specific, individ-

ualized inquiry is more likely to result in a well-informed judgment grounded in a careful and open-minded weighing of risks and alternatives.

Finally, public health regulation should be based on risks that are "significant," not speculative, theoretical, or remote. The level of risk needed to justify a regulatory response varies depending on the policy's economic costs and human burdens. If the costs and burdens are small, public health authorities need to demonstrate lower levels of risk to justify the intervention. As the policy's costs and burdens increase, public health authorities need to demonstrate ever-greater levels of risk. For example, where individual liberty is at stake, the risk justifying regulation should be substantial.

Four factors are helpful in risk assessments: the nature of the risk, the duration of the risk, the probability that harm will occur, and the severity of the harm if the risk were to materialize.

The Nature of the Risk.   As suggested above, populations face hazards from varying sources, each presenting different kinds of risk. For example, it matters whether the danger is from exposure to an environmental carcinogen, ingestion of genetically modified plants or animals, or infection with an organism. Assessing the risk of an environmental carcinogen requires understanding the toxicity of the particular substance, the dose, and the length of exposure.[33] The harm to any individual may be impossible to measure: Disease may not occur at all or it may take decades to develop, and even if the person does become ill, other causes cannot be eliminated. The risk, therefore, may be realized only in the aggregate based upon epidemiological investigations of various populations. Risk assessments for genetically modified plants and animals may be concerned not so much with the harm to those who ingest the food, but with difficult-to-measure effects on the ecosystem.[34] The potential harm may even be to future generations. Risk assessments for infectious diseases depend on the mode of transmission of the organism. Risks vary depending on whether the mechanism of transmission is sexual, airborne, bloodborne, waterborne, or foodborne. A significant risk would be established in cases involving a primary mode of transmission, not a mode that is unestablished or inefficient.

The Duration of the Risk.   Risks are rarely all-or-nothing events. Rather, risks change over time—a risk may remain constant, it may diminish or end, or it may increase. Assessments should take account of the risk as it exists at the moment and how it is predicted to change over time. Risks of radiation, radon, and tobacco smoke, for example, are cumulative and would be expected to increase the longer the person or population is exposed. Risks of infectious disease, however, exist only so long as the person remains contagious. A person should be subject to compulsory public health powers only if he is actually contagious and only for the period of time of contagiousness.

Public health authorities are often justified in averting future, as well as current, risks. Consider a population comprised of asymptomatic persons infected with *Mycobacterium* tuberculosis (M. TB) who are not currently contagious, but are likely to develop active disease in the future (e.g., persons dually infected with HIV and M. TB). Public health authorities may be justified in imposing directly observed therapy on the entire population to avert the threat of individuals relapsing and posing a serious risk of transmission of TB (see further chapter 9).[35]

The Probability of Harm. The probability of harm is an important aspect of risk assessment. Risk assessors seek to determine the chance that a particular harm will occur and, if so, when. The "probability of harm" standard involves a prediction of the future and, therefore, requires rigorous scientific evaluation. As the probability of a harmful event increases, so does the justification for a regulatory response.

The Severity of Harm. The seriousness of harm represents an important calculation in assessing public health regulation. The probability of a harmful event does not tell us a great deal about its severity if the harm were to materialize. Severity of harm may be measured by its effects on an individual: it matters when the disease or injury occurs (young or old age), whether the effects are debilitating (physically or mentally), how long the effects persist, and whether it will result in death. Severity of harm may also be measured by its effects on populations. The harm to any single individual may be relatively small, but if the harm occurs to large populations, the severity is greater. Finally, severity of harm may be measured by its detrimental effects on the things that human beings value. Degradation of the environment, the ecosystem, or animal life may, or may not, have measurable effects on human health. Yet, to the extent that people value intangible aspects of life, such as natural beauty, wilderness, or continuation and diversity of species, we count these harms in our risk calculations.

In assessing the validity of public health powers, a rough inverse correlation exists between the severity of harm and the probability of its occurrence. As the seriousness of potential harm to the community rises, the level of risk needed to justify the public health power decreases. Central to the understanding of the "significant risk" standard is the fact that even the most serious potential for harm does not justify public health regulation in the absence of a reasonable probability that it will occur.[36] Parents of school children, for example, have difficulty comprehending why children who are infested with lice may be excluded from school, but not those infected with HIV. The reason is that a very high probability exists that other children will become infested with lice, but the risk of contracting HIV in that setting is highly remote.

SOCIAL VALUES IN RISK ASSESSMENT

There are deep and fundamental and intuitively understood grounds for rejecting the view that confines itself
merely to checking the parity of outcomes, the view
that matches death for death, happiness for happiness,
fulfillment for fulfillment, irrespective of how all this
death, happiness and fulfillment comes about.
                                        Amartya Sen (1994)

The risk analysis offered so far is closely aligned to science. Science understands risk according to probabilistic assessments relating to the chance that a dangerous event will occur, and if it does, the severity of its effects.[37] The scientific risk assessor generally considers risk in an objective and narrow context. The lay public's understanding of risk, however, accounts for more than statistical likelihood; it includes personal, social, and cultural values.[38] The differences between lay and expert perceptions of risk lead to interesting questions about which perspective should prevail and, more importantly, the implications for democratic values: Should science trump popular judgment?

Scholars argue that lay judgments are prone to inaccuracy, leading to exaggerated perceptions of small risks and underestimations of larger risks.[39] The public often uses heuristics, or rules of thumb, to make judgments about risks; thus, lay persons make simplifying assumptions. For example, toxic waste is harmful to health, so *all* toxic material must be removed; or, nuclear disasters occur, so *all* nuclear power must be dangerous. People also perceive risks as more significant, the more these risks become salient. Thus, the public becomes concerned when the media draws attention to statistically low risks, such as streptococcus A infection ("flesh-eating" disease)[40] or the pesticide alar (in apples),[41] or when a dramatic event is reported (e.g., Love Canal, Three Mile Island, or Chernobyl).

Heuristics, salience, and other "unscientific" lay perceptions, it is argued, skew the regulatory agenda, resulting in selective attention to relatively remote risks.[42] While lay judgments are often "unscientific," they are not necessarily irrational. The public tolerates certain hazards because they voluntarily assume the risk, feel they can control the risk, or derive benefit from the activity. Lay persons, for example, may reject extensive regulation of grave risks that are voluntarily incurred, controllable, and enjoyable (e.g., smoking and automobile travel), but insist on extensive regulation of relatively low risks they feel are inescapable, unmanageable, and not tangibly valuable (e.g., hazardous waste sites and nuclear power).[43]

The public also adopts other values in risk assessments: Do the risks occur "naturally" or are they introduced by novel technologies (e.g., nuclear power, cloning, transgenic foods)? Does the behavior conform with community standards of morality (e.g., sexuality, drug use, abortion)? Are the risks fairly distributed among the population (e.g., disproportionate burdens on women or racial minorities)? If, as Amartya Sen suggests in the epigraph to this section, the scientific method of comparing "death for death" is deeply unintuitive, it may be because, on occasion, the public has a richer, more contextual understanding of risk that deserves attention in a democratic society. The public, therefore, need not routinely cede moral judgments to public health's claims of value-free science. Nor is it wrong for democratically responsive government to weigh benefits to public health against harm to traditional values.

I am emphatically not suggesting that lay perceptions should supplant risk assessments derived from scientific methodologies. Public health authorities gain their legitimacy by making sound scientific assessments. I am suggesting that, in a democratic society, public health has a political dimension that reasonably takes into account community values such as voluntariness, personal benefit, and fair distribution in risk assessments.

RISK–RISK TRADE-OFFS

Public health regulation entails trade-offs between competing risks to health. Frequently, when government intervenes to diminish one risk, it simultaneously increases another risk. Thus, drinking water standards requiring chemical disinfection decrease risks of *Cryptosporidium* but increase risks of cancer.[44] Universal precautions in medical settings decrease risks of bloodborne infection, but increase costs, and thus make health care less widely available. Nuclear power regulation reduces radiation risks, but drives the market toward coal- or oil-based energy, thus increasing other hazards to humans and the environment.[45]

Risk–risk trade-offs occur in several contexts, making the problem difficult to resolve. Most often, regulators are aware of the trade-offs, but have insufficient scientific data to choose the most serious risk among several hazards. It is not always possible, for example, to compare the immediate risk of a waterborne disease outbreak and the latent risk of introducing a carcinogen into the drinking water supply. Sometimes, regulators are simply unaware of competing risks. Since civil servants usually are responsible for one set of health problems, they may have "tunnel vision" and fail to notice other risks. Relatedly, agencies may have narrow regulatory authority that does not permit them to consider risks outside their jurisdiction. Environmental agencies, for example, may have jurisdiction to reduce exposure to lead or radon in homes, but lack authority to prevent an overall decrease in housing stock resulting from environmental regulation. Ideally, public health authorities should undertake a coordinating function among health and social services agencies so that they could consider aggregate rather than isolated risks.

THE EFFECTIVENESS OF PUBLIC HEALTH REGULATION: THE "MEANS/ENDS" TEST

As we have just seen, the objective of public health regulation is to avert or diminish a significant risk to health. While courts and the public readily understand the need for a substantial health objective, they pay less attention to the methods used to achieve the goal.[46] Instead, the intervention's effectiveness is simply assumed; or, more likely, the courts and the public trust the experts to develop, implement, and evaluate the intervention. It is unwise to assume that public health interventions are always effective. In fact, since the proposed regulation entails personal burdens and economic costs, government should affirmatively demonstrate, through scientific data, that the methods adopted are reasonably likely to achieve the public health objective. This is called the "means/ends test"—it is the government's burden to defend, and rigorously evaluate, the effectiveness of regulation. The fact that government regulates in a particular area does not necessarily mean that it is "doing something" about the problem. The better questions are whether public health authorities accurately measure the health hazard, effectively reduce the risk or ameliorate the harm, and rigorously evaluate the intervention.

Public health authorities should accurately measure relevant health risks as a prerequisite to meaningful action. If a regulatory response to radioactivity, magnetic fields, or lead paint is considered, public health authorities should understand the health risks posed—How much is known about the hazard? How much exposure, and of what duration, is safe? How much reduction in exposure is necessary to reduce the risk to acceptable levels? If the hazard is not well understood, then risk reduction strategies are unlikely to be successful.

Public health authorities should not simply measure the health risk but, in fact, reduce that risk or ameliorate the ensuing harm. Regulatory activities are frequently justified by historical convention. The need to demonstrate an intervention's effectiveness, therefore, requires ongoing evaluation.[47] The Institute of Medicine proposes the adoption of performance monitoring, a process of selecting and analyzing indicators to measure the outcomes of an intervention strategy for health improvement.[48] Admittedly, scientific evaluation is complex because many behavioral, social, and environmental variables confound objective measurement of the causal connection between an intervention and a health outcome. Nevertheless, asking public health authorities to demonstrate an intervention's effectiveness is necessary to ensure that the community health benefits outweigh the personal burdens and economic costs.

THE ECONOMIC COSTS OF PUBLIC HEALTH REGULATION

Public health regulations impose economic costs—agency resources to devise and implement the regulation, costs to individuals and businesses subject to the regulation, and lost opportunities to intervene with a different, potentially more effective, technique (opportunity costs). A major issue, much debated in the literature, is the relevance of cost in regulatory decisions designed to safeguard public health. Under standard accounts, government should prefer regulatory responses that provide the most health benefits (e.g., saving the most years of life, or quality-adjusted years of life)[49] at the least cost.[50] Health economists use this "cost-benefit" or "cost-effectiveness" analysis to estimate the net health effects of a regulatory program or intervention.[51]

Society cannot escape the role that cost plays. Few people question the premise that society has finite, and relatively scarce, resources available for public health regulation. Given the reality of scarcity, hard choices must be made between regulatory alternatives. Do we spend large sums to avert relatively trivial risks, or do we devote resources to rather more serious risks that can be ameliorated at significantly lower cost? Although society cannot tally up costs and benefits into a tidy number, it can make sensible choices in prioritizing regulatory expenditures.

THE STANDARD ECONOMIC ACCOUNT

Under the standard economic account, three serious problems exist with the regulatory state: inordinate costs for small health benefits (low cost-effectiveness), regulation carried to illogical extremes ("going the last mile"), and arbitrary selection of regulatory topics ("random agenda selection").[52] The principal critique of the regulatory process is that government often requires enormous expenditures to achieve relatively small health benefits. Focusing mostly on environmental regulations designed to reduce cancer risks, economists estimate that government spends, in some cases, millions of dollars to save a single human life.[53]

Regulators exacerbate the costs of intervention by "going the last mile"—insisting on near-zero risk from a particular hazard. Sometimes an agency is so single-minded in its pursuit of safety that it imposes high costs without achieving significant additional benefits. Trying to remove the last vestiges of risk often involves extraordinary technological measures, high cost, and legal fees. For example in one federal case, the EPA required an expenditure of $9.3 million to eliminate the last remnants of toxic material at a swamp site so that children could safely eat dirt for 245 days a year, rather than only 70 days.[54]

Finally, extreme disparities in regulatory decisions make the process appear arbitrary. Humans face innumerable hazards and only a small fraction are regulated. Even among those hazards that are regulated, little consistency exists in the costs incurred and the benefits achieved. When economists compare the resources that the government commits to eliminate different kinds of risk, the results are striking: Small risks, such as the carcinogenic effects of toxic substances, entail enormous regulatory cost, whereas large risks, such as injuries from unsafe product design, entail modest regulatory cost.[55] From a strict cost-benefit perspective, agencies devote dramatically different attention to different kinds of death.

While these economic critiques are powerful, cost-effectiveness analysis is highly controversial. First, market exchanges are not the principal measure of the value of a human life. Lives are not commensurate with dollars, and precise monetary valuation of human life cannot account for the hopes, fears, and fragilities of people, their families, and the things that humans value. Second, public health regulation cannot be compressed, through ever more complex economic methods, into one aggregate number, such as costs per quality-adjusted life saved.[56] Estimates of cost per life saved are not objective scientific facts susceptible to precise quantification.[57] Technical cost-benefit analysis is imbued with social values such as the worth of human lives, the appropriate policy response to scientific uncertainty, and the importance of intangible regulatory benefits, such as ecological improvements.[58] Yet regulatory costs do need to be considered because maximization of health benefits within a relatively fixed budget remains an important social value, as the following discussion of opportunity costs suggests.

OPPORTUNITY COSTS

Why is it a problem if public health regulations impose inordinate expense with relatively modest benefits? At least part of the answer is that whenever government regulates, it forgoes opportunities for other interventions that improve community health. It is helpful to look at both sides of the effectiveness-expense equation to understand opportunity costs. If government adopts an *ineffective* strategy, it loses opportunities to intervene with a different, potentially more beneficial, technique. There is usually limited political will and agency resources to adopt multiple methods of intervention simultaneously. Consequently, adoption of ineffective methods means that more beneficial strategies are either forgone or delayed, thus adversely affecting community health.

Now consider the *cost* side of the effectiveness-expense equation. A decision to devote extensive resources to avert trivial risks means that government is forgoing opportunities to regulate far more serious risks. Legislatures allocate limited resources to spend on public health regulation. Decisions to spend in one area mean that the money may not be available to spend in another, more problematic, area. Government can reduce morbidity and premature mortality more by concentrating on serious hazards that are amenable to reduction at a reasonable cost. When expensive regulations are seen as lost opportunities, it becomes clearer that the operable trade-off is not "money-for-lives," a choice that understandably generates public concern. Rather, the trade-off is "health-for-health" or "lives-for-lives," because a choice to spend excessively wastes not only dollars, but also opportunities to promote health and longevity.

PERSONAL BURDENS OF PUBLIC HEALTH REGULATION: THE LEAST RESTRICTIVE ALTERNATIVE

Public health regulations impose not only economic costs, but also human rights burdens. A public health policy may be well-designed, cost-effective, and likely to promote the health and well-being of the population, but still be unacceptable from an individual rights perspective. Table 3 lists many of the ways in which public health interventions invade personal rights such as autonomy, privacy, expression, association, and religion. It also lists many of the ways in which public health regulations interfere with proprietary interests such as the pursuit of trade and professional opportunities, the value of land or personal property, and commercial interests.

The following chapters offer a more detailed account of these personal rights and freedoms. For now, it is necessary to emphasize the importance of personal burdens in evaluating public health regulations. In each case, public health authorities should consider the (1) *invasiveness*—to what degree does the public health intervention intrude on the right in question? (2) *frequency and scope*—does the infringement of rights apply to one person, a group, or an entire population? and (3) *duration*—how long a period is the person or group subject to the infringement?

Public health authorities should adopt the policy that is most likely to promote health and prevent disease while incurring the fewest possible personal burdens. The least restrictive alternative does not require public health authorities to adopt policies that are less likely to protect the population's health. Rather, authorities should prefer the least intrusive and burdensome policy that achieves their goals as well as, or better than, possible alternatives.

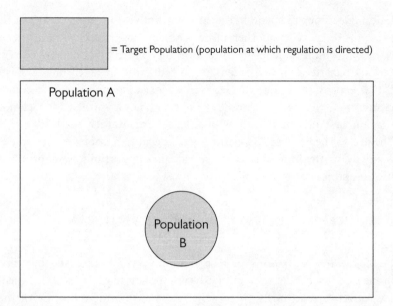

Population A = All people who fail to notify their sex partners of an STD
Population B = All prostitutes who fail to notify their customers of an STD

Figure 9a.   Underinclusion: policy imposing criminal penalties
against commercial sex workers. (Based on Lawrence Gostin and
Jonathan M. Mann, *Towards the Development of a Human Rights
Impact Assessment for the Formulation and Evaluation of Public
Health Policies*, 1(1) HEALTH AND HUMAN RIGHTS 59, 69 (1994).)

FAIRNESS IN PUBLIC HEALTH: JUST DISTRIBUTION OF BENEFITS, BURDENS, AND COSTS

Public health policy allocates benefits, burdens, and costs. Everyone realizes that, to achieve the common good, it is sometimes necessary to
confer benefits and impose regulatory costs and burdens. The mark of
a desirable public health policy is when benefits, burdens, and costs are
equitably distributed. But how are we to judge whether these distributions among populations are inherently just? The final step in a systematic evaluation of public health policy is an examination of fairness.

Public health policy is just where, to the extent possible, it provides
services to those in need and imposes burdens and costs on those who
endanger the public health.[59] Services provided to those without need
are wasteful and, given scarce resources, may deny benefits to those
with genuine need. Regulation aimed at persons or businesses where
there is no danger imposes costs and burdens without a corresponding
public benefit. Ideally, services should be allocated on the basis of need

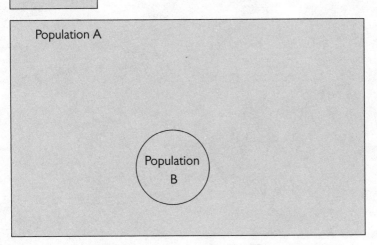

= Target Population (population at which regulation is directed)

Population A

Population B

Population A = All homeless persons with active TB
Population B = All homeless persons with active TB who actually will fail
                to take their medication and, as a result, are dangerous

Figure 9*b*.   Overinclusion: policy requiring directly observed therapy for
tuberculosis treatment.

and burdens should be imposed only where necessary to prevent a serious health risk.

Another way to think about equitable allocation is to consider the
policy's target population. Most policies target a particular population
by creating a class of people to whom the policy applies. Well-conceived
policies should avoid both under- and overinclusiveness (see Figure 9
and, for the constitutional implications, chapter 3). A policy is underinclusive when it reaches some, but not all, of the persons it ought to
reach. Thus, a policy is underinclusive if government provides services
to only a subgroup of those in need, or if it regulates only a subgroup of
those who are dangerous. By itself, underinclusion is not necessarily a
problem because government may tackle a public health problem gradually or in stages. For example, STD counseling and education targeted
to high prevalence urban areas, but not rural communities, simply
reflects reasonable government priorities. However, certain underinclusiveness masks discrimination, such as when government exercises coercive powers against politically powerless groups, but not others who engage in similar behavior. Suppose that government criminally penalizes

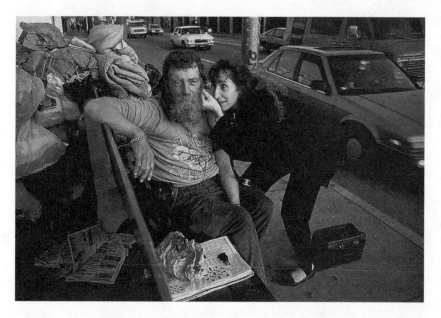

A physician conducts an examination of a homeless man in Los Angeles, 1995.
(Steve McCurry, Magnum Photos, Inc.)

prostitutes for engaging in sexual intercourse without informing their customers of the risk of an STD, but fails to prosecute all others engaging in the same behavior. Arguably, the underinclusion reflects animus toward commercial sex workers (see Figure 9a).

A policy is overinclusive if it extends to more people than necessary to achieve its purposes. The policy unnecessarily benefits or penalizes a group of people. Overinclusion in public health is often problematic. Overinclusiveness with regard to services is not cost-effective because some people receiving services are not in need. For example, HIV testing and counseling for all acute-care hospital patients is overinclusive since many children and elderly persons are not at risk. Overinclusiveness with regard to coercive regulation imposes economic costs and human rights burdens unnecessarily by penalizing persons who pose no health risk. Consider a policy that prohibits all physicians with a bloodborne infection from practicing medicine. The policy penalizes an entire class, even though most physicians in the class pose no risk to patients.

Public health policies can be both under- and overinclusive. Such policies burden individuals who do not pose a danger to the public (overinclusiveness), yet fail to include those individuals who do pose a danger (underinclusiveness). Suppose that public health authorities require homeless persons with M. TB tuberculosis to attend a clinic to receive compulsory treatment, but exempt all others with the same medical condition. The public health judgment is made on the unsupported premise that all those in the regulated group (homeless persons) pose a risk of not taking their medication, but those in the unregulated group pose no such risk. The policy is underinclusive because persons in the unregulated group may fail to take their medication, thus posing a risk to themselves and others. At the same time, the policy is overinclusive, since many people in the regulated group will take their medication, thus posing no risk (see Figure 9b).

In summary, public health authorities should justify regulation by demonstrating a significant risk, the intervention's effectiveness, reasonableness of economic costs and human rights burdens, and fundamental fairness. This proposed evaluation will not invariably lead to the best policy because any analysis is fraught with judgments about politics and values and is confounded by scientific uncertainty. Nevertheless, the evaluation at least requires public health authorities to think systematically and apply consistent standards when making policy.

THE SYNERGY BETWEEN HUMAN RIGHTS AND PUBLIC HEALTH

In this chapter I have argued that trade-offs between collective goods and individual rights are pervasive in public health, yet influential scholars have argued that these two values do not conflict. In fact, current public health literature suggests a synergistic relationship between public goods and individual rights.[60] The late Jonathan Mann famously argued, "The proposal that promoting and protecting human rights is inextricably linked to the challenge of promoting and protecting health derives in part from recognition that health and human rights are complementary approaches to the central problem of defining and advancing human well-being."[61] By this account, individual rights and public health are consistent objectives, even mutually reinforcing.

The public health literature offers three justifications in support of the conclusion that health and human rights are mutually reinforcing. First, government regulation that restricts personal freedom has unintended effects on health-seeking behavior. Individuals who fear the negative consequences of coercive government action are less likely to participate in public health programs such as testing for the presence of infection or disease, medical examination and treatment, partner notification, and so forth. Consider a statute, enacted in most states, that criminalizes sexual intercourse if the person knows she has a sexually transmissible infection and fails to inform her partner. The statute appears reasonably designed to prevent the transmission of disease, but it provides a disincentive for persons to seek testing or to confide in physicians. The unintended consequence of the statute is that it becomes better not to know one's serological status. As a result, proponents would argue, government should avoid coercive policies that drive epidemics underground.

Second, discrimination and invasion of privacy, resulting in social stigma and economic harms, provide similar disincentives for health-seeking behavior. Thus, if persons are concerned that they will suffer embarrassment, or discrimination in employment, insurance, or housing, they may avoid public health programs. As a result, government should take affirmative steps to protect individual rights, for example, by enacting and enforcing privacy and nondiscrimination laws.[62] The case for laws safeguarding privacy and nondiscrimination extends beyond the usual justifications of respect for persons and justice, and goes to the promotion of public health. For example, communities oppose named HIV reporting not only because it invades privacy (a consideration of autonomy), but also because it discourages testing (a consideration of public health).[63]

Third, the denial of social, economic, and political rights impedes the ability of persons to protect their own health and safety. In support of this view, scholars observe that traditional public health interventions do not alter risk behaviors unless populations are afforded human rights.[64] Consider women who are at risk of HIV infection within marriage. Public health authorities may test for HIV infection, counsel and educate about high-risk sex, and provide condoms as a means for behavior change. However, a woman's risk is her inability to control her husband's sexual behavior or to refuse unwanted or unprotected sex because of the fear of domestic violence or the economic ruination of divorce. Consequently, government efforts to reduce women's risk can be successful only by enhancing social and economic rights through violence prevention and laws improving women's status relating to property, marriage, divorce, and inheritance.[65]

Certainly, government can often improve the public health by safe-guarding civil and political rights and promoting social, economic, and cultural rights; however, it is not always possible both to ensure a full measure of rights and freedoms and to achieve all the goals of disease prevention and health promotion. Public and private goods can coexist in many cases, but hard cases remain that require careful analysis to re-solve the public-private tension.

To justify the assertion that public health and individual rights some-times cannot coexist, I turn to a series of classical conflicts between these two values. Part Two explores the collective benefits of a number of important public health strategies: surveillance, health communica-tion, case finding, immunization, mandatory treatment, criminal penal-ties, and a variety of powers directed toward businesses and the pro-fessions (e.g., inspections, zoning, nuisance abatement, and licensure). I also explore the public health benefits of indirect regulation through the tort system. Each chapter examines the trade-offs between public goods and individual costs and burdens.

PART TWO

Public Health and Civil Liberties in Conflict

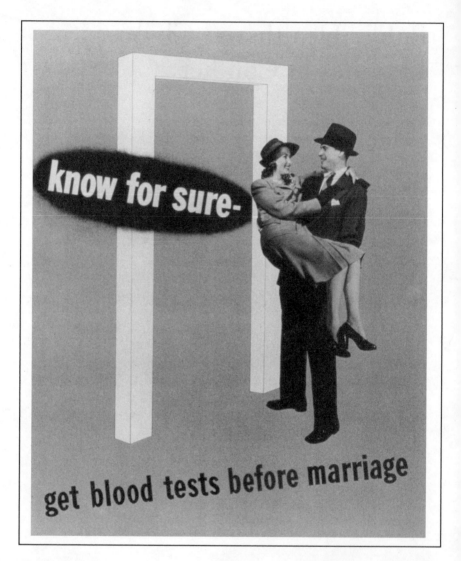

This 1940s poster was part of a Public Health Service campaign to encourage testing for syphilis before marriage. Many states enacted laws requiring premarital screening for sexually transmitted diseases.

5 Public Health Information

Personal Privacy

[H]alf the life is passed in infancy, sickness and dependent helpless-
ness . . . in exhibiting the high mortality, the diseases by which it is
occasioned and the exciting causes of disease, the abstracts of the
registers will prove that while a part of the sickness is inevitable and
a part may be expected to disappear by progressive social ameliora-
tion a considerable proportion may be suppressed by the general
adoption of hygienic measures.

William Farr (1838)

One of the core functions of the public health system is to gather health
information and to deploy those data for the welfare of the community.[1] Information concerning risk factors for—and the patterns, trends,
and causes of—injury and disease forms the basis for rational public
health decision-making. Health information is indispensable for virtually all public health activities including identifying, monitoring, and
forecasting health threats; response and intervention; program evaluation; and population-based research.[2] It is for this reason that biostatistics[3] and epidemiology[4] are the foundational sciences of public
health. Together, they supply the empirical evidence upon which public
health judgments are made and upon which public policy should rely.

I define the public health information infrastructure as the acquisition, use, retention, and transmission of data about the population's
health that supports the essential functions of the public health system
(for essential public health functions, see Table 4; for definitions of the
public health information sciences, see Table 5).[5] The development of
population-based information systems is not a distant concept, but an
emerging reality.[6] National, regional, and statewide databases are becoming vast reservoirs of public health information. Public health au-

TABLE 4
ESSENTIAL PUBLIC HEALTH FUNCTIONS

Function	Definition
Assessment	Identify needs, analyze causes, and find cases
Policy Development	Determine priorities, objectives, and means
Assurance	Ensure services to meet health needs

TABLE 5
THE SCIENCES AND PRACTICES
OF PUBLIC HEALTH: DEFINITIONS

Public Health Information Infrastructure	The acquisition, use, retention, and transmission of data about the population's health that supports the essential functions of the public health system.
Epidemiology (Originally, the Study of Epidemics)	The discipline concerned with the study of the distribution and determinants of health-related states or events in specified populations, and the application of this study to control health problems. Epidemiologists seek patterns, trends, and causes of morbidity and premature mortality, and proceed from two basic premises: (1) Disease is not randomly distributed in populations, and (2) subgroups differ in both disease frequency and contributing factors.
Biostatistics	The branch of statistics that analyzes data derived from the medical and biological sciences and is concerned with (1) the collection, organization, and summarization of data and (2) the drawing of inferences about a body of data when only a part of the data is observed.
Public Health Surveillance	The public health practice of continual watchfulness over the distribution and trends of risk factors, injury, and disease in the population through the systematic collection, analysis, and interpretation of selected health data for use in the planning, implementation, and evaluation of public health practice.

thorities can collect, reconfigure, identify patterns in, and disseminate health information with a speed and efficiency never before possible.

A sound public health information infrastructure can produce many social benefits:[7] early detection of microbial (e.g., Cryptosporidium, *Escherichia coli*, or drug-resistant M. TB), environmental (e.g., lead poisoning or radon), behavioral (e.g., iatrogenic injuries or gunshot wounds), and other health threats (e.g., abuse of a child, elderly person, or spouse); concentrate resources and focus interventions in areas of greatest need; promote behavioral, social, and environmental changes by identifying hazards and providing health information to persons at risk; assess public health measures by evaluations of efficacy and cost; and affect legislation and alter social norms by providing accurate health information to citizens and policymakers. In short, health data enable agencies to identify health risks, inform the public, intervene, and influence funding decisions, all of which are indispensable to the mission of public health.

The systematic acquisition of personal health data, however, poses serious privacy risks to individuals and groups. American society places a high value on individual rights, autonomous decision-making, and the protection of the private sphere from governmental or other intrusion. Health information can reveal intimate aspects about an individual's, or a family's, life and may affect the ability to hold a job, maintain custody of children, secure immigration status, or obtain access to insurance or public benefits. As vastly greater quantities of information are collected and transmitted to an increasing number of users, the ability of individuals to control access to personal information is sharply reduced.

Thoughtful scholarship in the area of informational privacy sometimes assumes that significant levels of privacy can coexist with the development of a modern public health information infrastructure.[8] To a certain extent, respecting confidences and promoting public health are consistent goals. Public health depends on the community's trust and cooperation, and failure to safeguard privacy discourages individuals from participating in programs such as screening, partner notification, and treatment. However, we cannot have it both ways; that is, society cannot fully protect privacy while still maintaining all the collective benefits of health information. Because privacy cannot realistically be assured, we confront a hard choice. Should we sharply limit the systematic collection of identifiable health data in order to achieve high levels of informational privacy? Alternatively, we may decide that the value of information is so important to the achievement of societal aspirations for health that government should not impede data flows with strong privacy safeguards.

This chapter first examines the major methods of information gathering undertaken by public health authorities: surveillance, reporting, partner notification, and public health research. Next, it takes a hard look at two forms of personal privacy—informational privacy and relational privacy—including major ethical dilemmas faced by public health and health care professionals, such as those occasioned by the "duty to warn" and the "right to know." Finally, it presents a model law designed to safeguard personal privacy while not unduly diminishing effective public health action.

PUBLIC HEALTH SURVEILLANCE

The French word *surveillance* was introduced into the English language at the time of the Napoleonic Wars and meant "a close watch or guard kept over a person."[9] Public health surveillance is the continued watchfulness over the distribution and trends of risk factors, injury, and disease in the population through the systematic collection, analysis, and interpretation of selected health data for use in the planning, implementation, and evaluation of public health practice.[10]

Historically, surveillance focused on identifying and controlling persons with communicable diseases. Mandatory reporting of diseases predated the founding of the Republic. A Rhode Island statute of 1741 required tavern keepers to report to local authorities any patrons known to harbor contagious diseases.[11] Systematic disease reporting at the state level was initiated in 1874 when Massachusetts instituted a voluntary plan for weekly physician reporting. In a letter to physicians, the State Board of Health enclosed a sample notification card to "reduce to the minimum the expenditure of time and trouble incident to the service asked of busy medical men."[12]

The federal government instituted national mortality data collection in 1850, the year of the first decennial census,[13] followed by morbidity data collection on plague, cholera, smallpox, and yellow fever in 1878.[14] The U.S. Public Health Service circulated a model law in 1913 to harmonize reporting requirements, but few states adopted it.[15] All states did not participate in national morbidity reporting until 1925, following the epidemics of poliomyelitis in 1916 and influenza in 1918–1919, which heightened public awareness of infectious diseases.[16]

Infectious disease surveillance assumed critical importance to public health in the mid-to-late twentieth century. In 1955, acute poliomyelitis among vaccine recipients threatened the program until surveillance data linked the problem to a single manufacturer. Globally, surveillance was the foundation for the control of malaria and the eradication of smallpox during the 1960s and 1970s.[17] In 1981, shortly after case clusters of unusual pneumonia and rare cancers among gay men were reported, epidemiologists described the acquired immunodeficiency syndrome (AIDS) and determined its likely mode of transmission.[18] Similarly, in 1993, after clusters of deaths among otherwise healthy residents of the Southwest were described, investigators identified a new strain of Hantavirus and devised a means of prevention.[19] At the turn of the twentieth century, surveillance to identify emerging infections[20] and to identify bioterrorism threats[21] have become national priorities.

Public health agencies gather data on more than just communicable diseases. In growing recognition of the effects of behavior on personal health, health authorities now collect and analyze behavioral information regarding, for instance, alcohol and drug use, seat belt and bicycle helmet use, smoking, exercise, and sexual practices.[22] To assess environmental risks, health agencies collect such data as pediatric blood lead levels and the incidence of cancers, birth defects, and pulmonary diseases. To assess genetic variations associated with disease, health authorities collect and evaluate genetic data among the population.[23] The public health system requires reliable information about communicable, behavioral, environmental, and genetic risks to reduce morbidity and excess mortality.[24] Despite its importance for the public's health, however, resources and priorities for surveillance are inadequate and the public health infrastructure is deteriorating.[25] (Table 6 presents current data systems used to monitor health status.)

MANDATORY REPORTING OF DISEASES AND OTHER HEALTH CONDITIONS

Morbidity registration will be an invaluable contribution
to therapeutics, as well as to hygiene, for it will enable
the therapeutists to determine the duration and fatality
of all forms of disease. . . . Illusion will be dispelled,
quackery. . . suppressed, a science of therapeutics
created, suffering diminished, life shielded from many
dangers.
                                        William Farr (1838)

States possess constitutional authority under their police powers to mandate reporting of a wide range of infectious diseases, injuries, and other health conditions to public health agencies. The Supreme Court has upheld reporting requirements against challenges that they violate personal privacy (discussed further below).[26] The states effectuate their police powers by

TABLE 6
CURRENT DATA USED TO MONITOR
HEALTH STATUS

Type of Data	Description
Vital Statistics	Registration system from records of live births, deaths, fetal deaths, and induced terminations of pregnancy
Morbidity and Mortality Reporting	Surveillance for selected diseases
National Health Interview Survey	National data on the incidence of acute illness and injury, chronic conditions and disabilities, and the utilization of health care services
National Health and Nutrition Examination Survey (NHANES)	Population-wide data collection by direct physical examination, clinical laboratory tests, and related measurements
National Electronic Injury Examination Survey (NEISS)	Surveillance of hospital emergency departments and investigation of representative cases of injury
Disease- or Purpose-specific	Data collection for diseases, such as HIV (sero-surveillance) or cancer (tumor registries), or to support functions such as childhood immunization
Genetic Databases	Research on stored tissue samples and systematic collection of population-based genetic information

enacting legislation that enumerates reportable health conditions (or classes of reportable diseases, such as "communicable" or "sexually transmitted") or delegates that task to state or local health agencies.[27] Where legislation delegates authority, courts afford health agencies considerable discretion in deciding how to classify particular diseases. For example, New York's highest court rejected a challenge by physician organizations that insisted the Commissioner classify HIV as an STD; the Commissioner refused to do so, and the court upheld his exercise of discretion.[28]

States vary in the diseases that are reportable, the conditions under which reports must be furnished, the time frames for reporting, and the agencies responsible for receiving reports.[29] Statutes also vary in the persons that owe a duty to report, but most impose the obligation on specified health care providers and laboratories.

All states and territories participate in a national morbidity notification system by regularly reporting aggregate or case-specific data to the CDC; reporting of data from states to the CDC is voluntary.[30] Currently, approximately sixty reportable conditions are included in the national morbidity reporting system.[31] The Council of State and Territorial Epidemiologists (CSTE), in conjunction with the CDC, annually proposes additions to and deletions from the list of diseases under national surveillance, and most states conform to these recommendations.[32] The CDC creates standardized case definitions for infectious diseases;[33] it is also developing case definitions for chronic, environmental, and occupational injuries and diseases. Standardized case reports contain extensive information such as demographics (e.g., patient's name, age, race, and address), laboratory analysis, risk behaviors, and clinical history.

THE JURISDICTIONAL PROBLEM: OUT-OF-STATE LABORATORIES

As explained above, states usually require reporting both by the physician and the laboratory. Laboratories are usually more reliable reporters of data and act as a failsafe system. This failsafe system can break down if large health care providers send their tests to laboratories outside the state. The out-of-state laboratory probably has no duty to comply with a reporting requirement in the originating state. Certainly, the in-state physician who receives a positive test result from the out-of-state laboratory must furnish a report to the health department but, if she fails to do so, there is no backup system of laboratory reporting.

There are imaginative state and federal remedies for this jurisdiction problem. At the state level, regulators could require managed care organizations (MCOs) and other providers to contract only with out-of-state laboratories that agree to report. Sanctions for failure to report would be directed at the in-state MCO rather than the out-of-state laboratory. At the federal level, Congress probably has the power under the Commerce Clause to require reporting. Infectious disease control is a problem that crosses state lines and reportable data may be viewed as articles of commerce. In the absence of some remedy, however, the jurisdictional problem can thwart efforts for complete reporting, particularly in an era of integrated delivery systems that operate regionally or nationally.

PHYSICIAN AND COMMUNITY RESISTANCE: A CASE STUDY ON NAMED HIV REPORTING

Despite its long traditions and current prevalence, reporting is politically controversial and socially divisive. Reporting is viewed very differently in the fields of public health and medicine.[34] Public health professionals see their first duty as protecting the population and justify reporting by invoking science and the ethics of collective responsibility. Private physicians, on the other hand, see their first duty as safeguarding patients and accord a higher priority to the sanctity of their therapeutic relationships.[35] Mandatory duties to report require physicians to notify government of their patients' names and other sensitive information, which are regarded as breaches of confidentiality. Patients, and the organizations that represent them, also sometimes oppose mandatory reporting because they do not trust the government to maintain sensitive case registries and are concerned about political retribution, invasions of privacy, and discrimination.

HIV case reporting has generated bitter political controversy and impassioned community resistance.[36] HIV reporting offers many public health benefits, including improved monitoring of the epidemic, more efficient targeting of prevention and support services, and improved clinical benefit by referring individuals for treatment.[37] Despite the importance of HIV surveillance, advocates fear government misuse of sensitive data.[38] A Florida health official, for instance, disclosed the names from an HIV registry to a dating service,[39] and Illinois enacted (but never implemented) legislation requiring cross-matching the state AIDS registry against health care licensure records.[40] Community representatives also express concern that HIV case reporting might deter people from being tested and seeking treatment,[41] although empirical research does not validate this concern.[42]

Because of their fears about privacy and discrimination, community organizations have urged public health authorities to implement a system of unique identifiers as an alternative to named surveillance,[43] yet studies of unique identifier systems have found that data collected often contain incomplete and difficult-to-match records.[44]

Here we have a classic illustration of a policy that produces important public health benefits but engenders fear and distrust within the community. Furthermore, less restrictive alternatives such as unique identifiers appear ineffective. No easy resolution exists: policies that meet public health objectives fail to satisfy community representatives, and policies that meet civil liberties objectives fail to satisfy public health authorities. The CDC's proposal is to promote named HIV reporting with alternative test sites and strong privacy and security assurances.[45] Under this policy, public health benefits appear to outweigh civil liberties concerns, particularly because states have strong records of privacy protection. The critical, unresolved question is whether, in a representative democracy, government should impose its view of the collective good on an unwilling community.

PARTNER NOTIFICATION

In no other respect is the [medical] practice in this
country more reprehensible than in the failure of
physicians, and even of public health clinics, to make
diligent inquiry as to sources of infection and to use
all available methods to bring these persons under
treatment.

Thomas Parran (1931)

Partner notification is a highly complex concept that has at least three distinct, if at times overlapping, meanings:[46] (1) *contact tracing*— statutory powers of public health agencies to identify and locate sexual partners and other "contacts" at risk of infection, and to notify them of their exposure; (2) *duty to warn*—the power or duty of private health care professionals to inform their patient's sexual or other partners of foreseeable risks; and (3) *right-to-know*—common law duty of infected persons to disclose their serological status to a sexual or other partner placed at risk. I discuss contact tracing here and the other two meanings later in this chapter.

Sexual contact tracing probably originated in the sixteenth century in Europe with the medical inspection of suspected syphilitic prostitutes through regulations that came to be known as reglementation.[47] The earliest reference to contact tracing in contagious disease law dates to mid–nineteenth century Europe.[48] "Contact epidemiology" became a central public health strategy in the United States during the syphilis epidemic in the 1930s.[49] The National Venereal Disease Act of 1938 adopted STD control measures proposed by the antivenereal disease campaigner, Surgeon General Thomas Parran.[50] Around the same time, states began enacting STD statutes giving public health authorities wide-ranging powers to control venereal diseases.[51]

From its widespread use during the 1930s, the notification of sexual partners remained an accepted part of the law and practice of STD control throughout the twentieth century.[52] This concept of tracking sexual contacts later would be called "partner notification," which has expanded over the years to include a range of support services, including counseling and medical treatment.[53]

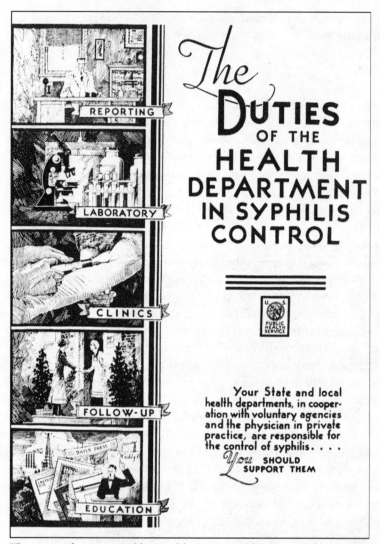

The cover of a 1940s Public Health Service publication emphasizing
the role of state and local governments in planning and conducting
campaigns for the diagnosis and treatment of persons with syphilis.
This poster illustrates a range of interventions to control syphilis.

Partner notification is a quintessential state and local function exercised through the police power. State statutes empower public health
agencies to implement partner notification as part of STD or HIV prevention programs.[54] The federal government does not require partner
notification but, as early as 1918,[55] through to the present day,[56]
Congress has influenced contact tracing policy through its conditional

spending power. Despite being classified as an STD since 1988, Congress has treated HIV separately from other STDs. The Ryan White Act of 1990 provides grants to states to implement partner notification programs for HIV-infected persons.[57] In 1996, the Act required states to notify spouses of persons infected with HIV as a condition of the receipt of partner notification funds.[58]

Public health authorities utilize two primary models of partner notification, namely, patient and provider referral. A hybrid of these two models is known as conditional referral.[59] With patient referral, index patients (infected patients identified in public health clinics or by physician referrals) are asked to contact their partners. Provider referral switches the responsibility for notification to trained public health personnel who inform contacts and offer counseling and treatment. Public health professionals protect confidentiality by declining to reveal the index patient's name (although contacts can often deduce the patient's identity).

Partner notification, like reporting, has generated bitter controversy. As members of stigmatized groups, commercial sex workers in the syphilis epidemic of the 1930s[60] and gay men in the AIDS epidemic of the late twentieth century[61] were suspicious of the true intentions of public health officials. These groups believed that partner notification, although nominally voluntary, had coercive elements because vulnerable persons may feel they have no choice but to cooperate with government officials. Providing the names of intimate sexual partners also was thought to be a gross invasion of privacy and left contacts susceptible to discrimination. Persons revealing the names of their partners also faced serious physical, sexual, and emotional abuse.[62] For example, a woman trapped in an abusive relationship may reasonably fear that she will be subject to a violent reaction if her partner discovers she is HIV positive.

While many in the community have opposed partner notification because of its intrusive qualities, persons in relationships with an infected person have claimed a right to be informed of the risk. Armed with adequate knowledge, the partners of infected persons could make reasoned judgments about sex and sharing drug injection equipment. Think about the situation of a woman who has been in a long-term sexual relationship and has never been apprized of the fact that her partner has an STD. She genuinely may feel wronged if health authorities are aware of, but fail to disclose, the risk.

Partner notification programs have sought mightily to straddle a fine line between the interests of infected persons and their partners. Partner notification, in theory, is warranted because only persons who are informed of their infected status can take steps to reduce risks and ameliorate harms. While partner notification is unexceptional in theory, empirical evidence of its cost-effectiveness is decidedly mixed.[63] On balance, partner notification remains a viable public health strategy. The traditions of voluntary cooperation, nondisclosure of names, and the provision of support services minimize social harms while still recognizing legitimate public claims to protection against undisclosed risks of infection.

POPULATION-BASED RESEARCH

Public health professionals engage in a great deal of population-based research, ranging from large field trials of candidate vaccines and pharmaceuticals to epidemiological studies and population surveys.[64] It is important for public health researchers to maintain the trust of communities and to ensure that research is conducted ethically. The trust of vulnerable communities has been strained by unethical research studies, such as the CDC-supported Tuskegee study initiated in the early 1930s to observe the natural course of syphilis among African-American men in Alabama. The men were not informed that they were research subjects and were not offered penicillin until the study became public in 1972.[65] Similarly, during the Cold War, vulnerable human subjects were exposed to radiation without their knowledge or consent.[66] More recently, the CDC sponsored a study in inner-city Los Angeles that administered an unlicensed measles vaccine to predominantly African-American and Latino children. The children's parents were not notified that the vaccine had not received FDA approval.[67]

Some commentators have also criticized international collaborative research conducted in developing countries. In 1997, ethical questions were raised about CDC/NIH-sponsored placebo-controlled trials of zidovudine (AZT) among pregnant women in Africa. A placebo-controlled trial would not have been ethically acceptable if performed in developed countries because AZT is known to be highly effective in preventing mother-to-infant transmission of HIV (see chapter 7). Comparing the African trials to the Tuskegee study, commentators argued that researchers knowingly permitted babies in their care to be born with preventable HIV infection.[68] However, the CDC and NIH observed that, far from harming African women, they were engaged in a search for an affordable regimen of AZT that would save hundreds of thousands of African children in the future.[69]

These kinds of ethical debates raise important questions about the salience of benefits to populations in public health research. For the most part, however, ethical principles stress the inherent worth and dignity of the individual rather than the benefits to communities. Under conventional theories, investigators should show *respect for persons,* which requires strict conformance with the choices made by competent persons and protection of vulnerable persons.[70] *Beneficence* (do good) and *nonmaleficence* (do no harm) impose affirmative duties on researchers to maximize benefits for subjects and minimize risks. *Justice* requires that human beings be treated equally unless there is a strong ethical justification for treating them differently. Thus, the selection of subjects, and the distribution of benefits and burdens in research, should be equitable.

These ethical principles have found expression in guidelines for the conduct of research, notably, in the United States, in the Belmont Report[71] and internationally, in the Nuremberg Code,[72] the Declaration of Helsinki,[73] and the Council of International Organizations of Medical Sciences' (CIOMS) Ethical Guidelines for Biomedical Research[74] and Epidemiological Studies.[75] Most of these ethical guidelines apply specifically to biomedical research and do not carefully consider population-based research.[76] Scholars have only recently begun to grapple with the complex problems of applying conventional ethics to population-based research.[77]

REGULATION OF HUMAN SUBJECT RESEARCH

Current legal regulations governing federally sponsored research adopt a biomedical approach and do not carefully consider population-based research. The Department of Health and Human Services (DHHS), in 1981, issued human subject regulations based on the *Belmont Report,* and in 1991, DHHS and sixteen additional executive branch agencies adopted a revised Federal Policy for the Protection of Human Subjects (the "Common Rule").[78] The Common Rule, which applies to human subject research conducted or supported by a federal agency, requires review and approval by an institutional review board (IRB) and the informed consent of human subjects. Despite providing important protection for research subjects, the Common Rule has significant gaps. The Common Rule applies only to federally funded studies, so purely private research remains unregulated. Furthermore, even with federally funded studies, the rigor with which IRBs review research protocols varies considerably.[79]

IRB Protection of Privacy.   The Common Rule, surprisingly, does not set minimum privacy standards. It does require IRBs to ensure that "[w]hen appropriate, there are adequate provisions to protect the privacy of subjects."[80] Furthermore, in seeking informed consent, the investigator must provide the subject with "[a] statement describing the extent, if any, to which confidentiality of records identifying the subject will be maintained."[81] Even if IRBs do take privacy seriously, the regulations themselves merely require safeguards when "appropriate." Although subjects must be informed whether their data are to be held confidentially, the regulations do not set minimum standards.

Court-Ordered Disclosure of Data (Confidentiality Assurance).   A "confidentiality assurance" under section 301(d) of the Public Health Service Act authorizes investigators to withhold the names or other identifying characteristics of research subjects.[82] Investigators who receive a confidentiality assurance cannot be compelled to identify research subjects in any civil, criminal, administrative, or legislative proceeding.[83] The certificate also appears to relieve researchers from the obligation to comply with state reporting requirements.[84] Although confidentiality assurances provide strong privacy protection, they are issued "sparingly," that is, "only when the research is of a sensitive nature where the protection is judged necessary to achieve the research objectives."[85]

DISTINGUISHING HUMAN SUBJECT RESEARCH FROM PUBLIC HEALTH PRACTICE

Federal and state health agencies have been wrestling with the problem of when routine state and local public health practice becomes a form of population-based research.[86] This is a vexing and important problem because, if routine public health practices (e.g., surveillance and outbreak investigations) were classified as "research," health departments would have to establish IRBs and obtain informed consent, which could impede a rapid and effective response to community health threats.

Since the Common Rule was never designed with population-based research in mind, it is difficult to tell as a matter of law when state and local health authorities must comply with research regulations. Research means "a systematic investigation, including development, testing, and evaluation, designed to develop or contribute to generalizable knowledge."[87] This definition is not satisfactory because many public health activities are systematic and generalizable; they use rigorous scientific methods to monitor and respond to health threats.

One way out of this morass is to focus on the word *design* in the Common Rule, which suggests that primary intent is important in classifying an activity as research or nonresearch.[88] If state and local health departments are serving populations for their own benefit (e.g., reporting, outbreak investigations, emergency response, and program evaluation), then the activity is public health practice.[89] If, however, public health authorities are seeking to answer a scientific question using methods such as random selection of subjects and experimental interventions, then the activity is research.[90]

The contemporary debates about the ethics of surveillance and public health research only underscore the importance of developing a code of public health research ethics or at least a well-articulated statement of principles. Minimally, such a code or statement would consider the material differences between public health practice and research, the salience of benefits to populations, the strength of individual interests in autonomy and privacy, and the role of communities.

DEFINITIONS OF PRIVACY, CONFIDENTIALITY, AND SECURITY

Public health professionals and researchers collect a great deal of personal information that invades the private sphere of human life. The following sections explore this private sphere, its philosophical underpinnings, and its legal status. Before examining privacy more closely, it will be helpful to offer some definitions (see Table 7).

Privacy, confidentiality, and security are sometimes thought to be identical concepts, but they are not.[91] The term *privacy*—an individual's claim to limit access by others to some aspect of her personal life—has acquired several different meanings in ethical discourse.[92] This chapter is not concerned with "decisional" privacy—the freedom claimed by individuals to make intimate decisions about their bodily integrity without interference. (Decisional privacy, asserted in contexts of medical treatment, is examined in chapter 8.) It is also not concerned with Samuel Warren and Louis Brandeis's conception of privacy as the "right to be let alone"—the freedom claimed by individuals not to be viewed, photographed, or otherwise inspected without their knowledge.[93]

This chapter refers primarily to "informational" privacy and, secondarily, to confidentiality (sometimes called "relational" privacy). I de-

TABLE 7

THE NATURE OF PRIVACY

Defining the Relevant Terms

Privacy	An individual's claim to limit access by others to some aspect of her personal life
Health Informational Privacy	An individual's claim to control the circumstances in which personal health information is collected, used, stored, and transmitted
Confidentiality	A form of health informational privacy that focuses on maintaining trust between two individuals engaged in an intimate relationship, characteristically a physician-patient relationship
Security	The technological, organizational, and administrative safety practices designed to protect a data system against unwarranted disclosure, modification, or destruction and to safeguard the system itself

fine health informational privacy as an individual's claim to control the circumstances in which personal health information is collected, used, stored, and transmitted.[94] Informational privacy, then, is concerned with an individual's claim to determine those persons or organizations that may access an identifiable health record. Confidentiality is a form of health information privacy that focuses on maintaining trust between two individuals engaged in an intimate relationship, characteristically a physician-patient relationship. Confidentiality is a person's claim to keep private the secrets exchanged in the course of that relationship, enforced not simply to respect the person whose confidences are divulged but also to underscore the importance of relationships of trust.

I define *security* as the technological, organizational, and administrative safety practices, policies, and procedures designed to protect a data system against unwarranted disclosure, modification, or destruction and to safeguard the system itself. For example, secure data systems require passwords or "keys" to access information, perform audit trails to monitor system users, and use encryption to scramble access codes. A secure data system will keep health records from unauthorized use. Invasions of privacy certainly occur, when, due to inadequate security, personal records are accessed without permission. No security measure, however, can prevent invasion of privacy by those who have authority to access the record. And many privacy scholars believe that the most serious threats to privacy come from authorized, systemic data uses.[95] Consequently, even the most technologically secure data systems do not ensure privacy.

THE NATURE OF THE PRIVACY INTEREST: PERSONALLY IDENTIFIABLE, CODED, AND ANONYMOUS DATA

A claim to informational privacy is generally valid only if the health record reveals private information about the subject of that record. Consequently, standards for disclosure should vary according to whether the record can be associated with a particular person (see Table 8). The most serious privacy concern arises when public health authorities use *personally identifiable data,* which has the following meaning: The person can be identified either by information contained in the record alone or with other information that is available to the record holder.[96] The inclusion of any uniquely identifiable characteristic, such as a name, social security number, fingerprint, or phone number, classifies data as identifiable. Even without a unique identifier, the data may provide sufficient evidence to make a connection to a specific person. Information about location, race, sex, date of birth, and other personal characteristics may make it possible to identify individuals within a small population (e.g., an STD study in a small, predominantly white school that identifies a cluster of syphilis infections among African-American females).

Release of *anonymous* data usually does not entail significant privacy concerns because individuals cannot realistically be identified. Data that have all identifiers stripped, with no reasonable means to associate the information with a specific person, are anonymous. Blinded epidemiologic research and statistical applications of aggregate data provide illustrations of anonymous research that affords substantial public health benefits with negligible effects on individual privacy. For example, collection and analysis of blood samples or other tissue that cannot be linked to any individual are anonymous; few, if any, restrictions need to be placed on research of this kind.[97]

Anonymous data can raise concerns about "group" privacy—the sometimes contested idea that ethnic, racial, or religious groups possess privacy interests. Suppose that a researcher does not collect personally identifiable data but publishes information that stigmatizes a particular group, as with genetics research on sickle cell anemia (African-Americans) or Tay-Sachs disease (Ashkenazi Jews). Or think about a

TABLE 8

THE NATURE OF PERSONALLY
IDENTIFIABLE INFORMATION

Personally Identifiable Data	Person can be identified either by information contained in the record or by other information that is available to the record holder
Anonymous Data	Data with all identifiers stripped, with no reasonable means to associate the information with a specific person
Linkable Data	Data that are not immediately identifiable to the record holder, but where the "key" unlocking the person's identity can be ascertained from a third party

study in a small Native American village finding that the population has extraordinarily high rates of drug abuse, mental illness, or STDs. In each of these cases, members of the group may feel that they have diminished reputation and social standing.[98]

Linkable data present an intermediate level of privacy concern. These data are not immediately identifiable but can be linked to a named person with the use of a highly confidential code. Linkable, or coded, data are not all the same for privacy purposes. If the data holder can readily obtain the key to decode the data, then privacy concerns are heightened; in this case, coded data can be viewed virtually as personally identifiable. However, if the holder cannot realistically decode the data to discover identifiable characteristics, then, for all practical purposes, these data may be viewed as anonymous. The major issue becomes whether the firewall between the holder of the data and the holder of the key is penetrable. For example, states send AIDS case reports to the CDC using a "soundex" code that the federal agency cannot decipher. The data held by the state health department are personally identifiable, but the data held by the CDC can be treated as anonymous for privacy purposes.

Public health professionals claim that identifiable, or linkable, data are often necessary for quality surveillance and research in order to assure accurate and complete records, avoid duplication of cases, and conduct follow-up investigations. Anonymous data complicate the task of obtaining useful information about risk behavior and natural history—the type of information that is available from interviews with physicians and patients and from medical records reviews that are currently accessed through the patient's name.[99]

Decisions to use identifiable, anonymous, or coded surveillance can be controversial. Recall the CDC's anonymous HIV seroprevalence study of newborns. The study provided scientifically valid, critically important surveillance data with negligible privacy risks. Nevertheless, this important study was criticized by Congress and ultimately withdrawn because, with anonymous records, health authorities lacked the capacity to inform mothers of an infant's infection status and need for treatment.[100]

HEALTH INFORMATIONAL PRIVACY: ETHICAL UNDERPINNINGS

Ethical justifications for privacy rely on the intimate nature of health data, the potential harm to persons, and the overall effect on the public health system if privacy is eroded.[101] Public health records contain significant amounts of sensitive information: public health officials are concerned about an individual's behavior (e.g., sexuality, smoking, and alcohol or drug use), genetic profile (e.g., genetic carrier states, predispositions, and disease), and social/racial/economic status (e.g., poverty, nutrition, and social relationships). Consequently, public health records contain a vast amount of personal information with multiple uses: demographics, public benefit eligibility, disabilities, sexual relationships, lifestyle choices, current and predictive health status, and much more. This information is frequently sufficient to provide a detailed individual profile. Traditional public health records, moreover, are only a subset of records containing substantial health or personal information held by other government agencies, such as social services, immigration, law enforcement, and education.

A variety of harms may result from unwanted disclosures of these sensitive health data. Intrinsic harms (sometimes called "wrongs") result from merely unwanted or unjustified disclosure of personal information. Many moral views recognize the desirability of protecting individuals against the insult to dignity and the lack of respect for the person evidenced by such disclosures.[102] Furthermore, a breach of privacy can result in economic harms such as loss of employment, insurance, or housing. It can also result in social or psychological harms; disclosure of some conditions can be stigmatizing and can cause embarrassment, social isolation, and a loss of self-esteem. These risks are especially great when the perceived causes of the health condition include the use of illegal drugs, socially disfavored forms of sexual expression, or other behavior that engenders social disapproval. Family members, neighbors, and work associates may withdraw social support from individuals known to have stigmatic diseases or physical or behavioral attributes that people find uncomfortable.

Privacy is important to the effective functioning of the public health system. Persons at risk of disease may not come forward for testing, counseling, and treatment if they are not assured that their confidences will be respected. They are also less likely to divulge sensitive information to health professionals. Failure to divulge communicable diseases may pose a risk to the health of sexual, needle-sharing, or other contacts. Informational privacy, therefore, is valued not only to protect patients' social and economic interests, but also their health and the health of the wider community.

HEALTH INFORMATIONAL PRIVACY: LEGAL STATUS

Thus far, I have suggested that health information affords meaningful public health benefits but also poses privacy risks. Legal protection of health information should, to the extent possible, facilitate use of health information to gain public benefits while still furnishing reasonable privacy protection.[103] Unfortunately, existing law—constitutional and legislative—neither promotes public goods nor satisfactorily protects privacy.

CONSTITUTIONAL RIGHT TO INFORMATIONAL PRIVACY

Judicial recognition of a constitutional right to informational privacy is particularly important since the government is the principal collector and disseminator of public health information.[104] Citizens should not have to rely on the government's choice to protect their privacy interests. Rather, individuals need protection from the government itself, and an effective constitutional remedy is the surest method to shield them from unauthorized government acquisition or disclosure of personal information. The problem with this approach is that the Constitution does not expressly provide a right to privacy.

Despite the absence of express constitutional language, the Supreme Court has found a qualified right to health informational privacy. In *Whalen v. Roe* (1977),[105] the Court squarely faced the question of whether the constitutional right to privacy encompasses the collection, storage, and dissemination of health information in government data banks. At issue was a New York statute requiring physicians to report to the state information about certain dangerous prescription drugs and to store the data in a central computer. The Court acknowledged "the threat to privacy implicit in the accumulation of vast amounts of personal information in computerized data banks or other massive government files."[106] It further noted that the supervision of public health activities "requires the orderly preservation of great quantities of information, much of which is personal in character and potentially embarrassing or harmful if disclosed."[107] However, the Court found no violation in *Whalen* because the state had adequate standards and procedures for protecting privacy: computer tapes were kept in a locked cabinet, the computer was run off-line to avoid unauthorized access, and the data were disclosed to a limited number of officials.

Most lower courts have read *Whalen* as affording a narrow right to informational privacy or have grounded the right on state constitutional law.[108] Courts have employed a flexible test balancing the invasion of privacy against the strength of the government interest. For example, the Third Circuit in *United States v. Westinghouse Electric Corporation* (1980)[109] enunciated five factors to be balanced in determining the scope of the constitutional right to informational privacy: (1) the type of record and the information it contains, (2) the potential for harm in any unauthorized disclosure, (3) the injury from disclosure to the relationship in which the record was generated, (4) the adequacy of safeguards to prevent nonconsensual disclosure, and (5) the degree of need for access (i.e., a recognizable public interest).

Judicial deference to government's expressed need to acquire and use information is an unmistakable theme running through the case law. Provided that the government articulates a valid societal purpose, such as protection of the public's health, and employs reasonable privacy and security measures, courts are unlikely to interfere with traditional surveillance activities.[110]

LEGISLATIVE AND REGULATORY PROTECTION OF INFORMATIONAL PRIVACY

A growing number of privacy statutes and regulations protect federal, state, and privately held records. Additionally, the Health Insurance Portability and Accountability Act of 1996[111] set an August 1999 deadline for Congress to enact privacy laws. Congress's efforts to enact a health informational privacy law failed, with interest groups on both sides refusing to compromise. As a result the Secretary for Health and Human Services issued proposed regulations on privacy and security standards in 1999.[112] However, the proposed rules do not regulate data held by public health agencies; public health data continue to be regulated under state law.

Federal Record Systems. The Privacy Act of 1974[113] requires federal agencies to utilize fair information practices with regard to "any record" contained in "a system of records." The statute gives individuals the right to consent to the disclosure of information and to review and correct inaccuracies in the record. Agencies can keep only relevant information and cannot "match" files through the use of a personal identifier. The Privacy Act, however, permits agencies to disclose information for "routine uses," meaning that they can use health records for any "purpose which is compatible with the purpose for which [the information] was collected."[114]

The Freedom of Information Act of 1966 (FOIA)[115] requires the disclosure of records that would otherwise have to be kept confidential under the Privacy Act. However, the Act contains several exemptions that permit agencies to withhold disclosure. The exemptions most important to public health are specific statutory exclusions from FOIA disclosure requirements (e.g., identifiable health statistics, drug abuse treatment records, and venereal disease records);[116] "privileged or confidential" data (federal health agencies rely on this exemption to resist judicial discovery of confidential patient or research records, for example, in cases involving toxic shock, Reyes syndrome, and cancer registry data);[117] and personnel and medical files (federal agencies can use this exemption to protect individuals from injury and embarrassment).[118]

State Health Records. States have enacted health information privacy protection in highly diverse ways, including statutes modeled after the federal Privacy Act and FOIA. A careful examination of the myriad state law protections of public health data is beyond the scope of this text, but national surveys are reported in the literature.[119] All states provide some statutory protection for governmentally maintained health data—public health data, in general, and communicable or sexually transmitted diseases, in particular. Many states provide specific protections for data reported to the health department or data held in state registries or databases (e.g., congenital birth defects, cancers, or childhood immunizations). Virtually all states permit disclosures of public health information for various purposes including statistics, partner notification, epidemiologic investigations, subpoena, or court order.

Privately Held Health Records (Including Disease-Specific Statutes).
Although many states have reasonably consistent standards for
government-held health information, the privacy protection afforded to
privately held data is widely regarded as inadequate. The law is fragmented, highly variable, and, at times, weak. Some states have comprehensive medical information statutes, others regulate the use of information by licensed professionals or hospitals, and still others regulate
the use of insurance information.[120] The Department of Health and
Human Services described this body of privacy legislation as "a morass
of erratic law."[121]

Federal and state law frequently single out particular diseases for
special status, so that data relating to these health conditions receive
high levels of privacy. For example, the law often affords extraordinary
privacy protection for data relating to drug and alcohol treatment,[122]
HIV/AIDS,[123] or genetic conditions.[124] These disease-specific privacy
statutes create inconsistencies in the rules governing the use of health
information. Different standards apply to data held by the same institutions depending on whether the patient is receiving treatment for a
protected disease. More important, the argument that certain diseases
deserve a special status rests on a weak foundation because many other
health conditions raise similar issues of sensitivity and intimacy.

The problem with existing health informational privacy protection is
that it does not adequately protect either of the major interests at stake.
That is, the law does not afford individuals reasonable privacy assurances,
nor does the law facilitate data uses for the collective good. At one extreme, health care providers in many states legally are able to use, transfer, or sell intimate health data for non-health-related purposes (e.g., commercial, employment, and criminal justice). At the other extreme, private
and public entities may not be able to use information for important
health purposes such as research and public health. For example, many
local health authorities are barred from matching TB, STD, and HIV registries for purposes of surveillance, prevention, and treatment. Privacy interests are certainly implicated in matching registries, but these epidemics
are interconnected, requiring an integrated public health approach.

CONFIDENTIALITY

In early shades of feminist theory, an ethical conundrum between medical secrecy and warning of risk
was evident in the views of a female physician:

> we have seen the wife murdered by syphilis
> contracted from an unfaithful husband and an
> innocent woman its victim for life.
>
> Marion C. Potter (1907)

As discussed earlier, confidentiality is a form of health informational privacy that focuses on maintaining trust between two individuals engaged in an intimate relationship. This section examines three different duties that arise from intimate relationships: the physician's duty of confidentiality, the physician's duty to protect third parties from harm (the "duty to warn"), and the duty of infected persons to inform their sexual or needle-sharing partners (the partner's "right to know"). The first two duties arise from special therapeutic relationships (e.g., physician-patient) and the third duty arises from sexual or other intimate relationships. The underlying tort concept of "duty" is important in understanding all three kinds of cases. A duty is a legal obligation to conform to a certain standard of conduct toward another person. Of the many factors that determine the existence of a duty, the most important is the foreseeability of risk of harm to another. If it is foreseeable that a person's behavior will cause harm, that person has a duty to take reasonable steps, or to exercise "due care," to avoid such behavior (see chapter 9).[125]

HEALTH CARE PROFESSIONALS' DUTY OF CONFIDENTIALITY

Most states recognize a common law duty of confidentiality between certain health care professionals (often physicians or therapists) and their patients. Thus, if a patient divulges personal information to a health care professional, the professional may be liable for disclosure without the patient's consent or another valid justification.[126] This can be described as the "breach of confidentiality" tort, although courts have relied on various theories of recovery, including invasion of privacy, implied term of contract, and breach of fiduciary relationship.[127]

The breach of confidentiality tort usually requires a special kind of relationship, one in which the patient has a clear expectation of privacy. When information is disclosed in the absence of a relationship or when the nature of the relationship itself is ambiguous (e.g., a doctor acting for an insurer[128] or employer[129]), a duty of confidence may not exist. Finally, a tort action usually will succeed only against the person who holds information in confidence.[130] Since the "holder" of the information can be unclear in an automated system, a tort duty may have questionable utility.

HEALTH CARE PROFESSIONALS' "DUTY TO WARN"

The duty of confidentiality poses a powerful dilemma for physicians and other health care professionals[131] when their patients pose a significant risk to others (for example, if the patient discloses an intention to harm a third party). If the physician reveals the risk, she breaches patient confidentiality; if she fails to disclose, she subjects known persons to danger. Most states impose on physicians a duty to protect third parties at risk, which may include a duty to warn. In such cases, physicians are held liable if they do not take reasonable care to protect third parties. Other states permit disclosures to protect third parties without creating a legal obligation. This approach creates a "privilege," but not a "duty," to inform third parties at risk.[132] In such cases, physicians have discretion to maintain confidentiality or to reveal a known risk; in either case, they do not face liability. These duties and privileges are created by statute[133] and/or by court decision.[134]

The duty to protect was famously recognized in *Tarasoff v. Regents of the University of California* (1976),[135] where a therapist was held liable for failing to warn a woman of the patient's intent to kill her.[136] Under *Tarasoff,* the duty to protect requires (1) *foreseeability*—the therapist must have determined, or reasonably should have determined, that her patient poses a risk to another;[137] (2) *a serious risk*—the risk posed to the third party must be genuine and not merely speculative or remote;[138] and (3) *an identifiable victim*—the person endangered should be known to the patient and therapist.[139] The *Tarasoff* line of cases is said to establish a "duty to warn," but this is technically incorrect. Rather, the physician has an obligation to use reasonable care to protect the third party placed in danger. This may require a "warning," but not in every case.

The duty to protect applies not only when patients pose a threat of physical harm, but also when they risk transmission of an infectious or sexually transmitted disease.[140] Courts usually require an identifiable person who faces a serious risk of contracting a disease, such as a known sexual or needle-sharing partner of a patient with HIV infection. For example, in *Gammill v. United States* (1984), a court held that an army physician had no duty to inform a nearby community of an outbreak of hepatitis B because he was not aware of specific risks to particular persons.[141]

The physician still may have duties to protect the public from an infectious disease, even if there is no identifiable victim. Some courts hold physicians liable if they fail to diagnose an infectious condition[142] or, if they do diagnose the condition, they fail to "instruct and advise" patients about the public risks they present.[143] Thus, physicians should advise patients of the nature of the infection, how it is spread, and precautions that can be taken. This may require explaining safer sex to persons with HIV infection or the importance of treatment and isolation for a person with infectious TB.[144]

DUTY OF INFECTED PERSONS TO INFORM

Persons who know they have an infectious condition have a duty to protect their close contacts or partners.[145] This duty ordinarily means abstaining from sexual relations or from sharing drug injection equipment. If a contagious person does expose another to infection, he may have to disclose the risk. For example, in the widely publicized case of *Christian v. Sheft* (1989),[146] a jury rendered a verdict against the estate of Rock Hudson because Mr. Hudson had engaged in "high-risk" sex and intentionally concealed his HIV status.[147] The duty to inform requires that the person knew, or should have known, that he was contagious. For example, a Michigan court found that Earvin "Magic" Johnson had no duty to inform his sexual partners of his HIV infection (of which he was then unaware), even though he had an extensive history of sexual relationships.[148] (As to the duty to inform sexual partners under the criminal law, see chapter 8.)

The physicians' and infected persons' duty to protect individuals at foreseeable risk raises fascinating public policy issues. Most people would not dispute that, at least in some circumstances, individuals have a valid claim to be informed of the risks they face. Whereas a person who visits a bathhouse for casual or anonymous sex may be said to assume the risk, the same probably cannot be said of a person in a stable long-term relationship. The so-called right to know is grounded on a person's need to make informed decisions and to take steps to protect himself.

Although individuals may have legitimate interests in knowing the risks they face, disclosure policies have heavy social costs. In the context of a physician's duty to warn, the consequence may be that patients are less likely to divulge their intimate secrets. In the context of a patient's duty to inform, the consequence may be that individuals refrain from getting tested for infectious conditions. (If there is liability only when a person knows his serological status, the law may create incentives not to know.) The duty to inform also presupposes that the infected person is solely "responsible" for assuring safety. Public health authorities, however, prefer to counsel that both infected and noninfected persons are responsible for safety (e.g., by using condoms when having sex and sterile syringes when injecting drugs).

In thinking about the duty to warn, therefore, policymakers have to balance the right to confidentiality against the "right to know." Beyond this conflict is the broader issue of the effects on access to testing, counseling, and treatment once the community realizes that health care professionals will disclose confidences. One way to balance these interests would be to create a narrow power, but not a duty, to inform. The power could be exercisable only where necessary to avoid a serious, prospective risk to an identifiable person, and no less intrusive measure could ameliorate that risk (e.g., the patient making the disclosure himself).

TOWARD A MODEL PUBLIC HEALTH
INFORMATION PRIVACY LAW

The collection of vast amounts of information in the course of public health practice and research yields substantial collective benefits for the public's health and well-being. At the same time, personally identifiable data pose serious privacy risks. As hard as they may try, policymakers cannot design a perfect method for reconciling these interests. Inevitably, individuals will have to give up some privacy to achieve public goods and society will have to forgo some benefits to afford individuals respect for their privacy. Despite these complex trade-offs, rational policy could be formulated to improve informational privacy and security while still facilitating legitimate uses of public health data. Elsewhere, my colleagues and I have proposed a Model State Public Health Privacy Act that balances collective and individual interests.[149] This section offers an abbreviated description of that proposed statute (see Figure 10).

The Model Act's approach is to maximize privacy safeguards where they matter most to individuals and facilitate data uses where necessary to promote the public's health. Consider the sequence of events when government collects, uses, and discloses public health data. First, the agency collects the data and, providing it has a strong public health purpose, most people believe that individuals should forgo this small privacy invasion for the communal good. For example, the reporting of infectious diseases and injuries by name is indispensable to the public's health, but not seriously invasive of individual privacy.

Second, the agency uses the data strictly within the confines of the public health system (i.e., within the agency itself or with other state or

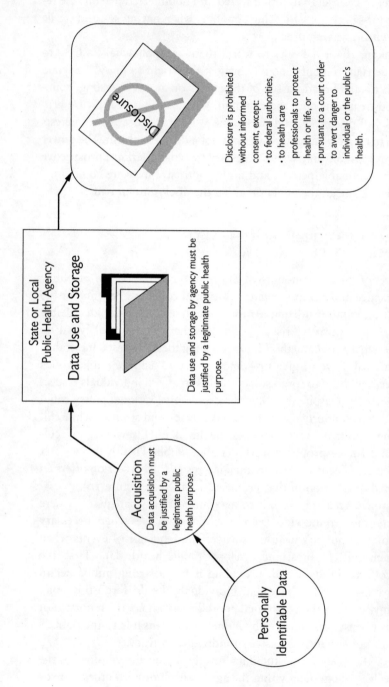

Personally Identifiable Data

Acquisition
Data acquisition must be justified by a legitimate public health purpose.

State or Local Public Health Agency

Data Use and Storage

Data use and storage by agency must be justified by a legitimate public health purpose.

~~Disclosure~~

Disclosure is prohibited without informed consent, except:
• to federal authorities,
• to health care professionals to protect health or life, or
• pursuant to a court order to avert danger to individual or the public's health.

A "legitimate public health purpose" is a population-level activity or individual effort primarily aimed at the prevention of injury, disease, or premature mortality or the promotion of community health.

Figure 10. Model Health Information Privacy Act.

local public health agencies). Again, provided the agency has a strong public health purpose and the data are shared only with public health officials who have a need to know, data uses should prevail over privacy. The reason for this conclusion is that when public health authorities acquire and use data strictly within the public health system, health benefits are at their highest and privacy risks are at their lowest. Public health authorities need the freedom to use the data to monitor and prevent health risks. If these data remain inside the public health system, patients face few social risks.

Third, the agency may seek to disclose the information to persons outside the public health system (e.g., to employers, insurers, commercial marketers, police, family, or friends). These kinds of disclosures are not very important for the public's health, but they do place patients at considerable risk of embarrassment, stigma, and discrimination. For these reasons, the law ought to provide maximum privacy protection. The Model Act would impose significant civil and criminal penalties for unauthorized disclosures to individuals or businesses outside the confines of the public health system.

In sum, the Model Act's approach is to give government flexibility to acquire and use data strictly within the confines of the public health system, providing it can demonstrate an important public health purpose. However, the Model Act affords public health authorities very little discretion to release data outside the public health system and imposes serious penalties for unauthorized disclosures without the patient's informed consent.

The Model Act also requires public health agencies to adopt a set of fair information practices with the following components:

Data protection review. An independent data protection authority should be established to review carefully privacy and security protocols and practices.

Data collection justification. Acquisition of health information cannot be regarded as an inherent good, so agencies should demonstrate that identifiable information is necessary to achieve an important public health purpose.

Information for persons and populations. Individuals and populations are entitled to basic information, such as the purposes for data collection and how personal information will be used, the length of time that data will be stored, and procedures for disclosure.

No secret data systems. Agencies should inform the public about all record systems maintained by the agency.

Access to, and correction of, information. Persons should have access to information about themselves, and there should be fair procedures for correcting and amending their records.

Security measures. Agencies should develop and distribute written security plans requiring physically and technologically secure informational environments.

These proposals, while not perfect, provide a balance between the social good of data collection (recognizing its substantial value to community health) and the individual good of privacy (recognizing the normative value of respect for persons). Perhaps citizens do not desire absolute privacy, but rather reasonable assurances that public health authorities will treat personal information with respect, store it in an orderly and secure manner, and use it only for important health purposes and in accordance with publicly accountable principles of fairness.

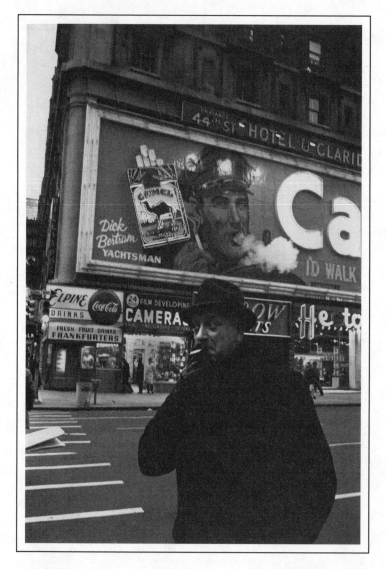

This billboard advertisement for Camel cigarettes in Times Square is one of the images of tobacco products that pervaded the country's visual landscape during the twentieth century. However, on April 23, 1999, cigarette billboards were dismantled as part of a Medicaid cost reimbursement settlement reached in 1998 between tobacco producers and forty-six states. (Eddie Hausner/New York Times, 1964)

6 Health, Communication, and Behavior

Freedom of Expression

In his American travels, Alexis de Tocqueville witnessed a multitude of public health activities—the temperance and women's rights movements, the discouragement of gambling and prostitution in the cities, and the public concern with education, housing, and nutrition. What astonished him was not the regulatory response, but rather the power of emerging mass communication: "the skill with which the inhabitants of the United States succeed in proposing a common object to the exertions of a great many men, and in getting them voluntarily to pursue it."

The field of public health is deeply concerned with the communication of ideas. Human behavior is a powerful contributor to injury and disease, so public health strives to influence behavioral choices. Public health authorities understand that many factors influence behavior, but information is a prerequisite for change.[1] The population must at least be aware of the health consequences of risk behaviors to make informed decisions. The citizenry is bombarded with behavioral messages that affect their health—by the media and entertainment, trade associations and corporations, religious and civic organizations, and family and peers.[2] Public health authorities strive to be heard above the din of conflicting and confusing communications. Consequently, the field of public health is a virtual battleground of ideas.

Public health agencies deliver messages to promote healthy behavior and restrict messages that encourage risk taking. Health authorities exert influence on behavior at various levels of intervention: at the individual level, they counsel individuals at risk for injury and disease (e.g., HIV prevention, genetic disease, or reproductive choice); at the group level, they inform and promote behavior change (e.g., hospital or HMO newsletters, or support groups for stress reduction or smoking cessation); at the population level, they educate the public and market healthy lifestyles (e.g., public service advertisements, health communication campaigns, or school-based health education).

Government not only delivers health messages but also regulates private sector communications. Government suppresses commercial messages deemed hazardous to the public's health and compels messages deemed essential to the public's health. However, governmental control of the informational environment raises profound social and constitutional questions. Substantial public health benefits can be achieved by reducing risk behavior, but regulation of communications can stifle freedom of thought, expression, and association.

TWO ANTITHETICAL THEORIES OF HEALTH COMMUNICATION

[T]he ultimate good desired is better reached by free
trade in ideas—that the best of truth is the power of
the thought to get itself accepted in the competition
of the market, and that truth is the only ground upon
which their wishes safely can be carried out. That at
any rate is the theory of our constitution.
                    Oliver Wendell Holmes (1919)

The First Amendment, as written, is simple and unqualified—but it is far from easy and certainly not absolute: "Congress shall make no law . . . abridging the freedom of speech, or of the press." First Amendment and public health theorists offer two antithetical visions of government's role in health communication: a "free marketplace of ideas" vision in which individuals are free agents with the ability to assess health messages and to make decisions in their own interests, and a "consumer protection" vision in which government actively intervenes to convey messages conducive to population health and constrain messages detrimental to that goal.[3]

First Amendment theory is grounded both on intrinsic and instrumental values.[4] Free expression is an end in itself, for it is essential to autonomy, self-fulfillment, and personhood. Free expression has intrinsic value because it provides a vehicle for self-realization in which individuals and groups define and proclaim their identity.[5]

Beyond its intrinsic value, the most familiar theories hold that free expression has instrumental value in that it enhances democracy or self-governance and advances truthful ideas. Freedom of expression is necessary for representative government. In the absence of the free exchange of ideas, the electorate cannot become informed, public officials cannot arrive at wise policy choices, and the public cannot exercise democratic control or insist on political accountability.[6] The self-governance theory emphasizes the importance of political speech,[7] which, in turn, may insufficiently value artistic, scientific, and other forms of expression.

Finally, and most important for our purposes, freedom of expression is thought necessary for the discovery of truth. On this theory, a robust discourse of all potential ideas will, ultimately, advance knowledge and "truth." Classic statements of the "truth-finding" function of free expression are offered by John Milton[8] and, later, John Stuart Mill,[9] who claimed that suppression of communication is always wrong: "[I]f an idea is true, society is denied the truth; if it is false, society is denied the fuller understanding of truth which comes from its conflict with error; and when the received opinion is part truth and part error, society can know the whole truth only by allowing the airing of competing views."[10] Oliver Wendell Holmes invoked the potent metaphor of the "marketplace of ideas" to capture the notion that truthful expressions will prevail in the competition of a free market.[11]

Public health authorities do not dispute the intrinsic value of free expression and promoting autonomy or personhood; nor do they quarrel with the instrumental value of political speech for enhancing representational democracy. Public health authorities, however, do not abide the theory that "truth" (in this context, a health-promoting idea) will necessarily prevail in a free market of communication. The field of public health, by its nature and design, is interventionist, taking as its starting point the necessity of behavioral change to enhance the well-being of the population.[12] Rigorous scientific investigation of behaviors that are safe, and those that are risky, is the ultimate arbiter of "truth." Therefore, "wise" communications are those that convey the best scientific evidence of health and behavior. For this reason public health authorities seek, more or less, to control the environment of health information—to disseminate health messages, to compel "truthful" disclosure of risks and hazards, and to constrain false or misleading statements.

Public health authorities are interventionist because they distrust the free market to inform the public objectively about risk behaviors or to persuade the polity to conform to guidelines for healthy living. A cacophony

of explicit and implicit messages and images about health exists. How can
the lay public identify science-based messages accurately? More important, the "marketplace" rationale assumes that all competing messages
possess a fair chance of being heard. In the real world, though, the managers of mass media, and those with economic resources or political
power, gain disproportionate access to the most effective channels of communication.[13] Laurence Tribe asks, "How do we know that the analogy
of the market is an apt one? Especially when the wealthy have more access to the most potent media of communication than the poor, how sure
can we be that 'free trade in ideas' is likely to generate truth?"[14]

How does the Constitution mediate between these antithetical visions of
health, communication, and behavior? In this chapter, I explore the parameters of government's role in controlling the informational environment:
first, in conveying health information (government speech); second, in constraining advertising that adversely affects the public's health (commercial
speech); and third, in requiring product health and safety disclosures or
counter-advertising (compelled commercial speech).[15] I conclude this chapter with a case study on the regulation of cigarette advertising.

GOVERNMENT SPEECH: PUBLIC HEALTH COMMUNICATIONS

"If there is any fixed star in our constitutional constel-
lation, it is that no official, high or petty, can prescribe
what shall be orthodox in politics, nationalism, religion, or other matters of opinion." . . . Under the
First Amendment the government must leave to the
people the evaluation of ideas. Bold or subtle, an idea
is as powerful as the audience allows it to be.

Frank H. Easterbrook (1985)
quoting Robert H. Jackson (1943)

[As part of the "Celebrate the Century" series, the
U.S. Postal Service issued a stamp of one of Jackson
Pollack's most important abstract expressionist works.]
The image, however, is missing something. In the original, . . . Pollack had a cigarette stuck in the left corner
of his mouth, and a cloud of smoke hung spectrally
over his outstretched hand. They're gone. . . . It's a
striking visual image that has been cleansed . . . for the
masses to see.

David Brown (1999)

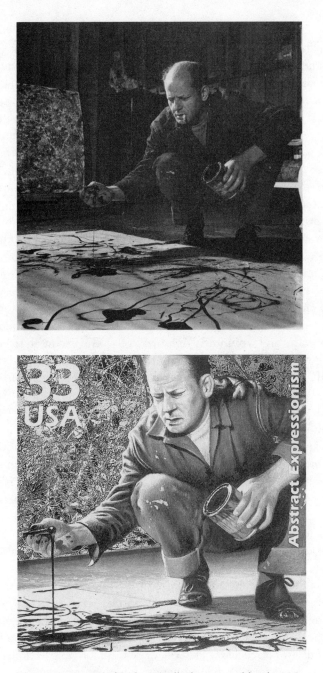

This 1960s image of Jackson Pollack was used by the U.S.
Postal Service for a stamp issued in 1999. Note that the
Postal Service removed the cigarette from the original
image. (Martha Holmes/LIFE Magazine © Time Inc.)

Government, as a health educator, uses health communication campaigns as a major public health strategy. Health education campaigns, like other forms of advertising, are persuasive communications; instead of promoting a product or a political philosophy, public health authorities promote safer, more healthful behaviors.[16] Consider some of the highly developed health education campaigns initiated by the National Institutes of Health: "Milk Matters" (strong bones for young girls), "Back to Sleep" (SIDS), "Sisters Together: Move More/Eat Better" (obesity control), depression awareness, and cancer survivorship.

Government is becoming highly sophisticated in its health educa-tion campaigns and employs a number of mass media technologies: radio and television (paid and public service advertisements), news-papers and magazines (press releases and briefings), telephone lines ("800" number hotlines and "broadcast" and "auto-response" faxes), and Internet (web sites, listservs, and e-mails). Government also subsidizes educational messages through grants and contracts with private and voluntary organizations. Government selects the funding recipient and the messages that the organization will convey. In its HIV prevention grants, for example, the government subsidizes health messages about safer sex but forbids encouragement of drug use or homosexuality.[17]

Health education is often a preferred public health strategy and, in many ways, it is unobjectionable. In health communication campaigns, government persuades individuals to alter risk behaviors. By imparting knowledge, government helps inform the polity about activities that promote health and well-being. When government speaks, citizens may choose to listen and adhere or they are free to reject health messages.[18]

We like to think that public health's concern with "healthy messages" is an inherent good, and we are prepared to give government considerable leeway in constructing a "favorable" informational environment. But the concern of public health authorities with health, communication, and be-havior frequently conflicts with other important social values. When pub-lic health authorities counsel individuals or educate groups or populations about the government's view concerning unsafe sex, abortion, smoking, a high-fat diet, or a sedentary lifestyle, there is no formal coercion. Yet, ed-ucation conveys more than information; it is also a process of inculcation and acculturation intended to change behavior. Even though they are not always particularly adept or successful, public health authorities routinely construct social norms or meanings to achieve healthier populations. Not everyone believes that public funds should be expended, or the veneer of government legitimacy used, to prescribe particular social orthodoxies.[19]

Although public health campaigns are well intended, they can cause social and psychological harm by making people feel responsibility (or shame) for their disease or associating ill health with socially undesirable characteristics.[20] As to the issue of responsibility, education campaigns can increase resentment of personal lifestyles that impose financial and other costs. The person who fails to lose weight or stop excessive drinking or smoking is burdened not only with health risks, but also with the loss of sympathy and support.

As to the issue of socially undesirable characteristics, consider two alternative ways of delivering a comparable health message. In the first, government conveys basic information about risk behaviors (e.g., smoking cigarettes causes cancer, or eating high-fat foods causes heart disease). In the second, government associates the risk behavior with unattractive features (e.g., people who smoke cigarettes have bad breath, develop aging effects of the skin, or may become sexually impotent; or people who eat high-fat foods or live sedentary lifestyles are lazy and become obese). The first message is socially acceptable but is unlikely to effect behavioral change. The latter message is more likely to alter behavior but can exacerbate social and psychological harms such as stigma (caused by teasing or ostracizing) and low self-esteem (among, for example, overweight girls or women).[21] Government may, understandably, claim that these images simply portray the real health effects of risk behaviors, and public health education does counteract misleading advertisements that associate attractive lifestyles with smoking cigarettes, drinking alcoholic beverages, or eating fast foods. Still, there is a line beyond which government should not go in constructing social meanings, especially when messages and images pose psychological risks for vulnerable populations.[22]

Despite their effects on freedom of choice and social relationships, health communication campaigns can be justified in several ways.[23] Arguably, government has a duty to protect and promote the population's health, independent of individual preferences. Certainly, failure to inform citizens of scientific information relevant to their health and safety would be objectionable. Most people want government to educate the public about healthy lifestyles, recognizing that existing information sources may be insufficient or unreliable. Health education campaigns can also appeal to third-party interests. To the extent that the behaviors at issue are primarily self-regarding (e.g., diet, smoking, and seat belts), the government can emphasize the collective harms such as the social and health care costs. To the extent that the behaviors are "other regarding" (e.g., drunk driving, and unsafe sex), the government can emphasize the harm to public health and safety, as well.

Justifications for health communication campaigns are weakest when government health claims are not based solidly on scientific research. Government cannot claim to be objectively informing citizens if the scientific evidence is unpersuasive or contradictory. In some cases, the scientific underpinnings of the public health message are weak or uncertain. Even the most enduring and credible health messages are based on observed associations rather than clinical trials. For example, large clinical trials refuted government health messages delivered for many years that a diet high in fiber prevents colon cancer.[24] In other cases, experts disagree on the correct health message. Think about the credibility of government pronouncements about obesity (health authorities changed the definition, thereby increasing the number of "obese" people by 27 million)[25] or mammography (expert panels disagreed on screening for 40-year-old women).[26]

Sometimes public health officials face intriguing ethical questions about "truth telling." Suppose government distorts scientific evidence to achieve desirable public health goals. Public health officials may overestimate the risk to secure healthy behavior or conceal the degree of behavioral change necessary to promote good health, if full candor may result in noncompliance.[27] Is the government's beneficent intention sufficient to warrant a misleading health message? For example, would it be ethical for public health officials to overstate or mischaracterize the risk of second-hand smoke in support of a ban on smoking in stadiums, restaurants, and other public accommodations?

Justifications for health communication are also weak if the campaigns are unlikely to alter risk behavior. Government cannot claim to promote the public's health if educational messages do not work, and, unfortunately, evaluations of education campaigns are inherently complex and infrequently undertaken.[28] Two related scientific issues, therefore, are important in thinking about health promotion: the scientific evidence underlying the health claim and the effectiveness of the campaign in preventing risk behaviors.

Like so many other public health activities, health communication campaigns entail difficult trade-offs between public goods and private choices. Effective communication campaigns reduce risk behaviors and enhance quality of life and longevity, but burden free choice and present social risks. At the same time, despite their complexity, government's public messages pose few problems from a constitutional perspective.

WHEN GOVERNMENT SPEAKS: A CONSTITUTIONAL PERSPECTIVE

Constitutional scholars distinguish government's addition of its own voice from government's silencing of others.[29] Generally, the former raises few, if any, serious constitutional concerns, while the latter requires careful reflection. Thus, government can add its own voice to the other opinions that it must tolerate, provided it does not drown out private communication.[30] Given the prolific health information generated in the private sector, government speech is unlikely to dominate the marketplace. The First Amendment, for example, does not prevent the government from promoting the "right to life" over abortion or restricted access to drug injection equipment over needle exchange. Those who object to these controversial positions cannot insist that government articulate their views, nor can they legally contest government's expenditure of considerable resources to enunciate controversial opinions.[31]

SUBSIDIZED HEALTH SPEECH: THE "UNCONSTITUTIONAL CONDITIONS" DOCTRINE

Government not only conveys health messages itself, but also funds private and voluntary organizations to deliver health information. Although it has considerable discretion in the messages it is willing to support financially, government may not grant a benefit on the condition that the recipient perform or forgo a constitutionally protected activity.[32] Known as the "unconstitutional conditions" doctrine, government cannot punish those who convey disfavored ideas by denying them benefits.[33]

The Supreme Court has not been wholly consistent in its jurisprudence regarding unconstitutional conditions.[34] For example, in *Rust v. Sullivan* (1991), the Court upheld a so-called gag-rule that forbids clinics receiving federal family planning funds from counseling or referring women for abortion and from encouraging, promoting, or advocating abortion. Chief Justice Rehnquist, writing for the Court, said, "The Government has not discriminated on the basis of viewpoint; it has merely chosen to fund one activity to the exclusion of the other. [This] is not a case of the Government 'suppressing a dangerous idea,' but of a prohibition on a project grantee or its employees from engaging in activities outside of the project's scope."[35]

In summary, government has near plenary constitutional authority to convey its own health messages or subsidize private health messages. Government, then, may add its own voice and funds to the marketplace of ideas about health and behavior. However, it has considerably less constitutional power to suppress ideas of which it disapproves.

COMMERCIAL SPEECH

[T]he task of the political sphere in a republican scheme is to oversee the market in order to protect the common welfare. Public health restrictions on liberty and property to limit the promotion of harmful or dangerous products, including restrictions on advertising, are a staple of public policy in a democratic republic.

> *Dan E. Beauchamp (1988)*

As to the particular consumer's interest in the free flow of commercial information, that interest may be as keen, if not keener by far, than his interest in the day's most urgent political debate.

> *Harry Blackmun (1976)*

No matter how much government educates the public, it is bound to have difficulty changing risk behaviors. The reason is that the private sector has a strong economic interest in influencing consumer preferences: manufacturers and retailers desire to sell products, the advertising industry strives to devise alluring campaigns, and the media compete for advertising revenue. Advertising commands ever-increasing resources and engenders ever-more-creative approaches to stimulate consumer demands.

As a result, government regulation of commercial speech is an important strategy to safeguard consumer health and safety. First, government is concerned with advertising that increases the use of hazardous products and services, such as cigarettes, alcoholic beverages, firearms, and gambling. For example, advertisements extol the virtues of handguns for home defense and safety, despite scientific evidence of increased risk of suicide, domestic violence, and unintended death.[36] Second, government is concerned with marketing "age-restricted" products to children and adolescents. For example, the Distilled Spirits Council lifted its 48-year-old voluntary ban on hard liquor advertising on radio and television, prompting concern about the targeting of young people.[37] Third, government is concerned with industry health claims that mislead the public. For example, government actively reviews food and dietary supplement labels[38] and direct-to-consumer pharmaceutical marketing for unsubstantiated health claims.[39] Regulation of commercial speech is becoming even more challenging as government monitors Internet marketing of the sale of hazardous products or the expression of deceptive health messages.

A DEFINITION OF COMMERCIAL SPEECH

Commercial speech is an "expression related solely to the economic interests of the speaker and its audience"[40] that "does no more than propose a commercial transaction."[41] The three attributes of commercial speech are that it (1) identifies a specific product (i.e., offers a product for sale), (2) is a form of advertising (i.e., is designed to attract public attention to, or patronage for, a product or service, by paid announcements proclaiming its qualities or advantages), and (3) confers economic benefits (i.e., the speaker stands to profit financially) (see Figure 11).[42]

None of these three factors alone provides a complete description of commercial speech, but the Supreme Court classifies an expression as commercial if it has a combination of them all. Thus, in *Bolger v. Youngs Drug Products Corporation* (1983), the Court found that "informational pamphlets" with titles such as "Plain Talk about Venereal Disease" and "Condoms and Human Sexuality" were "commercial" because they were advertisements, they referred to a specific product, and the publisher had an economic motivation.[43]

Many speakers stand to gain economically, including publishers, broadcasters, and film producers. The fact that a speaker will profit from a message is not conclusive, nor is the fact that the speaker must pay for the message definitive.[44] For example, the following advertisement in the *New York Times*, which was paid for by tobacco companies, is political, as opposed to commercial, speech: "Can We Really Make the Underage Smoking Problem Smaller by Making the Federal Bureaucracy Bigger? . . . Together We Can Work It Out."[45] The next advertisement, also found in the *New York Times* and paid for by the tobacco industry, is more difficult to classify: "'Of Cigarettes and Science': Why a Federal Study Failed to Prove the Causal Relationship between Smoking and Heart Disease."[46] Both advertisements express an opinion on a matter of public interest rather

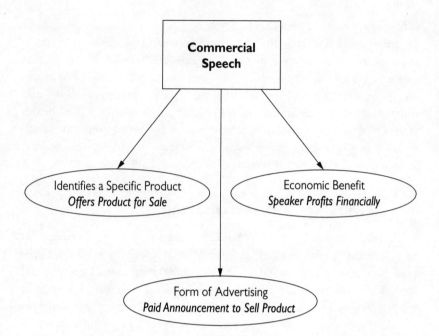

Figure 11.   Commercial speech: a definition.

than propose a commercial transaction.[47] Although the latter message is morally reprehensible, history informs us that it would be a mistake to suppress statements that cast doubt on scientific orthodoxies of the day because scientific "truths" are rarely stable and certain.

THE CONSTITUTIONALIZATION OF COMMERCIAL SPEECH

In 1942 the Supreme Court declared that the Constitution imposes "no such restraint on government as respects purely commercial advertising."[48] It was not until 1975 that the Court first found that commercial speech merited constitutional protection: "The relationship of speech to the marketplace of products or services does not make it valueless in the marketplace of ideas."[49] The early commercial speech cases involved instances where the message itself had public health value: abortion referral services,[50] advertisements for contraceptives,[51] or the price of pharmaceuticals.[52]

Nominally, commercial speech operates as a category of "lower-value" expression, deserving of less constitutional protection than social or political discourse.[53] Recognizing the "commonsense distinction[s],"[54] the Court finds that the Constitution "accords a lesser

1942	Valentine	Commercial speech deserves no First Amendment protection: "[N]o restraint on government [for suppressing] purely commercial advertising."
1950		For over three decades, there remained no constitutional protection of commercial speech.
1960		
1970		
1975	Bigelow	Commercial speech is afforded First Amendment protection for the first time in a case involving advertising abortion referrals. Commercial speech is "not valueless in the marketplace of ideas."
1976	Virginia Pharmacy	Commercial speech is protected: advertising the price of pharmaceuticals.
1977	Carey	Commercial speech is protected: advertising contraception.
1980	Central Hudson	Supreme Court announces criteria for evaluating commercial speech (see Figure 13).
1986	Posadas	Supreme Court takes a permissive approach to government regulation of commercial speech (gambling advertisements). "The power to ban a product includes the lesser power to regulate advertising."
1989	Fox	Supreme Court continues the permissive approach to government regulation of commercial speech (conducting product demonstrations in dormitory rooms).
1990		
1995	Coors Brewing Co.	Supreme Court adopts more careful scrutiny of commercial speech (analyzing "irrationality" of restriction on alcohol advertisements).
1996	44 Liquormart	Supreme Court continues closer scrutiny of commercial speech (advertising of the price of liquor): rigorous protection of truthful, non-misleading speech.
1999	New Orleans Broadcasting	Supreme Court continues closer scrutiny of commercial speech (advertising of private casino gambling).

Figure 12.   The constitutionalization of commercial speech: a time line.

protection to commercial speech than to other constitutionally guaranteed expression."[55] In reality, though, the level of scrutiny for commercial speech has changed over the years and is still in transition. Moreover, although it may not say so frankly, the Court does not afford all commercial speech the same level of protection (see Figure 12).

THE *CENTRAL HUDSON* TEST

In *Central Hudson Gas v. Public Service Commission* (1980),[56] the Supreme Court articulated a four-part test for government regulation of commercial speech. First, for commercial speech to be protected by the First Amendment, it must concern a lawful activity and not be false, deceptive, or misleading. Second, the government interest asserted must be substantial. Third, the regulation of commercial speech must directly advance the governmental interest asserted. Fourth, the regulation must be no more extensive than necessary to serve the government's interest. The four parts of the *Central Hudson* test are not discrete but are interrelated; in particular, the third and fourth parts of the test are complementary.[57] The Court reviews commercial speech under a standard of "intermediate scrutiny,"[58] and the government carries the burden of justification (see Figure 13).[59]

Step 1: Is the Activity Unlawful, and Is the Speech False, Deceptive, or Misleading?   The Court consistently holds that advertisements are not protected by the First Amendment if they promote unlawful activities[60] or if they are false, deceptive, or misleading.[61] The rationale for excluding such commercial expressions from constitutional protection is that they lack value in the commercial or ideological marketplace. False, deceptive, or misleading advertisements distort those markets by leading consumers into error, risk, or a disadvantageous position.[62] Yet it is not always easy to know if a commercial expression fits into one of these categories.

Unlawful activities. Government may prohibit commercial speech that promotes or portrays unlawful activities, such as illicit drug use; driving while intoxicated; or underage possession of tobacco, alcoholic beverages, or handguns. Certainly, a commercial message or image that expressly endorses unlawful behavior (e.g., children smoking cigarettes) is not constitutionally protected. However, it is less clear whether or not commercial speech that attracts children, but also appeals to adults, deserves First Amendment protection. For example, does a cigarette advertisement that presents a youthful image, such as a cartoon character, promote an unlawful activity?[63]

Falsity or deliberate concealment. Government may prohibit commercial messages, such as unsubstantiated health claims, that are false or that deliberately conceal or misrepresent the truth. The tobacco industry, for example, cannot assert that cigarettes have no effect on breathing or athletic abilities, or that they pose little risk to health. An advertisement stating that Liggett & Myers filters are "just what the doctor ordered" is unlikely to receive constitutional protection.[64]

Inherently deceptive or misleading. The Court holds that even true advertisements that promote lawful activities merit no constitutional

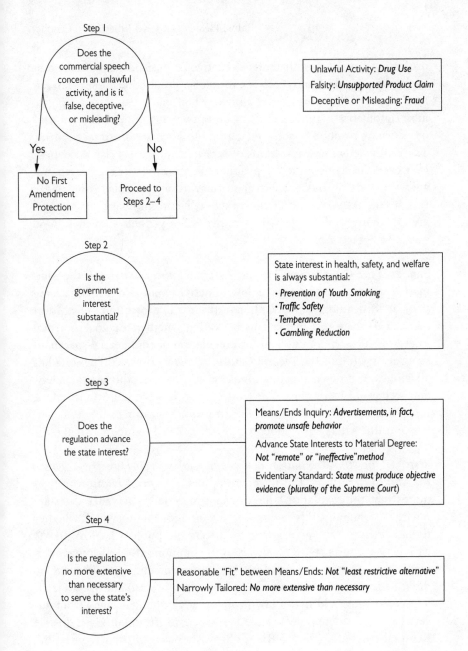

Figure 13. The *Central Hudson* test: a four-step assessment of commercial speech.

protection if they are inherently deceptive or misleading. Deceptive or misleading commercial speech is a form of fraud, undue influence, over-reaching, or other vexatious conduct.[65] For example, states may prohibit optometrists from advertising and practicing under trade names[66] or attorneys from in-person solicitation of patients in hospital rooms.[67] The rationale is that these kinds of activities inherently risk deception. However, the constitutional position of "puffery" (exaggerated imagery) or "glamorous" advertising of hazardous products is less clear. Despite the intuitive sense that attractive, healthful images of smokers are inherently misleading,[68] the Court has not yet held that they stand outside the First Amendment.

Step 2: Is the Government Interest Asserted Substantial?   If the commercial expression promotes a lawful activity and is not false, deceptive, or misleading, it warrants constitutional protection. The Court uses a balancing test that begins by asking whether the governmental interest is substantial. Public health regulation of commercial speech almost always fulfills this second *Central Hudson* criterion. The state has a significant, if not compelling, interest in protecting the health, safety, and welfare of its citizens. The Court recognizes the importance of injury or disease prevention and health promotion, for example, to enhance traffic safety,[69] promote temperance,[70] and reduce gambling.[71]

Step 3: Does the Regulation of Commercial Speech Directly Advance the State Interest?   The third prong of the *Central Hudson* test requires that the regulation "directly and materially" advance the state interest. Nominally, this requires a "means/ends" inquiry (i.e., whether the advertising campaign adversely affects the public's health). In the early cases, courts routinely deferred to commonsense legislative judgments that advertising stimulates consumer demand.[72] In *Posadas de Puerto Rico Associates v. Tourism Company of Puerto Rico* (1986), the Supreme Court held that a law prohibiting gambling casinos from advertising to residents of Puerto Rico was constitutional. Chief Justice Rehnquist noted: "[Puerto Rico] obviously believed [that] advertising of casino gambling aimed at [its residents] would serve to increase the demand for the product advertised. We think the legislature's belief is [reasonable]."[73]

    This permissive approach to the third prong of the *Central Hudson* test has turned into "close scrutiny" in recent cases. These cases suggest that government must have a clear and consistent policy and evidence to demonstrate that its regulation is likely to achieve the asserted public health objective. In *Rubin v. Coors Brewing Company* (1995), the Court unanimously invalidated a federal statute that prohibited beer labels from displaying alcohol content. The government defended the act as necessary to prevent "strength wars" among brewers who would compete in the marketplace based on the potency of their beer. Although the governmental interest was substantial, the act did not directly advance that interest, "given the overall irrationality of the Government's regulatory scheme."[74]

In *44 Liquormart, Inc. v. Rhode Island* (1996), the Court became even more insistent that government affirmatively demonstrate a relationship between means and ends. Rhode Island prohibited advertising the price of alcoholic beverages "in any manner whatsoever," except inside liquor stores, and asserted the goal of "temperance." Justice Stevens's plurality opinion declared,[75]

> [T]he State bears the burden of showing not merely that its regulation will advance its interest, but also that it will do so "to a material degree." . . . [T]he State has presented no evidence to suggest that its speech prohibition will significantly reduce market-wide consumption. . . . Thus, [any] connection between the ban and a significant change in alcohol consumption would be purely fortuitous. [Any] conclusion that elimination of the ban would significantly increase alcohol consumption would [rest on] "speculation or conjecture."

While none of the opinions in *44 Liquormart* garnered a majority, a strongly united Court in *Greater New Orleans Broadcasting Association v. United States* (1999) made clear its intention to use a more rigorous First Amendment standard.[76] The Court returned to a theme introduced in *Coors Brewing* that public health policy that lacked consistency and coherency is near fatal under its evolving commercial speech doctrine. Congress's policy on gambling (which proscribed private casino advertising but promoted gambling on certain Native American land and in state-run lotteries) was "so pierced by exemptions and inconsistency that the Government cannot hope to exonerate it."[77]

Some of the language in *Greater New Orleans Broadcasting* has troubling implications from a public health perspective. Recall that in *Posadas*, the Court acceded to the commonsense legislative assumption that advertising restrictions decrease demand for socially harmful products. While accepting this assumption, the Court in *Greater New Orleans Broadcasting* said it was also reasonable to assume that advertising would merely channel consumers to a different venue or brand.[78] This argument is worrisome because it is exactly the claim made by tobacco and advertising beverage manufacturers, who insist that they are advertising only to achieve greater market share, not to stimulate demand.

In the aftermath of *Coors Brewing*, *44 Liquormart*, and *Greater New Orleans Broadcasting*, government must demonstrate, most probably with credible evidence, that the regulation will, in fact, achieve the asserted public health goal,[79] and not be an "ineffective" or "remote" method.[80]

Step 4: Is the Regulation No More Extensive than Necessary to Serve the State's Interest?   The government must not merely show that its regulation directly advances a public health objective, but also that the means used are not more extensive than necessary to achieve that goal. Again, the early cases readily accepted legislative judgments that commercial speech restrictions were no broader than necessary to pursue the public health goal.[81] In *Board of Trustees of the State University of New York v. Fox* (1989), the Court held that the fourth *Central Hudson* criterion did not require government to use the least restrictive alternative. "The ample scope of regulatory authority [in commercial speech cases] would be illusory if it were subject to a least-restrictive-means requirement, which imposes a heavy burden on the State":[82]

> [What] our decisions require is a "fit between the legislature's ends and the means chosen to accomplish those ends"—a fit that is not necessarily perfect, but reasonable; that represents not necessarily the single best disposition but one whose scope is "in proportion to the interest served"; that employs not necessarily the least restrictive means . . . but a means narrowly tailored to achieve the desired objective.[83]

While not explicitly questioning the rationale offered in *Fox*, the Court in *Coors Brewing*, *44 Liquormart*, and *Greater New Orleans Broadcasting* conducted a more demanding inquiry. In these cases, the Court invalidated commercial regulations because less restrictive alternatives were, in fact, available to achieve the desired ends.[84] Commercial speech regulation, therefore, must be narrowly tailored and no more extensive than necessary.

THEORIES FOR THE FUTURE OF COMMERCIAL SPEECH

Earlier I asserted that the Supreme Court does not accord all commercial speech the same level of constitutional protection,[85] and that the

Court's jurisprudence is in a state of transition. Here, I discuss several theories that help predict future commercial speech decisions.

The Fair Bargaining Theory: Distinguishing Truthful from Deceptive Messages. The Court appears to subject two kinds of commercial speech—truthful and deceptive—to two different standards of review. The Court defers to regulation designed to assure a fair bargaining process between businesses and consumers. Thus, the Court characteristically approves government suppression of misleading, deceptive, or aggressive sales practices; or it approves government mandates to disclose truthful, beneficial consumer information. Regulation to assure fair market negotiations is consistent with the reasons (i.e., to safeguard consumer health and safety) for according to commercial speech a lower standard of constitutional review. The Court, however, vigorously reviews the suppression of truthful data, believing that consumers are rarely served by depriving them of information. The Court is suspicious of government policies designed to keep consumers ignorant.

The Informational Worth Theory: The Role of Image, Context, and Association. Closely related to "fair bargaining" is the "informational worth" theory. That is, the Court considers the informational value that the advertisement affords to consumers. Commercial speech that informs consumers objectively about the product's price, quantity, ingredients, and quality deserves stronger constitutional protection. Most advertising does not convey objective information, but rather uses imagery, context, and association. The Supreme Court once said that "the use of illustrations or pictures in advertisements serves important communicative functions: it attracts the attention of the audience to the advertiser's message, and it may also serve to impart information directly."[86] The Court, however, could find that advertisements that depict hazardous products as rugged, athletic, adventuresome, or sexual have little informational worth.[87] Alluring images and associations do not inform consumers but may induce them to act against their self-interest in maintaining health and vitality.

The Alternative Channels of Communication Theory: Distinguishing Blanket Prohibitions from "Time, Place, and Manner" Regulation. Since the Court does not desire to have consumers kept in the dark about relevant market information, it is particularly mistrustful of blanket prohibitions or content censorship. Justice Stevens's plurality opinion in 44 *Liquormart* emphasizes the "special dangers that attend complete bans on truthful, nonmisleading commercial speech."[88] Accordingly, the Court rarely permits government to prevent completely the dissemination of truthful messages or to select the messages it will, and will not, allow.[89] The Court is more likely to cede to government the power to control the "time, place, and manner" of expression. This kind of regulation is "content neutral," meaning that government does not intend to censor a particular idea, but only to control its method of dissemination. Thus, regulation that leaves open alternative channels for consumers to hear messages is more likely to conform to the Constitution.[90]

The Unlawful Practices Theory: Distinguishing Children from Adults. The judiciary gives greater deference to commercial speech regulation that is designed to effectuate a governmental interest to protect minors rather than adults.[91] This is particularly true if the regulation filters out messages harmful to minors while, to the extent possible, leaving adults with alternative means of acquiring the information.[92] The Supreme Court has repeatedly recognized an independent governmental interest in protecting minors from harmful materials for several reasons.[93] If children and adolescents have legally restricted access to a hazardous product (e.g., cigarettes, alcoholic beverages, or handguns), advertisements that target this population arguably promote an unlawful activity. Additionally, minors are not yet fully able to assess and analyze independently the value of the message presented.[94] By the time they are capable of making a mature judgment, their health may be harmed irrevocably and their decisional capacity impaired by the product's addictive qualities.

The Underlying Social Harm Theory: Taking Public Health Interests Seriously. First Amendment theorists understandably urge that harmful messages, even those that are most unpopular, deserve protection in a vibrant democracy. The Supreme Court, moreover, has rejected the notion "that legislatures have broader latitude to regulate speech that promotes socially harmful activities."[95] However, justifications for commercial speech regulation must inevitably take account of the serious underlying harms of the products being sold and to whom the products are sold.[96] The strength of the government's interests is classically relevant to constitutional analysis, even when the Court engages in "strict" or "intermediate" scrutiny. Thus, if the government's interest is compelling, such as a reduction in youth smoking, it should weigh heavily in the constitutional balance. In the case study at the end of this chapter, I revisit these commercial speech theories and apply them to the regulation of cigarette advertising.

COMPELLED COMMERCIAL SPEECH: HEALTH AND SAFETY DISCLOSURE REQUIREMENTS

There is certainly some difference between compelled
speech and compelled silence, but in the context of
protected speech, the difference is without constitutional significance, for the First Amendment guarantees
"freedom of speech," a term necessarily comprising
the decision of what to say and what *not* to say.

William J. Brennan (1988)

Federal and state regulations compel a great deal of speech for public health, or consumer protection, purposes. First, government requires businesses to label their products by specifying the content or ingredients (e.g., foods and cosmetics), the potential adverse effects (e.g., pharmaceuticals and vaccines), and the hazards (e.g., warnings on packages of cigarettes, alcoholic beverages, or pesticides). Second, government provides a "right to know" for consumers (e.g., performance of managed care organizations),[97] workers (e.g., health and safety risks), and the public (e.g., hazardous chemicals in drinking water).[98] Third, government mandates counter-advertising whereby industry or the media must provide health education as a counterbalance to advertisements of hazardous products (e.g., forced dissemination of anti-drinking[99] or antismoking[100] messages). The Food and Drug Administration (FDA), for example, proposed a rule to compel tobacco companies to establish a national education campaign to discourage young people from using tobacco products.[101] (For an interesting historical perspective on counter-advertising, examine the Federal Communications Commission's "fairness doctrine"[102] and its application to cigarette advertisements.[103])

Commercial disclosure requirements simply require businesses to provide more consumer information. The First Amendment, however, bestows not only a right to speak freely, but also a right to refrain from speaking at all.[104] The Court offers two complementary rationales for affording First Amendment protection to compelled speech. First, to compel a person to enunciate a view in which she does not believe violates the freedom of conscience or belief. This reasoning was used to invalidate state laws making flag salute and pledge compulsory[105] or requiring automobile owners to display license plates carrying the state motto, "Live Free or Die."[106] Second, government-compelled speech may deter the speaker from expressing his own views. The Court struck down state laws prohibiting anonymous handbills[107] or campaign literature[108] because they discouraged the person's underlying right to publish and disseminate his work.[109]

The Supreme Court's compelled-speech jurisprudence is concerned almost exclusively with political and social discourse, as opposed to product health and safety. Despite having an opportunity in at least two cases,[110] the Supreme Court has not definitively extended the doctrine of compelled political or ideological speech to mandatory commercial speech. However, the Court's current line of reasoning provide a few clear parameters for compelled commercial speech. The Court stresses that businesses have a fully protected First Amendment right to express truthful, non-misleading commercial messages about lawful products.[111] It is likely that the Court would support a corollary principle— that government has constitutional power to compel businesses to make accurate, nondeceptive disclosures for health, safety, or consumer protection purposes. Consequently, government labeling and product liability rules mandating content or ingredients, approved uses, potential adverse effects, or hazard warnings are almost certainly constitutionally permissible, and the Court is unlikely to subject these rules to exacting First Amendment scrutiny.[112]

When commercial speech first attained constitutional legitimacy in *Virginia Pharmacy*, the Court stated that government has the power to assure that "the stream of commercial information flows cleanly as well as freely,"[113] including the authority to compel businesses to issue disclaimers or additional information to render commercial messages nondeceptive.[114] The following year, the Court approved state requirements that attorney advertisements include "some limited supplementation, by way of warning or disclaimer, . . . to assure that the consumer is not misled."[115] Later, it upheld a disclosure rule mandating attorneys, who advertised contingent rates, to state that clients would be responsible for litigation costs:[116] "disclosure requirements trench much more narrowly on an advertiser's interest than do flat prohibitions on speech."[117]

Whereas government certainly can require truthful disclosures relevant to health, safety, or consumer protection, interesting issues arise when the state mandates disclosures purely to satisfy consumer curiosity. In

International Dairy Foods Association v. Amestoy (1996),[118] dairy manufacturers challenged a Vermont law requiring labeling of products from cows treated with recombinant bovine somatotropin (rBST) (a synthetic growth hormone that increases milk production). Vermont defended the regulation not on the basis of health or safety, but rather "strong consumer interest and the public's right to know."[119] The dairy products derived from herds treated with rBST are indistinguishable from products derived from untreated herds, and the FDA concluded that there are "no safety or health concerns." The Second Circuit Court of Appeals held that "consumer curiosity alone was not a strong enough state interest to sustain the compulsion of even an accurate, factual statement."[120]

In summary, the Supreme Court is likely to view two different kinds of commercial compelled speech quite differently. On the one hand, the Court will almost certainly permit government to compel disclosures of accurate, nondeceptive information—particularly if state justifications rely on a cognizable harm to health, safety, or a fair consumer/business bargaining process. On the other hand, the Court will more carefully scrutinize compelled commercial speech that fits within the rationale already articulated for political and ideological speech (i.e., regulation that undermines freedom of belief and chills the speaker's own desire and capacity to speak). The Court has already clarified that the right not to speak inheres in political and commercial speech alike[121] and extends to statements of fact as well as statements of opinion.[122] Thus, constitutional problems arise where government compels businesses to enunciate an objectionable message out of their own mouths, forces them to respond to a hostile message when they would prefer to remain silent, or requires them to be publicly identified or associated with another's message.[123] Under this rationale, compulsory counter-advertising may be harder to sustain if the manufacturer is forced to convey detailed educational content with which it disagrees.

REGULATION OF CIGARETTE ADVERTISING:
A CASE STUDY

Since the Surgeon General's first report was released in 1964,[124] government strategies to reduce cigarette smoking have focused on advertising restrictions and compelled disclosures.[125] Congress enacted the Cigarette Labeling and Advertising Act in 1965, requiring warning labels on all cigarette packages.[126] In 1971 Congress prohibited cigarette advertising on radio and television; the Supreme Court upheld the prohibition because, at that time, commercial speech did not receive constitutional protection.[127] A year later the Federal Trade Commission (FTC) required that all advertisements contain the same warning label used on cigarette packages.[128]

During the last decade, the government has explored more aggressive regulation to curb the estimated $5 billion advertising and promotional activities of the tobacco industry.[129] The FDA issued regulations on August 28, 1996, restricting the promotion and advertising of nicotine-containing cigarettes and smokeless tobacco to minors.[130] The tobacco industry and media challenged these regulations, claiming that the FDA lacked authority to regulate cigarettes as a "nicotine delivery" device and that the advertising restrictions were unconstitutional. In 2000, the Supreme Court held that the FDA lacked jurisdiction to regulate cigarettes; the Court did not address the First Amendment issue.[131] Previously, Congress had failed to enact the National Tobacco Policy and Youth Smoking Reduction Act of 1998 (the McCain Bill), designed to regulate cigarette advertising. However, on April 23, 1999, every cigarette billboard in America was dismantled as part of the $206 billion settlement agreement reached in 1998 between tobacco producers and forty-six states to resolve all state claims for excess Medicaid costs due to tobacco-related illnesses. The settlement agreement transformed the country's visual landscape, removing ubiquitous images that had become cultural touchstones.[132] (See chapter 10 for more on the settlement.)

Throughout this extensive national debate, the public health community proposed the following kinds of regulation:[133] manner of presentation (e.g., in print media, black and white text only, with no color and no use of human or animal images or cartoon characters, a so-called "tombstone" format); location of advertisements (e.g., ban on outdoor display in school or play areas or in stadiums); promotions (e.g., ban on offers of non-tobacco products, such as T-shirts, hats, and posters, that possess brand-identified symbols or messages); sponsorship (e.g., ban on support for sporting and other events with use of brand-identified symbols or messages); and compelled disclosures of health information (e.g., intended use and age restrictions, such as "this product is a nicotine delivery device for individuals aged eighteen years or older"). These kinds of advertising restrictions raise important, and controversial, First Amendment issues.[134]

IMAGERY IN CIGARETTE ADVERTISING HAS LOW INFORMATIONAL VALUE AND IS DECEPTIVE

Cigarette advertisements are replete with imagery that associates tobacco use with healthy, adventuresome, glamorous lifestyles. The industry is certain to fight hard to maintain the imagery and attractive features of its advertising campaigns; it will, therefore, strongly resist regulatory requirements of black and white text only and a prohibition on graphics. The current Supreme Court, moreover, may be sympathetic to the claim that equates image with message and informational content.

Despite the industry's protestations, government has strong justifications for curtailing images that do not convey truthful information useful to consumers. Images in tobacco advertisements have little informational value because they do not impart any objective information about the product. Imagery in tobacco advertisements is not merely devoid of useful information, but also misleads the public. It can deceive consumers into believing that cigarette health warnings are exaggerated and that smoking is consistent with a robust and active existence.

The Newport "Alive with Pleasure!" campaign, for example, used scenes of healthy outdoor activities, implying that tobacco use is safe and the choice of energetic people. Similarly, advertisements for low-tar cigarettes such as Vantage and True contained the implied message that they were a safe alternative to quitting. In both cases the FTC expressed concern about the "misimpressions" and "implied representations."[135] Government has the power to remedy the deceptive quality of cigarette advertisements by strictly controlling imagery, association, and context and by mandating additional health disclosures, such as a notice that the product is for purchase by adults only.

REGULATION OF CIGARETTE ADVERTISING LEAVES ALTERNATIVE CHANNELS OF COMMUNICATION

The tobacco industry claims that tobacco advertising regulations would impose special burdens on particular kinds of messages and close off vital channels of information. By proscribing imagery, for example, the industry argues that health authorities are targeting particular messages conveying the positive features of the product. Thus, by prohibiting many magazine advertisements, outdoor advertising, and sponsorships, the industry asserts that the regulations would choke effective methods of communication.

Despite the industry's arguments, good grounds exist for believing that the proposed regulations are narrowly crafted to comport with prevailing constitutional doctrine. First, they are content neutral because they do not select out particular commercial facts for suppression. Reasonable regulations would not prevent manufacturers from informing consumers about who is producing and selling what tobacco product, for what purpose, and at what price. For example, a requirement to use only black and white text would not dilute the factual quality of consumer messages. Second, regulations would impose reasonable "time, place, and manner" restrictions because they would merely regulate the placement, location, and visual presentation of tobacco advertising. Regulations would affect the forms and fora of presentation—not the substance—of the message. Finally, regulations would leave open alternative channels of communication. The government would not foreclose the plethora of newspaper, magazine, direct mail, Internet, point-of-sale, and other media available to tobacco advertisers.

CIGARETTE ADVERTISING ENCOURAGES THE UNLAWFUL PRACTICE OF YOUTH SMOKING

Perhaps the most persuasive public health argument is that advertising targets a youth audience despite the fact that promotion and sale of cigarettes and smokeless tobacco to people under eighteen years of age is unlawful in every state. Tobacco company documents reveal comprehensive strategies to capture the youth market. One internal R.J. Reynolds memo from the mid-1970s stated, "Evidence is now available to indicate that the 14- to 18-year-old group is an increasing segment of the smoking population. RJR-T must soon establish a successful new brand in this market if our position in the industry is to be maintained over the long term."[136] Canadian court documents also uncovered tobacco industry research on children, underscoring its strategic interest in the youth market.[137] Tobacco advertising, notably the "Joe Camel" campaign,[138] captured the attention of young people.[139] Similarly, promotional activities, including specialty items (e.g., free tobacco samples, lighters, apparel), reach large numbers of underage smokers.[140]

This marketing strategy has been successful in influencing young people to smoke cigarettes.[141] Adolescent smoking markedly increased during the 1990s.[142] Currently, at least 3 million daily smokers in the United States are under the age of 18,[143] and 1 million young males use smokeless tobacco.[144] Those who begin smoking by their early teens are more likely to be heavy smokers than those who begin smoking as adults,[145] with lung cancer mortality rates highest among those who begin smoking before the age of 15.[146] Children, like adults, suffer from the pharmacological effects of nicotine on dependency,[147] and there is evidence of slowed growth of lung function among adolescent smokers.[148]

THE UNDERLYING PUBLIC HARMS
OF CIGARETTE ADVERTISING

The public harms attributable to cigarette smoking are unprecedented and provide a strong justification for commercial speech regulation. Tobacco use is the single leading cause of preventable mortality and is associated with more than 430,000 premature deaths each year from tobacco-related illnesses, such as cancer, respiratory illnesses, and heart disease in the United States.[149] The morbidity and mortality attributable to cigarette smoking are greater than that caused by AIDS, automobile crashes, alcohol, homicides, illegal drugs, suicides, and fires combined.[150] Moreover, since some 50 million Americans smoke, even relatively small changes in behavior could benefit the public health.

Reduction in tobacco-related illnesses would also reduce the economic burdens on society. Direct medical care expenditures attributable to smoking are estimated at $50 billion per year,[151] and this does not include the indirect costs associated with premature morbidity and mortality, also estimated at $50 billion per year.[152] Sterile estimates of direct and indirect costs, however, do not begin to measure the value to individuals, families, and society if tobacco-related disease were diminished. The decrease in personal pain and suffering, enjoyment of more energetic lifestyles, and healthier parents and children are among the profound social benefits.

The constitutional debate over cigarette advertising will be contentious, and its outcome is surely in doubt. Nevertheless, in this case study I have presented the public health case for regulation. Cigarette advertisements have low informational value and a deceptive quality, they entice children and adolescents, and they result in profound social and economic harms. Strong grounds exist for asserting that the reasonable regulations would be narrowly tailored to comport with prevailing constitutional doctrine because they are content neutral, regulate the "time, place, and manner," of advertisements, and leave open alternative channels of communication.

CONCLUSION

The field of public health, in many ways, is a battleground of ideas—the government's strategy is to capture the public's attention and, ultimately, to change behavior. Its methods are to deliver health messages to inform and influence the public, suppress deceptive commercial messages, and mandate private disclosures of health and safety risks. Government has good reason for seeking tighter control of the informational environment because an unfettered marketplace of ideas can result in grave public health consequences, as the experience with smoking in America vividly demonstrates. But the government can go only so far in a constitutional democracy. When government acts as an educator or a censor, it intrudes on the freedom of expression, one of the most powerful and persistent ideas in Western thought. These antithetical social visions—a free market of ideas and a regulated market to defend health and safety—cannot be easily reconciled. In the end, society must grapple with a values question: Which goal, freedom or security, matters most and why?

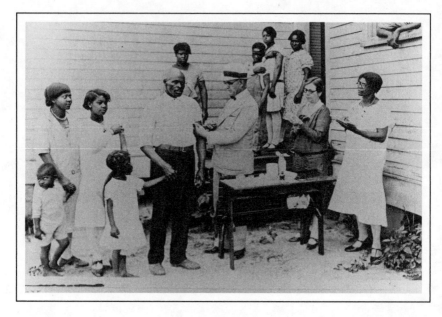

An entire family receives inoculation against typhoid fever, circa 1930.

7 Immunization, Testing, and Screening

Bodily Integrity

> "Now I know these rods are alive," breathed Koch. "Now I see the way they grow into millions in my poor little mice—in the sheep, in the cows even. One of these rods, these bacilli—he is a billion times smaller than an ox—. . . but he grows, this bacillus, into millions, everywhere through the big animal, swarming in his lungs and brain, choking his blood-vessels—it is terrible."
>
> *Paul de Kruif (1926)*

This chapter and the next are devoted primarily to infectious diseases. Infectious diseases preceded the development of humans on earth[1] and, throughout civilization, organized society has struggled—often without hope or success—to contain microbial threats to health.[2] For most of history, society did not understand the etiology of infectious disease or how to prevent it. The social response was largely confined to crude separation of the ill from the rest of society through isolation or quarantine (see chapter 8).

Despite the dearth of knowledge, European physicians were already devising methods of prevention a century before the discovery that germs cause infectious disease. In 1796, Edward Jenner observed that people who had cowpox rarely contracted smallpox. He induced cowpox in a young boy and later tried to infect the boy with smallpox, but the immunity provoked by the cowpox virus was effective against smallpox.[3] It was not until 1879 that Louis Pasteur advanced the theory of immunization. He discovered that neglected cultures of the bacteria that cause chicken cholera lost much of their ability to cause the disease, while fresh cultures failed to infect chickens previously inoculated with the old cultures.[4] Later, Pasteur established prophylactic inoculations for anthrax, swine erysipelas, and rabies; afterward, other researchers found vaccines for the bubonic plague and typhoid. By the close of the century, scientists had demonstrated that inoculation with organisms in attenuated live or dead form afforded resistance to communicable diseases, a practice known as active immunization.

It was also in the late nineteenth century that microbiologists such as Louis Pasteur, Robert Koch, and Gerhard Hansen discovered that microorganisms caused infectious diseases—anthrax, cholera, consumption, leprosy, and rabies.[5] They observed, moreover, that microbial disease could be spread from person to person. It was then possible to test persons for the presence of infection, even before the onset of symptoms. For example, in 1890 Koch developed the tuberculin skin test, which diagnosed tuberculosis infection. Tuberculin testing, as well as other forms of infectious disease testing (such as for syphilis and gonorrhea), would soon be administered to larger populations as part of public health screening programs.

In a speech on bacterial research the same year he discovered a test for tuberculosis, Koch stated, "Shortly after discovery of the tubercle bacillus, [I sought] substances that would be therapeutically useful against tuberculosis."[6] Although a treatment for tuberculosis had to await Selman Waksman's discovery of streptomycin in 1944, Alexander Fleming had noticed in 1928 that growth of the pus-producing bacterium *Staphylococcus aureus* had stopped around an area in which an airborne mold contaminant, *Penicillium notatum*, had begun to grow. Fleming determined that a chemical substance had diffused from the mold, and named it penicillin.[7] It was not until 1939 that a team of Oxford University scientists led by Howard Florey identified and isolated substances from molds that could kill bacteria. That observation led to the mass production of penicillin for treating wounds during World War II.[8] By the mid-1940s, however, microbiologists were already aware that antibiotics have an Achilles' heel. Fleming wrote in 1946 that "the administration of too small doses . . . leads to the production of resistant strains of bacteria."[9] Antibiotic-resistant strains of bacteria are a problem that vexes public health to this day.

The realization that it was scientifically feasible to immunize persons against infection, test for the presence of infection, and treat the infection (thereby reducing contagiousness) led to the ascendancy of biological strategies against infectious diseases. Public health law was closely modeled on the biological approach, and to this day, the law maintains a strong biological orientation. Indeed, it is relatively easy to summarize biological strategies that have, to a greater or lesser extent, been codified in state infectious disease laws throughout the twentieth century. These statutes authorize public health officials to compel vaccination against specified infectious diseases. For diseases that cannot be prevented by immunization, public health authorities are empowered to identify cases of infection by implementing a series of strategies known as case finding. Public health authorities "find" cases through medical testing, physical examination, and population screening. Positive cases are reported to state health authorities, who also engage in partner notification to identify new cases (see chapter 5). This chapter examines the public health powers of immunization, testing, and screening. For those who are found to have an infectious condition, public health authorities can exercise personal control measures: civil confinement (quarantine, isolation, and civil commitment), compulsory medical treatment, and criminal penalties for willful exposure to disease. The following chapter examines these restrictions of the person. Before we embark on a review of legal doctrine and public health practice, it will be helpful to think about the various theories that have informed our understanding of infectious diseases.

CONCEPTUALIZING THE DETERMINANTS OF HEALTH AND DISEASE

There are at least three ways of conceptualizing the determinants of health and disease: the microbial model, the behavioral model, and the ecological model. Despite considerable overlap, these three theories help explain the underlying rationales for the exercise of personal control measures and the political problems that result.

The microbial model, or "germ theory," of public health probably conforms best with the lay perception of disease, together with its causes and methods of control.[10] Under this view, disease is seen as a product of microbial infection, and the job of public health authorities is to identify the pathogen and to eliminate or contain it. This work can be done in a variety of ways. Vaccination controls microbes by denying them susceptible hosts. Mosquito abatement kills the vectors of insect-borne diseases, such as yellow fever and encephalitis.[11] Water purification[12] and meat inspection[13] help prevent harmful bacteria from entering the food chain. Case finding, medical treatment, and isolation curb transmission by people who are already infected. In each case, the intervention targets the pathogen. "Health" under this conception of "pathogen control" is secured by identifying cases and then intervening to break the cycle of infection.

The description of disease as being caused by contact with germs has a great deal of social acceptance. Nevertheless, restrictions placed on a person based on the microbial theory can be controversial. Although

few people object to disease reporting, partner notification, or even isolation of contagious persons in principle, resistance to such measures
arises from a combination of social vulnerability, mistrust of government, characteristics of the disease itself, and past practice. People living with HIV and their advocates, for example, perceive personal control measures as profoundly threatening and oppose them in the
language of constitutional rights, generally deployed when accusing the
government of overstepping its bounds. Germ-based interventions encounter the stiffest public opposition when identifying or controlling
the microbe means identifying or controlling the person who has it, and
the disease itself exposes its carriers to discrimination, ostracism, and
other social risks.

While the germ theory continues to undergird a great deal of public
health work, public health in the second half of this century has come
to recognize another important determinant of health—human behavior. While this notion of disease is reflected mostly in modern discourse
about the roles of smoking, diet, and sedentary lifestyle in the development of chronic disease, the influence of behavior in transmitting infection (e.g., sexual or needle-sharing behavior) is also well recognized.
Under the "behavioral theory" of disease control, public health assessment and interventions occur at the point of human conduct, whether
at the individual, group, or organizational level. The behavioral model
measures successful interventions or improvements in the "health" of a
population in reductions in risk behavior, so modern forms of surveillance do not merely "count" cases of disease but closely monitor the activities that give rise to morbidity and premature mortality.[14] From this
perspective, the germ is less important than the behavior that moves it
from one person to another or that makes people more susceptible to
becoming ill when they encounter a pathogen.

Seeing public health predominantly as the control of risky behavior
can quickly become, for cultural and political reasons, a warrant for
treating disease entirely as a matter of personal responsibility. Ill health
can be viewed, at least in part, as a just desert for wrongful behavior.[15]
Blame can feed the stigma of disease, adding to the social and psychological burdens.

A third account of disease control focuses on "ecological" understandings of health (i.e., the sources of disease in the social and physical environment). The ecological model conceives of illness not as an
external threat, such as a discrete pathogen, nor as a function of personal choices, but rather as a product of society's interaction with its

environment.[16] This understanding of public health does not see diseases that are listed on death certificates as "causes" of death at all, but merely as "pathways" along which more fundamental causes have exerted their effect. Ecological theorists do not ignore behavioral and microbial hazards; rather, they emphasize social institutions, environmental conditions, and human inequality as the major health risks in a population.[17] The poor are more susceptible to illness not simply because they encounter more microbes or engage in less healthy behavior, but because their access to health care and information on healthy living is blocked due to economic and social limitations.

Ecological approaches have gained favor in explaining emerging or resurgent infectious diseases such as streptococcus A, *E. coli,* and hantavirus.[18] These threats come from microbes, to be sure, and individual behavior also plays a role in their transmission. However, the ecological perspective offers a far broader view of the root causes, ranging from population growth, urban migration, and international travel to changes in the ecosystem, such as deforestation, flood, drought, and climatic warming.[19]

Understanding the ecology of health and disease helps to explain why public health activists are so torn between routine disease prevention and a more radical critique of present social and economic arrangements. Of course, when public health challenges conventional thought on the distribution of wealth, social structures, and the environment, it is likely to meet fierce political opposition and claims of overreaching.[20] It is important, however, to remember that public health began as a social reform movement[21] and continues to challenge accepted social practices by identifying the status quo as a fundamental determinant of health and disease. Because of this, public health never quite loses its potency as a force for political change.

Despite the attractions of the ecological model, public health statutes rely heavily on controlling and identifying pathogens through vaccination and screening.

COMPULSORY VACCINATION: IMMUNIZING THE POPULATION AGAINST DISEASE

The first experiment (14 May 1796) was made upon a
lad of the name of Phipps, in whose arm a little
Vaccine Virus was inserted, taken from the hand of a
young woman who had been accidentally infected by

a cow. Notwithstanding the resemblance which the
pustule, thus excited on the boy's arm, bore to vari-
olous inoculation, yet as the indisposition attending it
was barely perceptible, I could scarcely persuade
myself the patient was secure from the Small Pox.
However, on his being inoculated some months after-
wards, it proved that he was secure. This case inspired
me with confidence; and as soon as I could again furnish myself with Virus from the Cow, I made an
arrangement for a series of inoculations.

Edward Jenner (1801)

Edward Jenner called his cowpox inoculation a "vaccine," derived
from the Latin *vaccinus*, pertaining to cows. Louis Pasteur, in honor of
Jenner's work, extended the meaning to include all prophylactic inoculations. In modern scientific terminology, vaccination is the administration of a vaccine or toxoid used to prevent, ameliorate, or treat infectious disease.[22] A vaccine is a suspension of attenuated or noninfectious
microorganisms (bacteria, viruses, or rickettsiae) or derivative antigenic
proteins.[23]

Vaccinations are among the most cost-effective and widely used public
health interventions,[24] yet, since Jenner's time, vaccination has provoked
popular resistance. Although vaccination was generally accepted in early
America (actively supported by, among others, Thomas Jefferson), opposition arose in many quarters.[25] Some opponents expressed scientific objections about its efficacy, some worried that vaccination transmitted disease or caused harmful effects, and still others objected on grounds of
religion or principle. Finally, compulsory vaccination was seen as an unwarranted governmental interference with autonomy and liberty.[26] The
political, philosophical, and social struggles surrounding vaccination persist to this day. They are vividly reflected in legislative and judicial debates
on the powers, and limits, of government to compel vaccination.

STATE VACCINATION LAWS

In April, 1721, ships from the West Indies brought
smallpox to Boston. The Reverend Cotton Mather
proposed to the physicians of Boston that they undertake
inoculation. Only Dr. Zabdiel Boylston responded. . . .
[The following year] the selectmen of Boston had insisted

that Boylston should not inoculate without license and
the consent of the authorities. By 1760, legal safeguards
regulating the conditions under which inoculation could
be performed had been set up.

George Rosen (1993)

George Rosen's observations show that local government during colonial America regulated physician inoculation even before Jenner's historic discovery. Laws mandating immunization first appeared in the early nineteenth century,[27] and by the time of the landmark decision in *Jacobson v. Massachusetts* in 1905 (see chapter 3), many states required citizens to submit to smallpox vaccination.[28]

Modern immunization statutes were enacted in response to the transmission of measles in schools in the 1960s and 1970s. Legislatures at that time were influenced by the significantly lower incidence rates of measles among school children in states with immunization laws.[29] They were also influenced by the experience of states that strictly enforced vaccination requirements and school exclusions in outbreak situations without significant community opposition.[30] Rather than having health departments require immunization in emergency conditions, legislatures acted to prevent disease by mandatory immunization as a condition of enrollment or attendance in schools or licensed day care facilities.[31]

The CDC publishes a schedule of immunizations based on the recommendations of the Advisory Committee on Immunization Practices (ACIP) and others.[32] All states, as a condition of school entry, require proof of vaccination against a number of diseases on the immunization schedule, such as diphtheria, measles, rubella, and polio. These statutes often require schools to maintain immunization records and to report information to health authorities.[33]

Although the exact provisions differ from state to state, all immunization laws grant exemptions for children with medical contraindications to immunization. Thus, if a physician certifies that the child is susceptible to adverse effects from the vaccine, the child is exempt. Virtually all states also grant religious exemptions for persons who have sincere religious beliefs in opposition to immunization.[34] Some statutes require parents to disclose their religion, while others are more liberally worded. A minority of states also grant exemptions for parents who profess philosophical convictions in opposition to immunization.[35] These statutes allow parents to object to vaccination because of their "personal," "moral," or "other" beliefs. The process for obtaining an exemption varies depending on the specific state law. In practice, exemptions for all reasons constitute only a small percentage of total school entrants,[36] but disease outbreaks in religious communities that have not been vaccinated do occur.[37]

CONSTITUTIONALITY OF COMPULSORY VACCINATION: PUBLIC HEALTH AND RELIGION IN CONFLICT

The judiciary has firmly supported compulsory vaccination because of the overriding importance of communal well-being.[38] In the seminal case of *Jacobson v. Massachusetts,* the Supreme Court held that vaccination was squarely within the state's police powers.[39] The states' power to require children to be vaccinated as a condition of school entrance also has been widely accepted and judicially sanctioned.[40] In *Zucht v. King* (1922), the Supreme Court specifically upheld a local government mandate for vaccination as a prerequisite for attendance in public school.[41] Compulsory powers, however, must be exercised "reasonably," which means that states cannot impose vaccination on a person hypersusceptible to adverse effects, such as a severe allergic reaction.[42]

Antagonists of vaccination often frame their objections in terms of the First Amendment: "Congress shall make no law respecting an establishment of religion [the "establishment" clause], or prohibiting the free exercise thereof [the "free exercise" clause]." Does a law that requires people to submit to vaccination against their religious beliefs violate the free exercise clause? While all states currently grant religious exemptions, compelling a person to submit to vaccination against his religious beliefs would be constitutional.[43] The Supreme Court's jurisprudence makes clear that the right of free exercise does not relieve an individual of the obligation to comply with a "valid and neutral law of general applicability."[44] In *Prince v. Massachusetts* (1944), for example, the Court held that a mother could be prosecuted under child labor laws for using her children to distribute religious literature: "The right to practice religion freely does not include liberty to expose the community or the child to communicable disease or the latter to ill health or death."[45] The Supreme Court of Arkansas in 1965 explicitly upheld a compulsory vaccination law that did not exempt persons with religious beliefs: the "freedom to act according to religious beliefs is subject to a reasonable regulation for the benefit of society as a whole."[46]

States are not constitutionally obliged to grant religious exemptions, but are permitted to do so. State supreme courts (with the exception of Mississippi)[47] have permitted legislatures to create exemptions for religious beliefs.[48] Even so, courts sometimes strictly construe religious exemptions, insisting that the belief against compulsory vaccination must be "genuine," "sincere," and an integral part of the religious doctrine.[49] Furthermore, persons with ethical, but not religious, objections to vaccination are not always exempted.[50]

Legislatures often limit the scope of religious exemptions by applying them only to "recognized" and "established" churches or religious denominations. Individuals with sincerely held religious convictions that are not recognized or established have challenged these statutory provisions on two grounds. First, because they provide preferential treatment to particular religious doctrines, they argue that the provisions violate the establishment clause. Second, because these provisions discriminate against persons with nonestablished religious beliefs, they argue that the provisions violate equal protection of the law. Although these two claims have seldom been adjudicated, judicial precedent supports each of them.[51]

THE POLITICS OF COMPULSORY VACCINATION

From a public health perspective, state vaccination laws have been a great success. The rate of complete immunization of school-age children in the United States (more than 95 percent) is as high as, or higher than, those for most other developed countries. More important, common childhood illnesses, such as measles, pertussis, and polio, which once accounted for a substantial proportion of child morbidity and mortality, have been substantially reduced.[52] However, organized groups of parents have struggled against mandatory vaccination and actively lobbied for liberal exemptions.[53]

Public discourse about vaccination is often tense, with scientists and lay persons often talking at cross purposes.[54] Scientists dispassionately measure the population benefits against economic costs, concluding that vaccines are among the most cost-effective prevention strategies.[55] The lay public may mistrust expert claims despite the safety and efficacy of vaccination. Parents, in particular, may be concerned with the health of *their* child and may feel strongly that the risk of a catastrophic vaccine-induced injury should not be imposed by governmental fiat.

Perceptions differ sharply depending on whether the risk of vaccination is viewed from an individualistic or societal perspective. From the perspective of a single child, there may be greater risk if he is vaccinated than if he were to remain unvaccinated. For example, the only cases of polio in the United States are caused by the vaccine; an unvaccinated child's risk of contracting wild polio virus is negligible.[56] Government-imposed vaccination should be understood in this light. The state is explicitly asking parents to forgo their right to decide the welfare of their children not necessarily for the child's benefit, but for the wider public good. From a societal perspective, the choice not to immunize may be optimal to the individual if there is herd immunity, but in the aggregate this choice could lead to failure of that herd immunity.[57] Affording individuals the right of informed consent to vaccination, then, is not for the greatest good of the community. Rather, as Garrett Hardin suggests, informed consent can contribute to a "tragedy of the commons" if too many people make the decision not to immunize.[58]

GOVERNMENT VACCINE INITIATIVES: A RESPONSE TO EVENTS IN THE 1980s AND 1990s

Despite the vast potential of childhood immunization, the United States has struggled to ensure a stable vaccine supply, at reasonable cost, delivered efficiently to consumers. In particular, a series of events during the 1980s and 1990s threatened the viability of vaccine policy and stimulated legislative initiatives.

National Childhood Vaccine Injury Act of 1986.   In the early 1980s, manufacturers expressed concern that substantial tort costs would discourage research and innovation. At the same time, consumer groups felt that it was morally wrong to make parents prove that manufacturers were at fault before obtaining compensation for vaccine-induced injuries. As a result, Congress enacted the National Childhood Vaccine Injury Act (NCVIA) of 1986.[59] The NCVIA established four programs. The National Vaccine Program in the Department of Health and Human Services is responsible for most aspects of vaccination policy (e.g., research, development, safety and efficacy testing, licensing, distribution, and use). The Vaccine Injury Compensation Program compensates persons who suffer from certain vaccine-induced injuries according to values set in a vaccine injury table.[60] The Vaccine Adverse Events Reporting System requires health care providers and manufacturers to report certain adverse events from vaccines.[61] Finally, a vaccine information system requires all health care providers to give parents standardized written information before administering certain vaccines.

Comprehensive Childhood Immunization Act of 1993.   A second momentous event took place between 1989 and 1991 that refocused federal attention on immunization policy. Several major outbreaks of measles produced some 50,000 cases of disease, 11,000 hospitalizations, and 130 deaths, mostly among unvaccinated children.[62] These outbreaks led Congress to enact the Comprehensive Childhood Immunization Act of 1993. The Children's Immunization Initiative created an entitlement to free vaccine for eligible children, supported state efforts to deliver vaccines, increased community participation and provider education, enhanced measurement of immunization status, and developed combined vaccines to simplify the immunization schedule.[63]

State Immunization Registries.   Despite the Children's Immunization Initiative, vaccination rates among pre-school-age children stayed below the levels in many developed, and even some developing, countries.[64] As recently as the mid-1990s, approximately one-third of infants born annually in the United States had not received all of their recommended immunizations by age two.[65] Policymakers concluded that efforts to vaccinate children were being hindered by incomplete and inaccurate information. Immunization information that parents impart to health care providers was frequently incorrect or insufficient.[66] States began to develop immunization data systems to track children, identify those who needed to be vaccinated, and generate notices when a child's vaccinations were due or past due.[67] As a result of this and other initiatives, vaccination rates among pre-school-age children have improved significantly.[68]

THE SWINE INFLUENZA IMMUNIZATION
PROGRAM: A CASE STUDY

Just about everybody in public health knows something about 1976. . . . The swine flu program has become part of public health lore, with the moral of the tale depending on who is telling it and why it is being told. But the swine flu program is not the stuff of folklore. It is far too complex. There are no villains. It does not lend itself to easy analysis.
                        Walter R. Dowdle (1997)

After outbreaks of influenza among army recruits in 1976, the CDC discovered that the strain was swine flu, a virus transmitted easily through human-to-human contact.[69] The CDC feared the population would not have immune resistance to the disease. The media was already speculating that this epidemic would become as catastrophic as the 1918 swine flu pandemic, which caused 20 million deaths worldwide, including 500,000 in the United States.[70] David Sencer, the CDC director, advised President Gerald Ford to initiate mass immunization, reasoning that it was safer to gamble with money than lives. The president announced an ambitious public health program designed to immunize the American population at a cost of $134 million, and Congress followed with the requested appropriation.

As would be expected, there were massive logistical problems in manufacturing and distributing the vaccine, and political quarrels ensued. Liability risks posed perhaps the greatest challenge. The insurance industry, fearing massive liability exposure, informed pharmaceutical companies that it would not provide liability insurance for the swine flu vaccine, which posed a serious threat to the vaccine supply. Congress again acted quickly with a modified version of the Tort Claims Act that would underwrite liability costs. Despite waning support among top health officials, the program lurched forward. On October 1, 1976, the first vaccinations were given and, ten days later, three elderly people in Pittsburgh died shortly after receiving the vaccine. Despite health officials' claims that the deaths were not causally related to the vaccine, the media started a "body count" mentality. On October 14, the president and his family received immunizations on prime-time televison to reassure the public.

In November, a physician in Minnesota reported a case of ascending paralysis, called Guillain-Barré syndrome (GBS). After surveillance activities revealed an increased incidence of GBS, the swine flu immunization program was brought to an end on December 16, with the president's reluctant agreement; 45 million people had been vaccinated. The federal government changed hands in January 1977. President Jimmy Carter's Secretary of Health, Education, and Welfare, Joseph Califano, fired David Sencer and reimplemented the Victoria flu program (a component of the larger swine flu program) for high-risk individuals only.

The swine flu immunization program provides an intriguing account of policymaking in circumstances of uncertainty. Many commentators held government scientists primarily responsible.[71] For example, in a controversial report commissioned by Secretary Califano, Richard Neustadt and Harvey Fineberg found that health officials manipulated their constitutional superiors to comply with "expert" recommendations by their assumed air of arrogance: overconfidence among scientific experts spun from meager evidence, conviction fueled by personal agendas, and zeal by scientists to make their lay superiors do right.[72]

In retrospect, health officials did err in recommending a massive immunization campaign with substantial economic costs and potential harmful effects in circumstances of scientific uncertainty. The available data were inadequate to predict whether swine flu would be contained within narrow outbreaks or would become a more serious epidemic.[73] Nevertheless, the roles played by the media, industry, and politicians are also instructive. The media made swine flu salient in the public mind—exaggerating both the health effects of the disease and then the risk of vaccine-induced injury and death. The pharmaceutical industry convinced political leaders to hold it harmless against lawsuits while, at the same time, profiting from a massive vaccination program actively promoted by government. Politicians in both the executive and legislative branches wanted to position themselves to gain credit for a successful public health program (e.g., President Ford hoped to pin his reelection prospects on mobilizing the immunization program). At the same time, politicians wanted to avoid the blame for failure to respond to an emergent public health risk (e.g., Congress capitulated to demands for large expenditures first to fund the vaccination campaign and then to assume the liability costs).

The swine flu epidemic is instructive in many ways, but it still fails to answer the critical question of whether, in the face of scientific uncertainty, it is better to err on the side of excess caution or aggressive intervention. Consider the appropriate response to suspected bioterrorism with a microbial agent such as anthrax or smallpox.[74] In an emergency, to whom should vaccines be made available and under what circumstances would the government be justified in mandating vaccination? The costs both of action and of inaction are evident: the costs of inaction, if the risk materializes, are lost lives, but the costs of overreaction, if the risk is exaggerated, are wasted public funds and unnecessary burdens of vaccine-induced injury and diminished autonomy.

CASE FINDING: TESTING AND SCREENING

Disease screening is one of the most basic tools of modern public health and preventive medicine. Screening programs have a long and distinguished history in efforts to control epidemics of infectious diseases and targeting treatment for chronic diseases. . . .

In practice when screening is conducted in contexts of
gender inequality, racial discrimination, sexual taboos,
and poverty, these conditions shape the attitudes and
beliefs of health system and public health decision-
makers as well as patients, including those who have
lost confidence that the health care system will treat
them fairly. Thus, if screening programs are poorly
conceived, organized, or implemented, they may lead
to interventions of questionable merit and enhance the
vulnerability of groups and individuals.

Institute of Medicine (1999)

Although the terms are often used interchangeably, a distinction exists
between "testing" and "screening." Testing refers to a medical procedure that determines the presence or absence of a disease, or its pre-
cursor, in an individual patient.[75] Individuals are often selected for testing because of a history of risk or clinical symptoms. In contrast,
screening is the systematic application of a medical test to a defined
population.[76] Typically, medical testing is administered for diagnostic
or clinical purposes, while screening is undertaken for broader public
health purposes, such as case finding—identifying previously unknown
or unrecognized conditions in apparently healthy or asymptomatic persons.[77] At different times during the twentieth century, legislatures
screened for TB in schools and workplaces,[78] syphilis among newborns,[79] and HIV and TB among prison inmates.[80]

Screening is often fraught with political controversy. Legislatures
may wish to appear to be "doing something" about an urgent health
problem.[81] Screening, however, also reveals the identity of individuals
and subjects them to potential stigma and discrimination. Because it
can be costly and impose burdens, public health authorities should
evaluate screening programs under two broad criteria: Does screening
have adequate predictive value? Will screening achieve an important
public health objective?[82]

SCIENTIFIC MEASURES OF ACCURACY: POSITIVE PREDICTIVE VALUE

Careful policy assessments begin with an understanding of a screening
test's vital characteristics: its validity, determined by measures of sensitivity and specificity; its reliability (i.e., repeatability); and its yield, or

amount of disease detected in the population.[83] Validity is a screening test's ability to determine which individuals within a population actually have a disease and which do not. Validity has two components: sensitivity and specificity. Sensitivity is a test's ability to identify accurately those who have a particular disease, while specificity is a test's ability to identify accurately those who do not have that disease. Sensitivity and specificity are often inversely related; high sensitivity is generally achieved at the expense of low specificity, and vice versa. From a policy perspective, sensitivity and specificity pose difficult trade-offs. If a test has low sensitivity, a significant number of persons actually infected will escape detection (false negatives). Conversely, a test with low specificity will misclassify and mislabel many healthy people as having the infection (false positives).

Reliability is the consistency of a screening test's results when the test is performed more than once on the same individual under similar conditions. Two major factors affect consistency: methodological variation (e.g., inadequate quality control) and observational variation (e.g., insufficient operator training). Obviously, unreliable tests are of little value since clinicians and patients cannot depend on the results.

A screening program's yield is the amount of previously unrecognized disease that the test identifies. The most cost-effective screening programs achieve a high yield. However, programs that detect a nominal number of persons with disease can sometimes be justified if early detection and intervention can avert transmission (e.g., tuberculosis) or serious consequences (e.g., hyperthyroidism).

In summary, screening programs have value only if they are scientifically sound: high sensitivity and specificity, reliability, and yield. Thus, screening programs, in order to be effective, must use technically superior tests, trained test operators, and quality laboratories, and they must detect a significant number of cases that would not otherwise be identified. Even if a test is accurate in all these ways, it may still have low predictive value (PV). That is, the test may not be able to predict correctly the presence or absence of a disease in the population.[84] PV is determined not only by a test's validity, but also by the prevalence of disease in the population. Even highly valid tests have poor PV in a low-prevalence population. Consider a test with a sensitivity and specificity of 99 percent. If the prevalence of infection in the population is 10 percent, the positive PV is 92 percent, but if the prevalence is 1 percent, the PV is 50 percent. A PV of 50 percent means that a person with a positive test has an equal chance of being either infected or not infected. As the prevalence falls below 1 percent (which is common for diseases in low-risk populations), the positive PV is reduced still further. (See Table 9 for a worksheet explaining how to calculate PV.) The problem with applying a technically superior test to a low-risk population is that it is not cost-effective. The program is likely to identify few cases of infection because relatively few cases actually exist. The screening program, moreover, will produce many false positive cases. False positive results for serious conditions can have profound psychological effects, including suicidal behavior.[85]

The state of Illinois powerfully illustrated the problems with screening in a low-prevalence population by mandating premarital HIV screening. The legislature assumed that HIV could be prevented by screening marriage applicants, who would then be counseled on the risks of unprotected sex. However, during the first six months of the program, screening identified only eight HIV-positive persons at a cost of $2.5 million ($312,000 per infected individual). The annual cost was nearly 1.5 times the state appropriation for all other AIDS surveillance and prevention programs combined. At the same time, the marriage rate dropped in Illinois and rose in adjacent states.[86] This analysis suggests that policymakers need to think carefully about the likely costs and benefits of screening in low-prevalence populations.

PUBLIC HEALTH PURPOSES

Policymakers sometimes assume that acquisition of knowledge about a population's health status must promote the public's welfare. For example, legislators proposed screening as an immediate response to publicized cases of HIV transmission from health care workers to patients, mothers to infants, and rapists to victims. These legislative initiatives may appear to be appropriate responses to a health emergency, but screening should not be regarded as an inherent good. Policymakers should have an important public health purpose and demonstrate that the screening program will actually achieve the stated purpose. What is the marginal usefulness of the test? Given what is known about the population, does the test yield new information and, based on that information, are effective responses available?

One of the most important measures of a successful screening program is whether it is acceptable to the population.[87] Public acceptance is important because behavioral change is most likely if persons at risk participate in public health programs. Public acceptance is also important for political reasons since democratic support is crucial to the legitimacy of public

TABLE 9
POSITIVE PREDICTIVE VALUE WORKSHEET

The PV of a particular test is the number of persons who test true positive divided by the total number of persons who test true positive and false positive. Even highly valid tests have a poor PV in a low-prevalence population.

The following two-by-two table shows the possible results of testing on a person infected or not infected with a disease.

		Infected	Not Infected
Test Results:	Positive	True Positives	False Positives
	Negative	False Negatives	True Negatives

$$\text{Predictive Value (PV)} = \frac{\text{True Positives}}{\text{True Positives + False Positives}}$$

Consider a test with a sensitivity and specificity of 99%. This means that 99% of those who test positive are actually infected and 99% of those who test negative are actually not infected. Therefore, 1% of those infected will test false negative and 1% of those not infected will test false positive. In a population of 1000 with a prevalence of 10% infection in the population, 100 persons are infected with the disease. Of these 100, 99% will test true positive and 1% will test false negative. Of the remaining 900, 99% will test true negative and 1% will test false positive.

The resulting PV is 99/108, which is 92%. This means that persons who test positive have a 92% chance of really being infected.

		Infected	Not Infected	*Total*
Test Results:	Positive	99	9	108
	Negative	1	891	892
	Total	100	900	1000

PV = 99/108 or 92%

---

health activities. Public acceptance, of course, is far from simple—in urgent situations the public may clamor for strong measures, while persons at risk resist compulsion. Community acceptance of screening depends, in part, on the target population and on the voluntariness of the screening.

THE "TARGETING" PROBLEM

From a scientific and public health perspective, screening in higher-prevalence populations is preferable. High-prevalence screening finds more cases, at less cost per case, and generates fewer false positive results.

High-prevalence screening, then, is more cost-effective and less burden-some. Given its clear advantages, one would expect that public health authorities would almost always target populations at high risk of infection. However, this is not always the case, and there may be good reason. If the risk group is vulnerable, narrowly targeted screening may expose the population to social risk. Think about a disease that disproportionately affects minorities (e.g., tuberculosis among homeless persons, or HIV among gays, African-Americans, or Latinos). (Or, in the analogous field of genetics, think of the stigma associated with screening African-Americans for sickle cell or Ashkenazi Jews for Tay-Sachs or breast cancer.) Public health authorities face a dilemma. If they target the narrow, high-risk population, it reinforces existing bigotries, thereby creating harms to individuals and to the group itself (e.g., African-Americans targeted for HIV screening may become closely associated in the public's mind with disfavored behaviors such as homosexuality or drug use). Alternatively, public health authorities may choose to screen a much broader population that includes, but is not limited to, risk groups. This broad population-based approach, however, unnecessarily screens many individuals who are unlikely to be infected. There is no sure way to resolve this dilemma because it involves a values choice: Which is more important, the most efficient screening program or the program that is least burdensome to vulnerable communities? In the end, policymakers need to make a hard choice and will have to weigh public health against social justice.

Policymakers not only have to make difficult choices about how to target screening. They also have to decide what kind of screening program to initiate and whether to mandate compliance.

THE PROBLEM OF COMPULSION
AND CONSENT: A TAXONOMY

Ronald Bayer developed the idea of a "voluntaristic consensus" in the HIV epidemic, meaning that both public health authorities and community groups exhibit strong support in favor of cooperation rather than compulsion.[88] It was not always this way, and while voluntarism in public health may be currently fashionable, pressures for increased use of restrictions of the person are likely to reemerge. The politics of screening are particularly volatile since policymakers are often attracted to the notion that identifying contagious persons promotes the public's well-being. At the same time, groups that bear the burden of compulsion vigorously insist on maintaining their personal autonomy—a claim that civil liberties organizations strongly support. This section explores the problem of compulsion by offering a taxonomy of screening; the next sections examine screening from constitutional and disability rights perspectives.

The terms *voluntary* and *compulsory* appear simple enough: the former connotes unfettered freedom to choose and the latter the absence of freedom. Between these two extremes, however, is a gradation of different kinds of screening that warrants explanation. It is possible to identify at least five forms of screening: compulsory, conditional, routine with advance notification (opt-in), routine without advance notification (opt-out), and voluntary.[89]

Compulsory Screening.   Pursuant to their police powers, states may compel citizens to submit to medical screening without informed consent. Compulsory screening requires legislative authority, which many public health statutes provide. Compulsory screening is authorized in a range of statutes relating to communicable diseases, sexually transmitted diseases, or specific diseases such as tuberculosis and HIV.[90] This body of public health law contains a morass of confusing, sometimes contradictory, provisions that defy orderly characterization. First, statutes define a class of persons to which the compulsory power applies. The class may be generic, such as persons who are "suspected" of having an infection.[91] Alternatively, the class may be particular to certain groups, such as sex offenders,[92] migrant laborers,[93] prostitutes,[94] pregnant women,[95] newborns,[96] or inmates.[97] Second, statutes define a set of circumstances that triggers a screening requirement, such as when a person is "exposed" to bloodborne infection.[98] Third, statutes specify procedures that public health authorities must follow, ranging from unfettered discretion to requiring a judicial order prior to screening.[99] Finally, statutes impose a civil or criminal penalty on individuals who fail to comply.

Conditional Screening.   The government can make access to certain privileges or services contingent upon undergoing medical screening. For example, some statutes mandate STD screening to obtain a marriage license,[100] PPD tuberculin skin screening to work in a school or nursing home,[101] or HIV screening to immigrate to the United States.[102] Conditional screening is not mandatory in the strict sense of the term, because persons can avoid the test by forgoing the privilege

or service sought. However, if the privilege or service has high importance to the individual, the screening requirement may be perceived as
coercive.

Routine Screening with Advance Notification (Opt-In).   Few concepts are used with less care and precision than "routine" screening.
Routine screening is sometimes used simply to refer to population
screening: each member of a defined population is routinely tested.
However, this definition fails to explain the essential characteristics of
the screening—whether persons are informed that they are being tested,
how they are informed (e.g., individually or by public notice), when
they are informed (before testing or after the fact), and whether they
can withhold consent.

There are at least two forms of "routine" screening: with advance
notification (opt-in) and without advance notification (opt-out). In opt-
in screening, all individuals in the defined population are routinely "offered" testing (e.g., they are notified that a certain test is a standard part
of the treatment they are about to receive). As part of the informational
process, individuals are told that they have the right to give, or to withhold, consent; they are not actually tested until they have consented. A
clearer term for this kind of program is "routine offering" with informed consent.

Routine Screening without Advance Notification (Opt-Out).   In opt-
out screening, all individuals in the defined population are routinely
and automatically screened unless they expressly ask that the test not
be performed. This meaning of "routine" screening is a hybrid between
mandatory and voluntary. It verges on compulsory because individuals
may not be aware they are being screened and, even if they are aware,
they may not fully understand the purposes of the test or their right to
withhold consent. At the same time, opt-out screening does not expressly coerce because it theoretically respects a person's expressed desire not to be tested.

There are important policy implications in choosing between these
two forms of routine screening. Opt-in screening is far more respectful
of individual autonomy and the importance of informed consent. Opt-
out screening, however, reaches a larger population and is less expensive. In opt-out screening, health care workers do not have to provide
pretest counseling, which renders the program less time-consuming and
costly.

Voluntary Screening.   Voluntary screening is the norm in medicine and public health, and any deviation from the norm requires a careful justification. Voluntary screening requires information about the nature of the test in advance, full understanding by a competent person, and the freedom to choose to be tested or to decline. Nondirective counseling is thought to be the "best practice": individuals are informed of the options and the choice is left to them.

Even in the absence of legislation explicitly safeguarding voluntariness, the common law affords individuals a right to consent.[103] Since testing involves physical contact with the patient, physicians technically commit an intentional tort if they perform a test without consent or another legally sufficient justification; they are also negligent if they fail to provide adequate information so that the patient can make an informed decision.[104] Physicians sometimes bristle at such a stark legal requirement, arguing that hospitals routinely perform serological screening without asking each patient for permission. Physicians argue, by analogy, that it should not be necessary to seek the patient's consent before screening for a bloodborne disease, such as HIV or hepatitis B. The analogy does not hold because it assumes that the physician does not need consent for a routine serologic screening. In law, she does need consent but, because screening is sufficiently routine and expected, consent is implied. HIV screening, however, is far from routine or inconsequential; screening is essential to the diagnosis of a serious chronic disease so the patient would wish to be informed. A better analogy is to compare HIV screening with diagnostic tests for cancer or Huntington's chorea, where physicians usually respect patients' choices.

COMPULSORY SCREENING FROM A CONSTITUTIONAL PERSPECTIVE: UNREASONABLE SEARCH AND SEIZURE

Since the guarantees of the United States Constitution constrain principally actions by the state,[105] the legal battleground over screening has centered on government agencies, as well as private entities acting on federal or state rules that require or authorize testing. The primary constitutional impediment to testing is the Fourth Amendment's right of people to be "secure in their persons" and not subjected to "unreasonable searches and seizures."[106] The Fourth Amendment is popularly perceived as applying solely to personal or residential searches (as to administrative searches, see chapter 9), but the Supreme Court has long recognized that the collection and subsequent analysis of biological samples are "searches."[107] Privacy and security are threatened by the invasion of bodily integrity involved in collecting the sample and the ensuing chemical analysis that extracts personal information. The constitutional issue is whether the analysis of blood, urine, or other tissue is "unreasonable." In most criminal cases a search is unreasonable unless it is accomplished pursuant to a judicial warrant issued upon probable cause; if the warrant requirement is impracticable, the courts require, minimally, "reasonable suspicion" based on an individualized assessment.

The Supreme Court, in drug screening cases, has held that when the state has "special needs beyond the normal need for law enforcement," the warrant and probable or reasonable cause requirements may not be applicable.[108] Most screening programs are not conducted for law enforcement purposes, thus falling within the "special needs" doctrine; for example, even mandated STD screening for persons accused or convicted of sexual assault is considered "special needs" because the results are not used as evidence in a criminal trial. If screening is for public health—rather than criminal justice—purposes, the courts balance the governmental and privacy interests to determine the reasonableness of the search. On one side of the balance is the government's interests in public health, and on the other is the individual's expectations of privacy. The courts weigh the state's interests in public health and safety quite heavily, but perceive individual interests as nominal: "[S]ociety's judgment [is] that blood tests do not constitute an unduly extensive imposition on an individual's privacy and bodily integrity."[109] As a result, most courts have assumed a permissive posture when reviewing government screening programs.[110] Even for highly stigmatized diseases such as HIV, the courts have upheld screening of firefighters and paramedics,[111] military personnel,[112] overseas employees in the State Department,[113] immigrants,[114] and sex offenders.[115]

Screening that is scientifically accurate and achieves an important public health purpose is often justified even if it imposes a burden on vulnerable groups. Nevertheless, the Supreme Court's Fourth Amendment jurisprudence does not fairly balance the benefits and burdens. The judiciary tends to accept government assertions of a strong public health interest without a searching inquiry into whether the screening will, in fact, achieve those objectives. For example, public health guidelines have not supported any of the mandatory HIV screening programs upheld by the courts.[116] Compulsory screening, rather than furthering the government's interests, may dissuade individuals at risk from accessing the health care system. At the same time, by focusing on the physical intrusion of the blood test, the courts do not sufficiently weigh the informational privacy interests entailed in compelled disclosure of sensitive information.[117]

COMPULSORY SCREENING FROM A DISABILITY DISCRIMINATION PERSPECTIVE

Society's accumulated myths and fears about disability
and disease are as handicapping as are the physical
limitations that flow from . . . impairment. Few
aspects of . . . a handicap give rise to the same level of
public fear and misapprehension as contagiousness.
William J. Brennan (1987)

The Americans with Disabilities Act of 1990[118] (ADA) and the corpus of antidiscrimination legislation appear to be unlikely sources of law to fill the doctrinal void left by deferential constitutional standards. Disability law, however, is highly relevant to screening, because the information acquired can be used to discriminate based on health status. Screening programs are common in employment, public services (e.g., government-conducted or government-authorized screening), and public accommodations (e.g., hospitals and managed care organizations). Although the specific titles to the ADA have different provisions, a finding of discrimination requires adverse treatment of a person with a "disability" who is "qualified," or who would be qualified if reasonable "accommodations" or "modifications" were made.

A "disability" is defined as a physical or mental impairment that substantially limits one or more of the major life activities, a record of such impairment, or being regarded as having such an impairment.[119] The definition of disability covers most serious medical conditions ranging from communicable (e.g., hepatitis[120]) to chronic (e.g., cancer[121]) diseases. The Supreme Court, for example, found that all stages of HIV disease, including asymptomatic infection, are covered disabilities.[122] A person is disabled if she has a "record" of or is "regarded" as being disabled, even if there is no actual disability.[123] A "record" indicates that a person has a history of a disability and "regarded" as disabled means that a person is perceived as if she were disabled.[124]

The Supreme Court, in its 1999 term, strictly limited the definition of "disability." First, the Court emphasized that a person's disability must

create a "substantial" limitation on a major life activity; it is not sufficient if the disability makes the individual merely different.[125] Second,
the Court held that the determination of whether a person's impairment
substantially limits a major life activity must be made with reference to
mitigating measures (e.g., medication or other corrective devices).[126]
Consequently, if a person with an infectious disease, due to medication,
is not substantially limited in his major life activities, he is not "disabled," but a person may still be disabled due to limitations that persist
despite mitigating measures or due to the negative side effects of the
medication. Finally, the Court held that, in order to be regarded as substantially limited in the major life activity of working, an employer must
mistakenly believe the employee is unable to perform a class or broad
range of jobs utilizing the employee's skills. Thus, if an employee is perceived to be unable to perform only her particular job, she may not be
protected under the ADA. Advocates see these cases as an assault on the
civil rights of persons with disabilities because they significantly reduce
the number of people who can claim the ADA's protection.[127]

A person is "qualified" if he is capable of meeting the essential performance or eligibility criteria for the particular position, service, or
benefit. Qualification standards can include a requirement that a person does not pose a "direct threat" to the health or safety of others.[128]
The "direct threat" standard means that persons can be excluded from
employment, public accommodations, or public services to prevent a
significant risk of transmission of infection. The ADA, however, requires reasonable accommodations or modifications[129] that do not impose undue hardships.[130] To accommodate persons with an infectious
condition, the entity might have to provide infection control, training,
or a leave of absence for treatment.

Employment Screening.   The ADA's prohibition against discrimination in employment (Title I) specifically includes medical screening,
physical examinations, and inquiries.[131]

Pre-offer: An employer is not permitted to screen applicants before
offering a job.

Post-offer: An employer is permitted to screen after a job offer is
made, provided that all entering employees are screened and the medical information is kept confidential.

Current employees: An employer may screen current employees only
if the screening is job related and consistent with business necessity.

Even where employers are permitted to screen, they may not withdraw a job offer or adversely treat a current employee if the person is qualified.

Government-Conducted or -Authorized Screening.   The ADA's prohibition against discrimination applies to all government-conducted or -authorized screening. For example, health department screening of its own employees (Title I), patients in public clinics (Title III), or populations pursuant to public health powers (Title II) are all covered by the ADA.[132]

Health Care Screening.   The ADA's prohibition on discrimination covers screening in public accommodations (Title III), including hospitals, managed care organizations, and physicians' offices.[133] For example, hospital decisions to test patients for hepatitis B, HIV, or syphilis would be viewed through the lens of disability discrimination.

CASE STUDY: HIV SCREENING OF PREGNANT WOMEN AND INFANTS

Screening policy for HIV was transformed in 1994 with the scientific discovery that perinatal transmission could be significantly reduced with treatment. AIDS Clinical Trials Group (ACTG) 076 determined that a regimen of zidovudine (AZT) during pregnancy and childbirth could reduce the risk of transmission from mother to infant by approximately two-thirds.[134] The Public Health Service responded to ACTG 076 by issuing guidelines for treatment of pregnant women in 1994[135] and for counseling and screening in 1995.[136] By 1996, Congress required the Secretary of Health and Human Services to determine whether HIV screening of infants was "routine practice" and, if so, Ryan White Treatment funds would become contingent upon the states demonstrating that perinatal transmission had declined by half, 95 percent of women are screened during prenatal care visits, or a program of mandatory newborn screening had been instituted.[137] During the same year, New York enacted legislation mandating HIV screening of all newborns.[138]

   The political response to the deaths of babies from HIV disease was as predictable as it was unscientific. The sponsor of the New York statute, Assemblywoman Nettie Mayersohn, reasoned that it was "criminal" to allow the suffering of "innocent and helpless victims."[139] However, knowing the HIV status of infants would not reduce perinatal transmission and, at the time, the benefit of early treatment of newborns was yet to be proven. It became apparent to public health authorities that perinatal transmissions could be reduced only by screening pregnant women and treating those who were seropositive. While screening was imperative, how could the problems of targeting and compulsion be overcome?

The Institute of Medicine (IOM) made a bold proposal for universal screening of pregnant women, but was faced with a classic dilemma about how to target the screening program. From a public health perspective, screening of groups at greatest risk would result in the highest yield, the best predictive value, and the least cost. On the other hand, narrowly targeted screening would starkly acknowledge differences of class and race (as well as the existing gender differences in all prenatal screening), separating women by skin color and socioeconomic status, separating fashionable suburbs from inner cities, and separating rural from urban America. The symbolic value of broad, rather than narrow, screening was obvious. Screening the entire population would convey the message that AIDS should concern everyone and that public health measures, by design, would apply universally. Targeted screening would convey a much different message—that AIDS was a disease of color and the underclass—singling out these groups and creating stigma and low self-esteem. Even though the epidemiologic evidence had long demonstrated that HIV indeed was a disease primarily among racial minorities, the IOM preferred population-based screening.

The IOM also faced the problem of compulsion and consent. The civil liberties paradigm had been set for a generation: informed consent, with pre-test and post-test counseling. This rights-oriented paradigm, however, had genuine deficits from a public health perspective. How would it be possible to assure that all, or most, pregnant women were screened if an elaborate pretest process were established? Such a process would incur considerable costs in counseling, training health care professionals, and creating incentives for hospitals. At the same time, would women decline testing or, worse, stay away from prenatal care? The IOM recommended a national policy of universal HIV screening with patient notification as a routine component of prenatal care. This proposal had natural attractions because it would maximize women's participation but nominally recognize their right to consent. At the same time, the proposal omits essential details about the theory and practice of notification. How would women be notified—individually or by public notice, orally or in writing, with or without the opportunity to ask questions? What safeguards would be instituted to ensure that women were competent, understood the information, and gave voluntary consent? The IOM proposal, by abandoning explicit written consent, appears to violate HIV-specific testing statutes in several states.

Women and infant screening programs demonstrate that case finding is far from a neutral scientific pursuit.[140] Rather, screening is political—elected officials perceive some groups as blameworthy and some as innocent. Screening is also rich in symbolism—the public health response helps socially to construct diseases on dimensions of race, gender, nationality, and socioeconomic status. Finally, screening is fraught with complex choices and weighing of values—cost, efficiency, autonomy, and justice. Perhaps the lesson is that tidy evaluative criteria are only part of a textured understanding of screening. Politics, symbolism, and values appear to be just as important as science in clarifying the complexities of case finding.

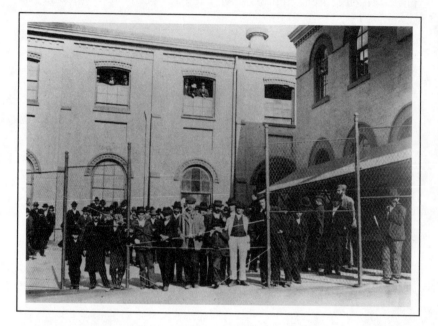

Arriving immigrants detained in quarantine on Hoffman Island, New York, circa 1900.

8 Restrictions of the Person

Autonomy, Liberty, and Bodily Integrity

Everybody knows that pestilences have a way of recurring in the world, yet somehow we find it hard to believe in ones that crash down on our heads from a blue sky. There have been as many plagues as wars in history; yet always plagues and wars take people equally by surprise.

Albert Camus (1948)

The previous chapter examined vaccination to prevent communicable disease and case finding to identify those who are infectious. This chapter explores the breadth of legal regulation intended to curtail communicable disease by controlling those who have the disease. Government engages in a broad range of restrictions of the person to reduce the spread of infection—civil confinement (isolation, quarantine, and compulsory hospitalization), mandatory treatment, and criminal penalties for knowing or willful exposure to disease.

It is interesting to observe that the social response to epidemic disease through civil confinement and criminal punishment has remained essentially the same throughout history. The obvious explanation is that people with disease are seen as vessels of transmission, justifying restraint, but this does not seem entirely consistent with the fact that civilizations have had vastly different understandings of the causes of diseases and their methods of transmission. In fact, many societies have actively rejected theories of contagion.[1] Despite the lack of a simple explanation for the persistence of personal control measures, it may have something to do with how communities organize themselves to ward off threats to health and safety and how they view those who are perceived as public menaces. Government measures to separate the ill from society are deeply complex, imbued with the social meanings of "community" and "the other," economic interests, and political controversy.

A BRIEF HISTORY OF PERSONAL CONTROL MEASURES

If the bright spot be white in the skin of his flesh, and
in sight be not deeper than the skin . . . then the priest
shall shut up him that hath the plague seven days. . . .
And the priest shall look on him again the seventh day
and, behold, if the plague be somewhat dark, and the
plague spread not in the skin, the priest shall pronounce him clean. . . . But if the scab spread much
abroad in the skin . . . and if the priest see that,
behold, the scab spreadeth in the skin, then the priest
shall pronounce him unclean: it is a leprosy.

                                                    Leviticus 14:4–8

Command the children of Israel, that they put out of
the camp every leper, and every one that hath an issue,
and whosoever is defiled by the dead.

                                                    Numbers 5:2

The story of the legal regulation of the person is interwoven with the great contagious maladies of leprosy, syphilis, and pest.[2] The Old Testament describes the inspection and sequestration of lepers. The crusaders found "lazarettos," places of isolation, still in existence outside the walls of Jerusalem and incorporated the word into their language to mean a house for the reception of diseased persons.[3] Lazarettos were built outside the gates of principal European cities, often under the religious name of St. Lazarus. These places of asylum confined not only persons with infectious diseases, but also the insane and others whose separation from society was deemed beneficial to the populace.[4]

Governmental edicts separated those with disease from the community during the early Middle Ages: Emperor Justinian's order in 532 that persons arriving from plague-contaminated localities should be "cleansed" in places set aside for that purpose, the Council of Lyons' policy in 583 for the restriction of association of lepers with healthy persons, and the Lombard King Rothari's edict in 644 for the isolation of lepers.[5]

Multiple methods existed to exclude the contagious from society. The ill were confined in their homes for the duration of their illness and, upon death, were passed through the windows and removed from the city. Lepers had to forbear communicating with the healthy; they wore special costumes, sounded a clapper, and could not appear in markets, inns, or taverns. Sanitary cordons were established along borders, whereby countries isolated themselves from their neighbors during periods of epidemic, leaving only special passages of egress.[6]

These were all variations of land sanitary laws, but much of the history of personal control was exercised through maritime laws. Overseers of public health were thought to regulate seafaring vessels as far back as the year 1000. Certainly by the fourteenth century, Venetian overseers were authorized to spend public funds to quarantine ships, goods, and persons at an island in the lagoon. Soon after, Venice appointed a public bureau of sanitation, and neighboring city-states that were engaged in Mediterranean commerce established sea lazarets.[7]

From these beginnings, the quarantine system began. The first compendium of Venetian legislative acts on the plague, around 1127, required merchants and travelers to remain for a period of forty days in the House of St. Lazarus before entering the city.[8] Sanitary Bulletins were incident to quarantines and cordons. When persons and ships were proclaimed free of disease, they were given official bills of health indicating they were free to enter or leave a geographic area. Health officials had considerable powers and duties, including inspection, disinfection (e.g., by fire or lime), and isolation of people, animals, and goods (e.g., garments, food, and merchandise) thought capable of carrying disease. Offenses against quarantine, both land and maritime, were severely punished—with whipping, forced service on sick galleys or hospitals, and even exile or death.[9]

EARLY QUARANTINE LAWS IN THE UNITED STATES

Quarantine has been practiced in the United States, mostly at a local level, since the early colonial period.[10] The earliest municipal ordinances were enacted in Boston in 1647; East Hampton, Long Island, in 1662; and New York in 1663.[11] During the next century, states such as Massachusetts[12] and New York[13] enacted quarantine statutes and, by the time the Constitution was drafted, quarantine was well established.[14] Persons with infectious diseases have been detained for prevention or treatment from the framing era up until the present day. The last "leper home" closed as recently as 1998,[15] and many states still maintain places for the treatment of tuberculosis.

Although it is principally a state and local power, the federal government also has a long history of quarantine regulation. A national presence was established in 1796 with the enactment of the first federal quarantine law that authorized the president to assist in state quarantines.[16] Several years later, the act was replaced by a federal inspection system for maritime quarantines.[17] Thereafter, the federal government became more active in regulating the practice of quarantine. The conflict between federal and state quarantine regulation sparked a federalism debate in the courts during the nineteenth century.[18] The courts determined that, while the states have authority to quarantine,[19] state power is preempted by federal law pursuant to the commerce power.[20] Currently, federal law provides for cooperation among national and state authorities in the enforcement of quarantine.[21]

INTERNATIONAL QUARANTINE REGULATIONS

For most of recorded history, nations acted alone, using quarantine for self-survival. The First International Quarantine Rules were adopted in 1852 and, between that year and the end of the century, nine international sanitary conferences were convened.[22] Presently, international sanitary regulations are promulgated under the auspices of the World Health Organization.[23]

SOCIETY AND POLITICS

It is difficult to exaggerate the dread caused by disease epidemics and the destabilizing effects on people and their communities.[24] A pestilence was a scourge, decimating the population and presenting a threat to the common security as momentous as war.[25] Society, through its institutions, felt justified in taking whatever measures necessary to defend itself. The prevailing social response was to exclude sufferers from the community to safeguard healthy members. The measures taken were harsh and punitive, subjecting individuals to indefinite periods of restraint, unbearable isolation from human companionship, and total deprivation of liberty.

Persons suffering from, or exposed to, disease came to be viewed as more than public menaces. They were loathed and reviled, often blamed for their own condition. Sufferers were shut out from normal social discourse, and boundaries were created between them and the wider community. It was not simply a matter of expelling, isolating, or separating sufferers. They were outcasts, socially dead. The awful finality of exclu-

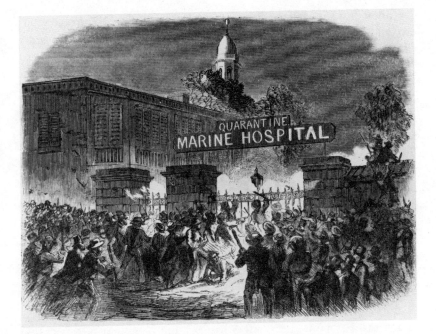

In the summer of 1858, an angry mob attacked and burned the quarantine hospital on Staten Island, New York.

sion from the human community was symbolized by a funeral service for lepers: "He was clad in a shroud, the solemn mass for the dead was read, earth was thrown upon him, and he was then conducted by the priests . . . outside the confines of the community."[26] Disease bred fear and provoked punitive actions. The community could justify this harsh treatment, in part, by blaming sufferers and branding them as "the other," deserving of ostracism.

Even in relatively more enlightened times, personal control measures have been applied in ways that may be better explained by animus than by science. Several campaigns of restraint in nineteenth- and twentieth-century America demonstrate the influence of prejudice:[27] isolation of persons with yellow fever, despite its mode of transmission by mosquitoes;[28] arrest of alcoholics, especially poor Irishmen, in the false belief that cholera arose in part from intemperance;[29] mass confinement of prostitutes "suspected" of having syphilis in state-run "reformatories";[30] and house-to-house searches and forced removal of children thought to have poliomyelitis.[31]

Tuberculosis during the post-bacteriologic era and AIDS in the modern era provide interesting illustrations of social intolerance. "Lungers" (the diseased organ representing their persona) were exiled to "Bugsville." Health officials, moreover, exercised their authority almost exclusively against the vagrant, the poor, and the immigrant, who were thought careless in their hygiene and "fractious and intractable" in their behavior.[32] Public health campaigners, such as Hermann Biggs and Charles Chapin, insisted that "autocratic," "radical," and "arbitrary" powers encroaching on liberty were necessary for the common weal.[33] However, in retrospect, the reduced incidence of tuberculosis probably was due to medical treatment and vastly improved sanitary conditions rather than to segregation of the ill.[34]

Persons with HIV were spared systematic sanctions; nevertheless, the community had exaggerated fears of contagion and segregationist instincts during the first decade of the epidemic (e.g., burning the home of Ryan White because his mother insisted he attend school[35]). Persons with HIV, particularly those associated with disfavored subgroups, such as gays and injecting drug users, were blamed for their disease— in contrast to "innocent" "AIDS babies" and hemophiliacs.[36] (This is reminiscent of *venereal insontium*, or venereal disease of the innocent in the early twentieth century.)[37] Popular indignation was evident in proposals for punitive measures, such as branding with a tatoo,[38] isolating,[39] and establishing special institutions.[40] Both tuberculosis and AIDS earned their own sobriquets: phthisiophobia[41] and AIDS phobia (often associated with homophobia).[42]

In summary, public health powers to control infectious diseases present vexing problems of cultural fear and misapprehension, blame and ostracism of marginalized individuals and groups, and political controversy. A discussion of government powers and constitutional limits on the exercise of personal control measures follows.

CIVIL CONFINEMENT: ISOLATION, QUARANTINE, AND COMPULSORY HOSPITALIZATION

Investigations by the Department of Human Services
have revealed that you have been engaged in activities which are potentially harmful to the public
health. You have been counseled as to the nature
and risk of these activities. Nevertheless, there is evidence to suggest that you have continued to partici-

pate in these activities. Now, therefore, I,
Commissioner of the Department of Human
Services, order you, [name], to cease and desist from
activities which are deemed to constitute a threat to
public health, effective immediately. If you fail to
honor this order, a court injunction may be sought
to compel your compliance.

State of Maine, Department of
Human Services (1993)

Public health authorities possess a variety of powers to restrict the autonomy or liberty of persons who pose a danger to the public.[43] They
can direct individuals to discontinue risk behaviors ("cease and desist"
orders),[44] compel them to submit to physical examination or treatment,
and detain them temporarily or indefinitely. This section will discuss
three different, but overlapping, powers of detention—isolation of
known infectious persons, quarantine of healthy persons exposed to
disease, and civil commitment (compulsory hospitalization) for care
and treatment. All of these powers are civil measures designed to prevent risks to the public. They are not intended to punish individuals for
morally culpable behavior as with criminal prosecutions. Civil remedies, therefore, are forward looking, aiming to prevent harm and improve health, while criminal penalties are backward looking, aiming to
punish wrongdoers.

MODERN DEFINITIONS: QUARANTINE, ISOLATION, AND CIVIL COMMITMENT

Although the terms *quarantine, isolation,* and *compulsory hospitalization* are often used interchangeably, both in public health statutes and
in common parlance, there are technical distinctions among them.

Quarantine.   Historically, quarantine was the detention, under enforced isolation, of persons suspected of carrying a contagious disease,
especially travelers or voyagers before they were permitted to enter a
country or town and mix with inhabitants.[45] Deriving from the Italian
quaranta and the Latin *quadragina,* the period of observation was forty
days, which was assumed to be the maximum duration of acute, as opposed to chronic, forms of disease.[46] The forty-day period was also
symbolic (e.g., Christ fasted for forty days in the desert *(quarentena)*

and Noah's flood lasted forty days and nights). The modern definition of quarantine is the restriction of the activities of healthy persons who have been exposed to a communicable disease, during its period of communicability, to prevent disease transmission during the incubation period if infection should occur.[47]

Isolation.   In contrast, isolation is the separation, for the period of communicability, of known infected persons in such places and under such conditions as to prevent or limit the transmission of the infectious agent.[48] Modern science usually can detect, through testing and physical examination, whether a person actually has an infectious condition. Accordingly, *isolation* is the appropriate term. Two different kinds of isolation statutes exist: those that authorize confinement of infected persons on the basis of disease status alone ("status-based" isolation) and those that authorize confinement of infected persons who engage in dangerous behavior ("behavior-based" isolation). The distinction between status-based and behavior-based isolation is pivotal, because one is concerned with an immutable health status while the other is directly targeted to those who engage in risk behaviors.

Civil Commitment.   Civil commitment is the detention (usually in a hospital or other specially designated institution) for the purposes of care and treatment. Civil commitment, like isolation and quarantine, is both a preventive measure designed to avert risk, and a rehabilitative measure designed to benefit persons who are confined.[49] Consequently, persons subject to commitment usually are offered, and sometimes are required to submit to, medical treatment. Civil commitment is normally understood to mean confinement of persons with mental illness or mental retardation, but it is also used for containing persons with infectious diseases, notably tuberculosis, for treatment.[50]

CIVIL CONFINEMENT UNDER PUBLIC HEALTH STATUTES

The power to detain is given to state and local health departments by legislation, and varies in its breadth from state to state. In some places, the legislature identifies the diseases subject to detention; in others, that determination is left to health authorities as a matter of professional judgment. Typically, powers of detention are found in three kinds of infectious disease law: sexually transmitted diseases, specific diseases, and communicable diseases (a residual class of conditions ranging from measles to malaria).[51] Notably, modern public health statutes authorize detention, under different circumstances, of persons with tuberculosis,[52] sexually transmitted diseases,[53] and HIV/AIDS.[54]

CONSTITUTIONAL REVIEW OF CIVIL CONFINEMENT: PRE–CIVIL RIGHTS ERA

States undoubtedly have power to detain individuals as necessary for the public's health. The Framers raised no objection to the prevalent use of quarantine at the time the Constitution was drafted. The Constitution does not explicitly mention quarantine. However, in discussing imports and exports, it does recognize the right of states to execute inspection laws, which are incident to quarantines.[55] Chief Justice John Marshall, as early as 1824, suggested that states have the inherent authority to quarantine under their police powers.[56] Since Marshall's time, numerous courts have found that states have sovereign authority to exercise a wide range of detention powers.[57] Most of the cases were decided in the late nineteenth[58] and early twentieth[59] centuries. Their hallmark was the deference consistently shown by the courts to the will of the legislature. Legislatures were given substantial latitude in authorizing civil confinement, and their actions were regarded as presumptively valid.[60] Indeed, litigation during this period usually did not challenge states' constitutional authority to detain, but inquired whether statutes delegated too much discretion to executive branch health officials or, alternatively, whether health officials acted *ultra vires* (i.e, outside of the scope of their statutory authority).[61] In other litigation, plaintiffs sought damages against state or municipal governments not for deprivation of personal liberty, but for deprivation of property. For example, if health officials confiscated a hotel,[62] apartment,[63] or vehicle[64] for purposes of quarantine, litigants pressed for economic damages.

The major impetus for judicial activity in the public health field was the sporadic occurrence of epidemics of venereal disease,[65] tuberculosis,[66] smallpox,[67] scarlet fever,[68] leprosy,[69] cholera,[70] and bubonic plague.[71] In this context, private rights were subordinated to the public interest, and individuals were seen as bound to conform their conduct for society's good.[72] As one court put it, quarantine does not frustrate constitutional rights because there is no liberty to harm others.[73] Even when courts recognized that personal control measures cut deeply into private rights, they would not allow the assertion of those rights to thwart public policy.[74] This preference for social control over individual autonomy emerged as a major characteristic of judicial rulings of the period.[75]

The judiciary, even during this early period, did assert some control over civil confinement. The courts, following the "rule of reasonableness" established in *Jacobson,* insisted that states must not act in "an arbitrary, unreasonable manner."[76] The Illinois Supreme Court said that isolation must be based upon "public necessity" and "must be exercised within reasonable limits, for the purpose of suppressing diseases."[77] In practice, however, this standard left basic questions unanswered: How was "rationality" or "necessity" to be judged? For example, a New York court left the question of necessity to "the people."[78] In examining the case law of this period, three limitations on civil confinement can be identified, although the courts have not always been clear or consistent (see chapter 3).

The Subject Must Be Actually Infectious.   Health authorities had to demonstrate that individuals were, in fact, exposed to disease and posed a public risk.[79] The courts appeared hesitant to stigmatize citizens in the absence of reasonable proof.[80] Even here, however, social prejudice often provided the principal basis for action. The Ohio Supreme Court upheld a quarantine regulation that "all known prostitutes and people associated with them shall be considered as reasonably suspected of having a venereal disease." "Suspect conduct and association" were deemed sufficient to justify imposing control measures, and the court did not appear unduly concerned with whether the woman actually had venereal disease.[81] An Illinois court accepted similarly unfounded assumptions: "suspected" prostitutes were considered "natural subjects and carriers of venereal disease," making it "logical and natural that suspicion be cast upon them."[82]

A Safe and Healthful Environment for Civil Confinement.   The courts periodically have insisted on safe and habitable environments for persons subject to civil confinement on the theory that public health powers are designed to promote well-being, and not to punish the individual.[83] On this theory, the quid pro quo for loss of autonomy or liberty on grounds of public health is that the state must take reasonable steps to avert harm through sanitary conditions as well as safe and adequate treatment. This theory of habitable and healthful conditions is illuminated in the mental health context, where courts have placed duties on government to protect and provide minimal levels of habilitation for patients within the care of the state.[84] For example, the Supreme Court in *Youngberg v. Romeo* (1982) held that persons who are civilly confined have constitutionally protected Fourteenth Amendment liberty interests in "conditions of reasonable care and safety," "freedom from bodily restraint," and "adequate food, shelter, clothing and medical care."[85] Although *Youngberg* was concerned with persons with mental retardation, its holding should extend to persons with infectious disease.[86] Since infectious disease powers are nonpunitive in nature and designed to safeguard public health, persons confined should not be harmed.[87]

The Power Must Not Be Exercised on Racial or Other Discriminatory Grounds.   One of the most invidious measures in public health history was struck down in *Jew Ho v. Williamson* in 1900.[88] Public health officials had quarantined an entire district of San Francisco containing a population of more than 15,000 persons, ostensibly to contain an epidemic of bubonic plague. The quarantine was made to operate exclusively against the Chinese community. The court held the quarantine unconstitutional on grounds that it was unfair—health authorities acted with an "evil eye and an unequal hand."[89] *Jew Ho* serves as a reminder that quarantine can be used as an instrument of prejudice and subjugation of vulnerable individuals or populations.

CONSTITUTIONAL REVIEW OF CIVIL CONFINEMENT:
POST–CIVIL RIGHTS ERA[90]

Constitutional doctrine changed markedly during the 1960s and the following decades (see chapter 3). In fact, the changes were so pronounced that they cast doubt on the precedential value of the vast number of early cases on civil confinement.[91] This was a time that the Court devised its "tiered" approach to constitutional adjudication and began to scrutinize state action strictly based on race or that invaded an important sphere of liberty or privacy. Most important, the Court found that deprivations of liberty, or "the right to travel," were "fundamental rights" deserving the highest standard of judicial review.[92]

The power to detain persons with infectious disease would be put to a strict legal test.[93] Civil confinement is a uniquely serious form of restraint because it constitutes a "massive curtailment of liberty."[94] Detention is justified not on a finding that a person has committed a criminal offense, but because of a prediction of future dangerousness.

Individuals, moreover, are not detained for a finite period based on the seriousness of past behavior. Rather, they are confined indefinitely, particularly if the condition is not susceptible to treatment. Under contemporary constitutional standards, the state must demonstrate a compelling public health interest, a "well-targeted" intervention, and the absence of a "less restrictive alternative."[95] The state must also provide procedural due process (see chapter 3). The following analysis uses civil commitment of the mentally ill as an analogy because, like detention of persons with infectious disease, the intervention is nonpunitive and is based on the health and safety of the individual and the community.[96]

A Compelling State Interest in Confinement.   Under the Supreme Court's "strict scrutiny" analysis, the state must have a compelling interest that is substantially furthered by the detention.[97] Consequently, only persons who are truly dangerous (i.e., pose a significant risk of transmission) can be confined.[98] In *O'Connor v. Donaldson* (1975), the Supreme Court held that, without providing treatment, the state could not confine a nondangerous mentally ill person who is capable of surviving in the community.[99] Lower courts have gone further by requiring actual danger as a condition of civil confinement in both mental health[100] and infectious disease[101] contexts. For example, in *City of New York v. Doe* (1994), the court required clear and convincing evidence of the person's inability to complete a course of TB medication before permitting restraint.[102]

A "Well-Targeted" Intervention.   Public health authorities sometimes order the detention of a large group of people (e.g., everyone in a geographic area). If some members of the group would not, in fact, transmit infection, the state action is overbroad. The Supreme Court finds overinclusive restraint constitutionally troubling because it deprives individuals of liberty without justification. For example, civil confinement of all homeless persons with tuberculosis on the theory that the entire class would fail to take their medication would restrain the liberty of those who would, in fact, comply. The Supreme Court is more tolerant of underinclusive interventions (i.e., those that restrain some, but not all, dangerous persons). However, if the underinclusion is arbitrary, or worse, purposefully discriminatory, it could be constitutionally invalid.[103] For example, confinement of gay men with HIV, but not others who engage in unsafe sex, would be prejudicial and, arguably, unconstitutional.

The Least Restrictive Alternative.   Given the strict standard of review in cases involving deprivation of liberty, the state would not be
permitted to resort to confinement if it could achieve its objectives
through less drastic means.[104] For example, if the state could avoid deprivation of liberty by directly observed therapy, it could be required to
do so. However, the state probably does not have to go to extreme, or
unduly expensive, means to avoid confinement.[105] For example, the judiciary would be unlikely to require the government to provide economic services, benefits, and incentives to persuade individuals to take
their medication;[106] nor must the state adopt less effective measures. In
the context of tuberculosis, New York City health officials aptly argued
that they could not be required "to exhaust a pre-set, rigid hierarchy of
alternatives that would ostensibly encourage voluntary compliance . . .
regardless of the potentially adverse consequences to the public
health."[107]

Procedural Due Process.   Persons subject to detention are entitled to
procedural due process. As the Supreme Court recognized, "there can be
no doubt that involuntary commitment to a mental hospital, like
involuntary confinement of an individual for any reason, is a deprivation
of liberty which the State cannot accomplish without due process of
law."[108] The procedures required depend on the nature and duration of
the restraint.[109] Certainly, the state must provide elaborate due process
for long-term, nonemergency, detention.[110] Noting that "civil commitment for any purpose constitutes a significant deprivation of liberty"[111]
and that commitment "can engender adverse social consequences," the
Court has held that, in a civil commitment hearing, the government has
the burden of proof by "clear and convincing evidence."[112]

In *Greene v. Edwards* (1980), the West Virginia Supreme Court
reasoned that there is little difference between loss of liberty for mental health reasons and the loss of liberty for public health rationales.[113] Persons with an infectious disease, therefore, are entitled to
similar procedural protections as persons with mental illness facing
civil commitment. These procedural safeguards include the right to
counsel, a hearing, and an appeal. Such rigorous procedural protections are justified by the fundamental invasion of liberty occasioned
by long-term detention, the serious implications of erroneously finding a person dangerous, and the value of procedures in accurately determining the complex facts that are important to predicting future
dangerous behavior (see Table 10).

TABLE 10
CIVIL CONFINEMENT

Form of Detention	Definition
Quarantine	Confinement of *healthy* persons during period of communicability
Isolation	Confinement of *known* infected persons during period of communicability
Civil Confinement	Confinement in a hospital or other institution for purposes of care and treatment

Constitutional Review

Pre–Civil Rights Cases	Post–Civil Rights Cases
Person actually infectious Conditions of confinement safe and healthful Power must not be used in an arbitrary or discriminatory manner	*Compelling state interest:* significant risk of transmission *Narrowly tailored intervention:* not under- or overinclusive *Least restrictive alternative:* no less drastic, but equally effective, interventions available *Procedural due process:* a fair hearing

In summary, provided they conform with procedural due process, public health authorities have ample power to detain persons to prevent transmission of infectious disease. The person or group confined must pose a significant risk to the public, and the state must exhaust less restrictive alternatives. Beyond these procedural and substantive standards, public health authorities retain considerable discretion. However, health authorities do not always exercise their discretion in value-neutral, scientifically sound ways. They are executive branch officials influenced by public opinion and political pressures. Consequently, societal misapprehensions and prejudices do affect public health judgments. It has always been this way in the great epidemics of the past, and it is likely to be so in the future.

COMPULSORY PHYSICAL EXAMINATION AND MEDICAL TREATMENT

No right is held more sacred, or is more carefully guarded, by the common law, than the right of every

individual to the possession and control of his own
person, free from all restraint or interference of others,
unless by clear and unquestionable authority of law.
Horace Gray (1891)

Medical treatment for an infectious disease affords both individual and
collective benefits. Treatment benefits individuals by ameliorating
symptoms and sometimes providing a cure. Treatment also benefits society by reducing or eliminating infectiousness. But these dual advantages of treatment are placed at risk if individuals do not take the full
course of their medication. Inconsistent treatment can result in drug resistance, so that modern therapies become less effective. Because of the
benefits to individuals and the community, and the problem of drug resistance, public health authorities have an abiding interest in compulsory treatment. However, mandatory treatment (as well as physical examinations that are antecedent to treatment)[114] represents a serious
intrusion into a person's bodily integrity. Mandatory physical examinations and treatment, therefore, require careful justifications.[115] This
section discusses common law, statutory, and constitutional rights to
refuse infectious disease treatment. It also examines the primary justifications for imposing treatment without consent.

COMMON LAW RIGHT TO REFUSE TREATMENT: INFORMED CONSENT

As the epigraph by Justice Horace Gray suggests, patients have a deeply
rooted common law right to refuse treatment that is embodied in the
concept of informed consent.[116] Absent a statutory power to impose
treatment, public health authorities are bound to respect the wishes of
competent patients. The doctrine of informed consent includes the following components.[117]

Information. Physicians have a duty to disclose the material benefits,
risks, adverse effects, and alternatives of treatment.[118] Thus, health authorities have a duty to disclose relevant information in ways that patients can comprehend (i.e., methods of disclosure should be educa-
tionally, linguistically, and culturally appropriate).

Competency. In order to give legally valid consent, individuals must be
capable of understanding the nature and purposes of the treatment.[119]
Persons who lack competency cannot provide valid consent, but this does

not mean that treatment can be imposed. Treatment can be authorized only by a person who is legally empowered to consent on the person's behalf, such as the parent of a minor or a judicially appointed guardian.

Voluntariness. The patient must make a free choice, without undue influence, fraud, or duress.[120] Consent sought by using a threat of restraint is not voluntary.

Specificity. The patient must consent to the actual treatment provided. Thus, patients should not be asked to give a "blanket" consent that covers a broad range of treatments.

MANDATORY TREATMENT UNDER PUBLIC HEALTH STATUTES

Public health statutes frequently authorize mandatory treatment, which has the effect of overriding common law. For example, most sexually transmitted disease[121] and tuberculosis[122] laws grant health officials the power to compel physical examination and medical treatment. Statutes often impose certain conditions for mandatory treatment, such as being a danger to the public; others may require a violation of some rule or order, such as noncompliance with a health directive or refusal to be treated. Still others limit treatment to active, or contagious, cases of infection; if the individual is not currently infectious (e.g., nonsymptomatic M. TB), public health authorities may lack authority to impose treatment.[123] Some public health statutes are designed to expand access to health care rather than to authorize compulsory treatment. For example, sexually transmitted disease statutes characteristically empower "mature" minors to consent so that they can obtain treatment without informing their parents.[124]

THE CONSTITUTIONAL RIGHT TO REFUSE TREATMENT

The right to refuse treatment, most importantly, has been grounded in the federal and state constitutions.[125] In a series of cases during the last two decades, the Supreme Court has recognized that a competent person has a constitutionally protected "liberty interest" in refusing unwanted medical treatment. The Court embraced the principle of bodily integrity in cases involving abortion[126] and the rights of persons with terminal illness[127] and mental illness.[128] The Court's jurisprudence provides ample reason to believe the Constitution safeguards treatment decisions which are among "the most intimate and personal choices a person may make in a lifetime, choices central to personal dignity and autonomy."[129]

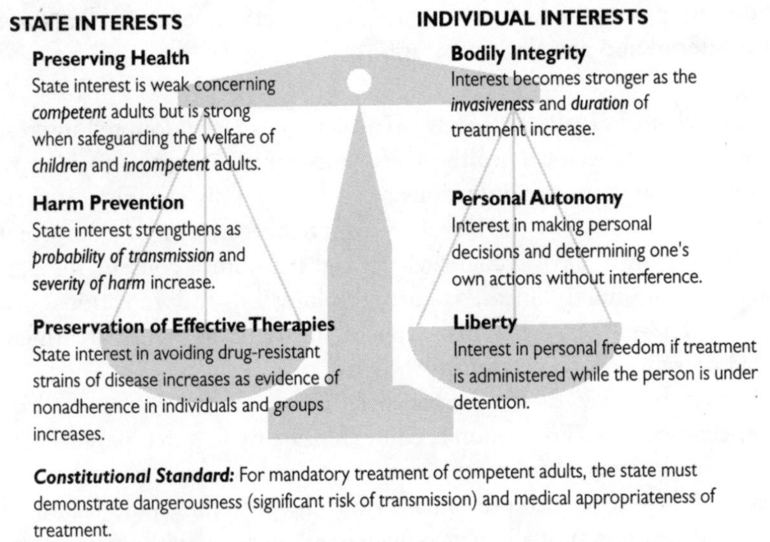

STATE INTERESTS

Preserving Health
State interest is weak concerning competent adults but is strong when safeguarding the welfare of children and incompetent adults.

Harm Prevention
State interest strengthens as probability of transmission and severity of harm increase.

Preservation of Effective Therapies
State interest in avoiding drug-resistant strains of disease increases as evidence of nonadherence in individuals and groups increases.

INDIVIDUAL INTERESTS

Bodily Integrity
Interest becomes stronger as the invasiveness and duration of treatment increase.

Personal Autonomy
Interest in making personal decisions and determining one's own actions without interference.

Liberty
Interest in personal freedom if treatment is administered while the person is under detention.

Constitutional Standard: For mandatory treatment of competent adults, the state must demonstrate dangerousness (significant risk of transmission) and medical appropriateness of treatment.

Figure 14. Mandatory treatment: balancing individual and state interests.

The Supreme Court's recognition of a right to bodily integrity does not mean that the right is absolute.[130] Outside the context of reproductive freedom, the Court has not viewed the right to refuse treatment as "fundamental." Instead of "strict scrutiny," the Court balances a person's liberty interests against relevant state interests. In fact, where it adopts a balancing test, the Court usually supports state interests over individual "liberty" interests.[131] In the context of infectious diseases, as the following discussion suggests, the courts have consistently affirmed the constitutionality of compulsory treatment. Despite the deference shown to public health judgments, it is still important to evaluate the justification for overriding the person's consent (see Figure 14).

JUSTIFICATIONS FOR MANDATORY TREATMENT

The state has three interrelated interests in compulsory treatment.[132] The first—"health preservation"—relates to the threat posed by infectious diseases to the health and life of persons who become infected. The second—"harm prevention"—relates to the threat posed by infected persons to the health of others. The third—"preservation of effective therapies"—relates to the effect that multidrug-resistant forms of disease pose to society by threatening the effectiveness of standard antibacterial and antiviral medications.

Preservation of Health or Life. The state has an undoubted interest in preserving a person's health or life, and might assert this interest to compel treatment for an infectious disease. Generally speaking, preservation of health does not justify unwanted treatment of competent adults.[133] Courts have recognized the right to refuse consent for persons with terminal illness,[134] mental illness,[135] and infectious disease.[136] The judiciary has also upheld the right to refuse treatment based on religious convictions.[137]

Courts, however, do permit beneficial treatment for children and incompetent persons. For example, courts repeatedly find that parents may not withhold medical treatment from their children, especially when the treatment is necessary to prevent a serious threat to the child's health.[138] Similarly, courts do not allow incompetent adults to go without necessary treatment. If an adult is incompetent, courts will often empower a surrogate decision maker to make the choice that the person would have made if he were competent (substituted judgment) or the treatment choice that is in the person's best interests.[139] For example, if an incompetent person has tuberculosis, health authorities may seek a court order to treat the person under a theory of substitute judgment or best interests.

Harm Prevention. The most telling justification for imposing infectious disease treatment is to prevent harm to others. Since persons with infectious disease can transmit the infection through casual contact (e.g., measles) or behavior (e.g., herpes simplex), the state has a substantial interest in treatment that reduces contagiousness. The Supreme Court has held that health authorities may impose serious forms of treatment, such as antipsychotic medication, if the person poses a danger to himself or others.[140] The treatment must also be medically appropriate so that the person benefits.[141] Lower courts, using a similar harm prevention theory, have upheld compulsory physical examination[142] and treatment[143] of persons with infectious disease. Conversely, courts have found compulsory treatment unconstitutional where the person was not dangerous[144] or the treatment was not medically appropriate.[145] Consequently, public health authorities (if authorized by statute) can require individuals to submit to medical treatment only if they pose a significant risk of transmission and the treatment is beneficial.

Preservation of Effective Therapies (the Problem of Drug Resistance).
As explained above, the state has an interest that is connected to public safety but can be stated separately for the sake of clarity. That interest is in preserving the therapeutic effectiveness of standard infectious disease medications. Drug resistance has been a major problem with antibiotic treatment ever since the discovery of penicillin.[146] It has become a transcending problem in the treatment of many bacterial infections,[147] notably common staph infections in hospitals,[148] M. TB,[149] and, more recently, HIV.[150] As the incidence of multidrug-resistant disease increases, society faces the specter of revisiting a pretherapeutic era when infectious disease was a scourge.

Patients develop drug-resistant disease in two ways. First, transmitted or primary drug resistance occurs when a person becomes infected with organisms that are already resistant to one or more drugs. Second, acquired or secondary drug resistance occurs when drug-resistant mutants multiply as a result of ineffective therapy. If persons with disease take their medication in an incomplete or sporadic fashion, or if they receive a suboptimal dosage, then organisms mutate and multiply to produce drug resistance.[151]

Drug resistance has many causes, including prescribing patterns of physicians (e.g., overuse of antibiotics) and patient dislocation (e.g., homelessness and inadequate access to health care).[152] The government's interest in reducing drug-resistant disease, therefore, can be accomplished, in part, by providing incentives for, or regulating, physician prescribing and by providing compliance-enhancing services for vulnerable patients. These remedies, however, are often seen as costly and sometimes ineffective, so public health authorities may resort to compulsory measures to ensure that "nonadherent" patients take the full course of their medication. One method of accomplishing that goal has already been discussed—civil commitment; another, less restrictive, measure is discussed next—directly observed therapy.

DIRECTLY OBSERVED THERAPY

The state's interest in ensuring the completion of treatment may not always require compulsory hospitalization. Treatment in the community can often be assured through directly observed therapy, commonly used in the management of tuberculosis.[153] Directly observed therapy (DOT) is a compliance-enhancing strategy in which each dose of medication is observed by a family member, peer advocate, community worker, or health care professional.[154] Supervised therapy can take place in a variety of locations, ranging from a personal residence or place of employment to a clinic, physician's office, or even a street corner. Supervised therapy can be either voluntary, which requires informed consent, or mandatory.

Legal and policy analysis of compulsory DOT requires a careful balancing of public health and individual interests. Directly observed therapy is frequently thought to be relatively unintrusive because it does not involve confinement. However, its imposition does affect an individual's liberty, dignity, and privacy. Individuals may have to show up for treatment at specific places and times, interfering with freedom of movement. Moreover, treatment may take place in public places known for infectious disease treatment, resulting in stigma or discrimination, or treatment may occur at the individual's home, interfering with privacy.

Public health interests must be sufficiently strong to override these personal interests. A significant proportion of persons who self-administer anti-tuberculosis medication do not complete the full course of treatment.[155] DOT appears to be effective in securing higher rates of completion of treatment. Although the empirical evidence is mixed,[156] many DOT programs achieve treatment completion rates of over 90 percent.[157] Moreover, DOT substantially reduces the rates of primary and acquired drug resistance and relapse, effectuating the state's interests in harm prevention and preservation of effective medications.[158]

Universal DOT.   If individuals with infectious disease have a history of nonadherence to treatment regimens, and if they pose a significant risk, then public health interests in DOT are sufficiently substantial to justify the restraint. The more difficult question is whether public health authorities should apply DOT to a large population, absent individualized risk assessments (universal DOT). International[159] and United States[160] public health agencies, as well as expert committees,[161] all recommend universal supervised therapy. Their reasoning is that it is very difficult to predict which persons will, and which will not, take the full course of their medication, so that a population-based approach is fairer and more effective. If DOT were to be applied only to groups assumed less likely to cooperate (e.g., persons with mental illness or drug dependency or without stable housing or access to private health care), it would be prejudicial and stigmatizing.[162]

The best public health policies often require a nuanced approach. Universal DOT may well be preferable in locales with low treatment completion rates but may be unnecessarily burdensome where rates are already high.[163] Experiences in high-incidence areas, moreover, suggest that comprehensive approaches work best using a combination of DOT and compliance-enhancing services—rigorous surveillance, access to health care (e.g., drug dependency and mental health treatment), support services (e.g., transportation and child care), and monetary incentives.[164]

BALANCING INDIVIDUAL AND COLLECTIVE INTERESTS

In constitutional litigation, the courts weigh collective interests in societal health and safety against individual interests in bodily integrity. However, it is not always easy to balance these interests, particularly when the person is a competent adult. On one side is the state's interest in preventing harm: What is the probability of the risk and the severity of the harm? On the other side is the individual's interest in bodily integrity: How intrusive is the treatment both in terms of its invasive quality and its duration? (See Figure 14.) This analysis may help explain why one injection of an antibiotic to eliminate a syphilis infection is constitutional, as is a short course of anti-tuberculosis medication. But would compulsory treatment for HIV pass constitutional muster?

Think about two hypothetical mandatory HIV treatment statutes— one targeted to pregnant women to reduce perinatal transmission and the other to individuals engaging in multiple, unprotected sexual relationships. Strong evidence already exists that antiviral medication reduces perinatal transmission,[165] and research also suggests that treatment may reduce sexual transmission.[166] Mandatory treatment of pregnant women probably does not represent good public health policy,[167] but the constitutionality is harder to predict. The state has an undoubted interest in protecting fetal health.[168] At the same time, the woman's interest in bodily integrity may be strong because the treatment regimen is arduous and lasts for months.[169]

The second hypothetical—compulsory treatment to reduce sexual transmission—is also complex. The state's interest in preventing HIV transmission is compelling, but the treatment regimen only reduces the risk and does not eliminate it. The person's interest is equally strong because antiviral treatment may have to be administered indefinitely, throughout the lifespan, in order to maintain a reduction in infectiousness. Arguably, the treatment regimen would be so physically intrusive that the patient's liberty interests would outweigh the state's public safety interest.

THE CRIMINAL LAW: KNOWING OR WILLFUL EXPOSURE TO INFECTION

Certain acts obviously calculated to prejudice the public health are, on grounds of policy, indictable. Thus it has been held indictable to expose in a public thoroughfare a person labouring under a contagious disease; or to bring a glandered horse into a public place at the risk of causing infection to the queen's subjects; and it is a misdemeanor at common law to give to any person injurious food to eat.

Herbert Broom and Edward A. Hadley (1869)

In 1997, public health authorities in Chautauqua County, New York, discovered that a man infected with HIV had sexual intercourse with fifty to seventy-five women over a two-year period. Authorities further discovered that he had infected thirteen women, and they, in turn, infected others.[170] Similar cases have been documented in Tennessee,[171] Missouri,[172] Pennsylvania,[173] as well as other states.[174] Countless additional detected and undetected cases of knowing or willful exposure to infectious disease likely exist. Research suggests that a substantial minority of persons infected with HIV engage in unprotected sex or needle sharing without disclosing the risk to their partners.[175]

There is a powerful appeal in using the criminal law in response to the problem of willful or knowing exposure. The public views individuals who engage in this behavior as morally blameworthy[176] and supports criminal sanctions for aberrant and irresponsible conduct.[177] The criminal law deters risk behavior and sets a clear standard for behaviors that society will not tolerate. The Presidential Commission on the HIV Epidemic said that criminal liability is "consistent with society's obligation to prevent harm to others and the criminal law's concern with punishing those whose behavior results in harmful acts."[178]

The attraction of the criminal law as a public health measure is also based on its clarity, objectivity, and safeguards.[179] Whereas civil confinement often uses broad standards, such as "dangerousness," the criminal law must specify the behavior that is prohibited. If its language is vague, a criminal statute fails to forewarn, and is for that reason unconstitutional.[180] Whereas civil confinement authorizes detention based on predictions of the future, the criminal law focuses on behavior that has already occurred. Whereas "dangerousness" need be proved only by clear and convincing evidence, each element of a crime must be proved beyond a reasonable doubt. Whereas the period of civil confinement is indefinite, the period of criminal confinement is usually finite and proportionate to the gravity of the offense.

Despite its social and political appeal, the use of the criminal law against persons with infectious disease is highly complex, raising fundamental issues of fairness and effectiveness as a public health measure. This section will first explain criminal law theory. Next it will survey the two main approaches—traditional crimes of violence and public health offenses.[181] Finally, it will evaluate the criminal law as a tool of public health.

CRIMINAL LAW THEORY

The legal definition of a crime is an act performed in violation of duties that an individual owes to the community.[182] It includes both harmful conduct (*actus reus*) and a culpable state of mind (*mens rea*). This section covers particular kinds of criminal offenses, namely, risking transmission of an infectious disease. The underlying assumption is that persons with infectious conditions owe a public duty to avoid transmission of the infection. These offenses, however, are far more complex and varied than they first appear because they incorporate a wide variety of behaviors and culpable states of mind.

Individuals with an infectious disease (principally sexually transmitted and bloodborne) have been prosecuted for acts that range from the trivial to the highly dangerous and from the common to the rare.[183] At one end of the spectrum are acts that are common and not usually dangerous, such as donating blood. However, if the person has a bloodborne infection, the act carries risk; the probability of the risk depends on the whether the blood supply is screened for the infectious agent. Persons with infectious disease are also prosecuted for assaults, such as biting, spitting, and splattering of blood. Although these acts are harmful in themselves, they often do not pose significant risks of transmission of infection. Finally, some acts are not usually harmful but become so if persons with infectious disease engage in those acts. For example, having unprotected sex and sharing drug injection equipment become potentially harmful acts if the person has a sexually transmitted or bloodborne infection.

Harmful acts, in and of themselves, do not constitute an offense. The individual also must have a culpable state of mind. States of mind in the criminal law are highly complex but, generally speaking, persons may act purposefully, knowingly, or recklessly.[184]

Persons act purposefully when they have the objective of causing a harmful result (i.e., they desire the consequences of their act). A person who actually seeks to transmit an infection acts purposefully.

Persons act knowingly when they are aware that their conduct will cause harm. For example, a person who tests positive for a sexually transmitted infection and understands the mode of transmission acts with knowledge. Persons can also act with constructive knowledge when they reasonably *should* know that their behavior poses an unreasonable risk. For example, a person who has had a long-term relationship and has persistent symptoms may be assumed to know his serological status even though he has never been tested. Persons who act with knowledge, or constructive knowledge, are deemed blameworthy because they understand the consequences of their harmful behavior.

Persons act recklessly when they consciously disregard a substantial and unjustifiable risk. Individuals who blatantly disregard risks to others deviate from the standard of conduct to which reasonable, law-abiding persons placed in similar situations would adhere. For example, a person with an STD who has unprotected sex with numerous partners grossly deviates from acceptable conduct and may be thought of as criminally reckless.

In summary, persons with infectious diseases are subject to prosecution for a wide range of behaviors and states of mind. Behaviors range from blood donations and simple batteries (e.g., spitting or biting) to sexual intercourse and sharing drug injection equipment. Depending on the infectious agent, each of these behaviors carries very different probabilities of transmission. Individuals may also engage in these behaviors with varying states of mind, each with its own degree of culpability (e.g., purposeful, knowing, and reckless). To understand the complexity of the criminal law, consider a hypothetical involving persons with HIV who engage in the same behavior (i.e., sexual intercourse), but with different states of mind: one woman is a prostitute who is paid for sex, another is a victim in a physically abusive relationship, and a third seeks revenge. Now consider a hypothetical involving the same state of mind (i.e., intent to kill), but different behaviors: one man jabs his victim with a contaminated needle, one has sex with her, and a third spits in her face. Each of these cases poses different risks of harm and different degrees of culpability. Ideally, the criminal law would be able to identify the truly harmful and blameworthy cases but, as we will see, it has difficulty doing so.

TRADITIONAL CRIMES OF VIOLENCE

The traditional crimes of violence that can be read to apply to the transmission of an infectious disease are homicide (actual and attempted) and assault.[185]

Homicide.   Murder prosecutions resulting from transmission of an infectious disease are very rare because they require the death of the victim. Infectious diseases often do not result in death and, if they do, the length of time from infection to death usually precludes prosecution; either the defendant has already died from the infection or there is a statutory requirement that death must occur within one year of the act. Additionally, homicide requires proof of causation, and it may be difficult to demonstrate that the person contracted the infection from the defendant.

Attempted Homicide.   Prosecutions for attempted murder also should be rare and difficult to prove. As Kathleen Sullivan and Martha Field observe, "having sex or sharing needles is a highly indirect modus operandi for the person whose purpose is to kill."[186] Nevertheless, attempted homicide charges have been brought for a broad range of conduct, but with mixed results. For example, the Maryland Supreme Court held that, even in the context of a rape by a person with HIV infection, intent to kill could not be inferred.[187] An Oregon court, however, convicted a man of ten counts of attempted murder for having consensual unprotected sex with multiple women after he had been counseled to refrain from sex or, minimally, use a condom.[188]

The criminal law uses a subjective standard for a criminal attempt so that if the facts are as the person believes them to be, it is an offense.[189] This is important in the infectious disease context because a person could be convicted of attempted murder if her intent is to kill, regardless of whether the method used poses a significant risk of transmission. Indeed, courts have determined that if the defendant believed her actions could transmit a lethal infection, it is irrelevant if the actual risk is negligible.[190] Under this theory, persons with HIV infection have been convicted of attempted murder for conduct that has exceedingly low risks: biting,[191] spitting,[192] and splattering of blood.[193]

If a person with HIV plans to kill for revenge or greed, and uses a primary mode of transmission, that person should bear full criminal responsibility. For example, most people believe that the following actors are culpable: a father who injects his child with an HIV-contaminated needle, hoping to avoid making child support payments,[194] and a physician who exacts revenge on his ex-lover by injecting her with HIV and hepatitis C.[195] But would it be contrary to public policy to punish nondangerous behavior? Think about an inmate who spits at a prison guard, hoping to harm him.[196] Should he be subject to prosecution for attempted murder because of his mistaken belief that his saliva will kill? Finally, what is the preferred public policy if a person acts in ways that appear more to be a cry for help than a malicious attempt to kill? In *State v. Haines* (1989), an HIV-positive defendant attempted suicide by slashing his wrists. When police and emergency workers came he pleaded with them, "Let me die, I have AIDS." When they continued to intervene, he splattered his blood on the officers. Mr. Haines was convicted of attempted murder.[197]

Assault and Aggravated Assault.   A simple assault is a purposeful, knowing, or reckless causing of bodily injury.[198] Defendants with infectious diseases who engage in harmful behavior, such as biting[199] or throwing "body waste,"[200] have been convicted of assault instead of attempted murder. The crime becomes aggravated assault if the person causes a "serious" bodily injury or uses a "deadly weapon."[201] Two federal courts of appeal have convicted inmates of aggravated assault, holding that teeth, under certain circumstances, can constitute a deadly weapon.[202] Certainly, persons who engage in assaultive behavior deserve criminal punishment. However, should individuals be convicted of more serious offenses (e.g., assault with a deadly weapon) *because* of their infectious state? From a public health perspective the answer would be no, because prevention of negligible risks would be a low priority.

Despite the spate of prosecutions for traditional crimes of violence, the mental elements of "purpose" or "knowledge" can be difficult to prove. A person acts with purpose only if she actually desires to transmit the infection. A person acts knowingly only if she is "practically certain" that her conduct will cause harm.[203] Since risks of disease transmission are highly variable, and frequently low, a person cannot realistically know that any single act will transmit the infection. The most common behavior that is subject to prosecution is sexual intercourse. Sexuality is a highly complex behavior involving many different passions, desires, and fears. Usually, neither partner wants to harm the other, but is willing to take risks. In order to establish beyond a reasonable doubt what the person knew or intended, it may be necessary to discover what went on and what was said in the privacy of a sexual encounter. Did the person know he was infected? Did he inform his sexual partner? Was a condom used? Did his partner assume the risk?[204] The answers to these questions are difficult to ascertain and, even if they could be known, police surveillance of intimate behaviors may be so intrusive that it would not be worth the cost.

PUBLIC HEALTH OFFENSES

Partly in frustration with proving intentionality or knowledge, and partly in response to political pressure, legislatures have sought other avenues to criminalize the risk of transmission. Infectious disease statutes create public health offenses that vary from state to state. A few states have broad provisions that criminally punish behavior that risks transmission of *any* contagious disease.[205] Most statutes, however, create "disease-specific" offenses that were often enacted in waves in response to public misapprehensions about epidemics of the day. In the early twentieth century states enacted statutes directed at TB, followed by STDs, and, in the latter part of the century, HIV/AIDS. In each case, politicians vilified persons who had the disease, both blaming them for their own affliction and holding them morally accountable for placing the public at risk (see Figure 15).[206]

Tuberculosis.   States provide for an array of public health offenses for risking transmission of TB. The most common is failure to comply with a public health order or knowingly or willingly exposing others to infection.[207] Other states make it an offense to allow a "child or irresponsible person" to expose others to disease; to expose others to a bodily secretion; to "wantonly or negligently" contribute to, or promote, the spread of TB; to conceal an infection in one's self or a child; to transport an infected person; and to willfully introduce the disease into the city.[208]

Sexually Transmitted Disease.   More than half the states have statutes that make it a criminal offense to knowingly risk transmission

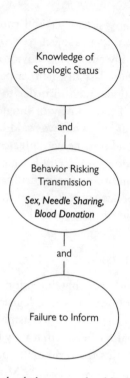

Figure 15. Standard elements of public health offenses.

of a sexually transmitted or venereal disease.[209] Most of these statutes have a common form, so that a person is criminally liable if he knows he is infected (e.g., tests positive for an STD), engages in sexual intercourse, and fails to disclose the risk to the partner. STD statutes usually are misdemeanors, levying a fine or a very short prison sentence.

HIV/AIDS.   Most statutes do not define HIV/AIDS as a sexually transmitted or venereal disease, so the statutory offense does not apply.[210] The highest court in New York, for example, upheld the Commissioner's determination not to add HIV to the list of sexually transmitted diseases.[211] Although a few states have explicitly defined "venereal disease" to include HIV,[212] most have enacted HIV-specific statutes modeled on older STD offenses.[213]

The federal government has enacted an HIV-specific offense relating to blood and tissue donation[214] and conditioned receipt of AIDS-related funding on state certification that its criminal laws are adequate to prosecute persons who risk transmission of HIV.[215] HIV statutes generally take the same form as STD statutes but have important differences: The person must know he is infected, engage in specified risk behavior (not always limited to sexual behavior), and fail to inform his partner of the risk.[216] While a few states require proof that the defendant tested positive for HIV[217] and/or had been informed of the risk,[218] most do not define "knowledge." It is unclear whether HIV statutes cover only actual knowledge or extend to "constructive" knowledge.

State statutes often list a range of prohibited behaviors carrying widely varying levels of risk. The great majority of HIV statutes proscribe primary modes of transmission, such as having sex or sharing of drug injection equipment. Some define sex quite broadly to include a variety of sexual activities.[219] Many also proscribe low-risk behaviors, such as donation of blood, body organs, semen, breast milk, or other tissue, or, more generally, "exposure to bodily fluids"[220] or "intimate contact."[221]

Since most statutes specify "failure to inform" as an element of the offense, informed consent is a defense.[222] Under a strict reading of the statutes, use of a condom would not excuse the failure to inform.[223] HIV-specific offenses, therefore, undermine the "safer sex" ethic, held by many in the gay community, that people are not required to disclose their HIV status so long as they use a condom.[224] Those adhering to this ethic would be liable to prosecution under modern HIV-specific statutes. It is important also to emphasize that while STD statutes tend to impose mild "public health" sanctions, HIV/AIDS statutes impose punitive sentences, often creating a felony.[225]

Courts have upheld the constitutionality of HIV-specific statutes against challenges based on vagueness,[226] overbreadth,[227] and the absence of a *mens rea* or specific intent requirement.[228] In particular, courts have found that HIV statutes are not impermissibly vague as applied to persons who engage in unprotected sexual intercourse, particularly after being counseled about safe sex.[229]

Evaluating Public Health Offenses.   Public health offenses have advantages over traditional crimes of violence. They are favorable to prosecutors because, if each of the elements is present, they do not need to prove specific intent or knowledge to harm. If narrowly written, they also can be more precise than the traditional criminal law: individuals are forewarned of the prohibited behaviors, and prosecutors are vested with less discretion. Finally, public health offenses declare a public interest in responsible behavior and encourage disclosure to persons at risk of infection.

Despite these benefits, public health offenses may not actually improve the public's health, and actually may be detrimental. First, because these statutes often apply to low-risk behaviors, any deterrent value may be misplaced. Public health authorities should set priorities for risk prevention activities; public resources devoted to conduct that poses little or no risk of transmission represent an opportunity cost. Second, to the extent that laws create incentives of *any* kind, they may create the wrong incentives. Persons at risk may be better off not knowing their serologic status because only those who are aware of their status can be prosecuted. Similarly, public health offenses encourage people to disclose their status, but the disclosure must take place prior to the first sexual encounter. If an infected person fails to disclose at first, the incentive thereafter would be not to inform her partner. Late disclosure, as a matter of public health, of course, is preferable to no disclosure at all.[230] Finally, by creating a specific offense, legislatures implicitly invite the interest of police, prosecutors, and the apparatus of the criminal justice system. This, in turn, engenders concerns about intrusive surveillance, selective enforcement, and loss of privacy, undermining the public education approach to disease prevention.[231]

EVALUATING THE CRIMINAL LAW AS A TOOL OF PUBLIC HEALTH

In thinking about the value of the criminal law in the context of infectious disease, it is helpful to inquire whether prosecution would achieve any of its traditional goals: deterrence, retribution, incapacitation, and rehabilitation. The answer is not simple, but depends on the severity of the case prosecuted. Most everyone would agree with prosecuting a person who truly intends to kill and who uses a means reasonably calculated to achieve that end (e.g., the father who injects his son with a contaminated needle to avoid paying child support). So, too, would most people agree with prosecuting a person who, knowing he has a serious infection, exposes many people (e.g., the person in Chautauqua County who hid his HIV status from multiple sexual partners). In these cases, society legitimately holds people with infectious disease criminally accountable for the same reasons it holds anyone accountable: the person has a culpable state of mind and poses a significant risk that is outside the socially acceptable range of conduct. In these cases, prosecution achieves several of the objectives of the criminal law—deterrence of high-risk behavior, punishment of morally blameworthy individuals, and incapacitation and rehabilitation of dangerous persons.

It is much more difficult to judge the utility of prosecutions in the majority of cases that involve minimal risks and behaviors that are common in society. After all, many prosecuted cases involve epidemiologically low risks, such as biting, spitting, or donating blood; and defendants, in fact, very rarely transmit infection. The criminal justice system does not achieve its goals if the behavior deterred involves negligible risk and the effect is to incapacitate and rehabilitate a minimally dangerous person.

A related problem is that many of the behaviors are common and resistant to change. As discussed above, most adults engage in sexual behavior, and studies show that a substantial minority of persons with sexually transmitted infections have had sex without disclosing the risk.[232] The result is that persons who engage in socially common behaviors are subject to serious criminal sanctions. Arguably, it is not in society's interest to seek retribution against persons who behave like many other people and who, in any event, are suffering from a serious, sometimes life-threatening, disease.

Suppose that policymakers want to use the criminal law as a tool of prevention rather than retribution. They might reason that criminal sanctions will promote the public health by deterring individuals from risk behavior. Although there is little empirical evidence to draw upon, it is conceivable that criminal law is antithetical to public health for the following reasons.

The criminal law may discourage individuals from being tested, providing accurate information to health professionals, and participating in clinical and public health programs. As explained earlier, criminal sanctions provide an incentive not to be tested because, legally, it is better not to discover one's serologic status. If individuals are not tested, they may be more likely to engage in risk behavior. Similarly, if having sex while infected is a crime, individuals may be less likely to disclose reliably their symptoms and behavior or to seek access to services. Failure to disclose impedes counseling and education. Moreover, if fewer people receive clinical treatment, the risk to the public increases. Treatment for some diseases virtually eliminates (e.g., syphilis) or reduces (e.g., HIV) infectiousness. Finally, if persons believe that discussions with public health authorities place themselves or their partners at risk of criminal prosecution, they may not cooperate. For example, persons may not participate freely in partner notification services for fear that their partners will be implicated in a crime. The criminal law, therefore, breaks down the trust that is vital to the success of clinical and public health programs.

Even if the criminal law could effectively deter risk behavior, it may be overly intrusive and unfair. As explained above, once the criminal law makes intimate behavior unlawful, it legitimizes police surveillance of deeply private activities. Further, police and prosecutors may selectively enforce the law by targeting vulnerable, and visible, populations, such as prostitutes, gays, the poor, and minorities. Indeed, since the targeted behavior is so common, it opens the door to discrimination in enforcement (e.g., white, middle-class individuals who have sex without disclosing the risk are seldom prosecuted, while disfavored classes are prosecuted for the same behavior).

In summary, the criminal law allows society to place a boundary around behavior it will, and will not, tolerate and to express its moral outrage at egregious conduct. The criminal law is justifiably applied to cases involving truly dangerous behavior and culpable states of mind. However, the generalized use of the criminal law is unlikely to become an effective tool for public health. It discourages exactly those behaviors necessary for the collective good—testing, disclosure, and participation in clinical and public health programs. The criminal law also invites intrusive surveillance, selective enforcement, and discrimination.

Sanitary Privies Are Cheaper Than Coffins

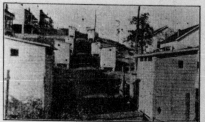

For Health's Sake let's keep this Privy CLEAN. Bad privies (and no privies at all) are our greatest cause of Disease. Clean people or families will help us keep this place clean. It should be kept as clean as the house because it spreads more diseases.

The User Must Keep It Clean Inside. Wash the Seat Occasionally

---

How to Keep a Safe Privy:

1. *Have the back perfectly screened against flies and animals.*
2. *Have a hinged door over the seat and keep it CLOSED when not in use.*
3. *Have a bucket beneath to catch the Excreta.*
4. *VENTILATE THE VAULT.*
5. *See that the privy is kept clean inside and out, or take the blame on yourself if some member of your family dies of Typhoid Fever.*

Some of the Diseases Spread by Filthy Privies:

Typhoid Fever, Bowel Troubles of Children, Dysenteries, Hookworms, Cholera, some Tuberculosis. The Flies that You See in the Privy Will Soon Be in the Dining Room.

Walker County Board of Health

A poster for a county campaign for sanitary privies, circa 1920. In the early twentieth century, the Public Health Service cooperated with state and local health authorities to promote rural sanitation. The incidence of typhoid fever and hookworm diminished in areas where active sanitary measures were taken.

9 Economic Behavior and the Public's Health

Direct Regulation

We think it settled principle, growing out of the nature of well ordered civil society, that every holder of property, however absolute and unqualified may be his title, holds it under the implied liability that his use of it may be so regulated, that it shall not be injurious to the equal enjoyment of others . . . nor injurious to the right of the community. All property . . . is held subject to those general regulations, which are necessary to the common good and general welfare.

Lemuel Shaw (1851)

The sovereign power in a community may and ought to prescribe the manner of exercising individual rights over property. . . . The powers rest on the implied rights and duty of the supreme power to protect all by statutory regulations, so that, on the whole, the benefit of all is promoted. . . . Such a power is incident to every well regulated society.

John Woodworth (1827)

I have discussed a series of conflicts between public interests in health and well-being and private interests in freedom from governmental interference. Thus far, the private interests I have examined involve primarily personal freedoms: autonomy, privacy, bodily integrity, and liberty. A great deal of the history and regulatory content of public health, however, has involved private economic interests: freedom of contract; unrestricted property uses; and the right to pursue businesses, trades, and professions. This chapter, on direct economic regulation by public health agencies, and the next, on indirect regulation through the tort system, examine the conflicts between health and safety standards and economic freedoms.

Commercial regulation creates a tension between individual and collective interests. In a well-regulated society, public health authorities set clear, enforceable rules to protect the health and safety of workers, consumers, and the population at large. Yet regulation impedes economic freedoms and business interests. It is not surprising, therefore, that public health regulation of commercial activity, like the regulation of personal behavior, is highly contested terrain.

Industry and commerce are widely, and legitimately, thought to be essential to social progress and economic prosperity. Business and trade create greater productivity, more employment, and higher living standards. These benefits are highly relevant to healthy populations because of the positive correlation between health and socioeconomic status.[1] Community well-being, to a large extent, is determined by improved standards of living and increased general wealth.

Important and influential economic theories (e.g., laissez-faire and, more recently, a market economy or free enterprise) support private enterprise as a means of economic growth. These theories favor free markets and open competition; regulation that hampers private initiative is often seen as detrimental to social progress.[2] Commercial regulation, if it is desirable at all, should redress market failures (e.g., monopolistic and other anticompetitive practices) rather than restrain free enterprise. Modern proponents of laissez-faire stress the importance to economic growth of the profit incentive and the undeterred entrepreneur.[3]

Public health advocates are opposed to unfettered private enterprise and suspicious of free-market solutions to social problems.[4] They are concerned more with the manifest harms to the community posed by an industrial economy and resulting urbanization. It is not difficult to identify the public health risks of unbridled commercialism. Manufacturers can create significant risks to the health and safety of employees who may be exposed to toxic substances or unsafe work environments. Businesses may produce noxious by-products, such as waste or pollution, or sell contaminated foods, beverages, drugs, or cosmetics. Property owners may create public nuisances, such as unsafe buildings, accumulations of garbage, or dangerous animals. Persons engaged in trades, occupations, or professions may pose harms to consumers due to lack of qualifications or expertise. At the same time, migration to the cities for jobs brings the manifest health risks of overcrowding, substandard housing, rodents, infestations, and squalor.

The deep-seated problems of industrialization and urbanization pose complex, highly technical challenges that require expertise, flexibility, and deliberative study over the long term. Solutions cannot be found within traditional government structures such as representative assemblies or governors' offices. As a result, governments have formed specialized entities within the executive branch to pursue the goals of population health and safety. These administrative agencies form the bulwark for public health activities in America.

Agencies have developed numerous regulatory techniques and decision-making processes to identify and respond to health and safety risks. Agencies can control entry into a field by requiring a license or permit to undertake specified activities; set health and safety standards, inspect to assure compliance, adjudicate violations, and impose penalties; abate nuisances that threaten the public; dispense grants, subsidies, or other incentives; and influence conduct through a wide variety of informal methods.

This chapter first presents a brief history of public health regulation of commercial activities, showing the long-standing and pervasive interest of state and local public health authorities in regulating trades and professions, public health institutions, and businesses. Second, it examines the structure and powers of public health agencies particularly (but not exclusively) at the state and local levels. This section explains the expansive authority of public health agencies as well as the constitutional and administrative constraints on agency power. Third, this chapter reviews the law relating to three of the most common forms of commercial regulation: licenses and permits, health and safety standards and inspections, and nuisance abatements. Finally, it explores some of the complex trade-offs between the benefits of regulation to advance collective well-being and the resulting retardation of economic growth. This section examines the politically charged issue of economic liberty: economic due process, freedom of contract, and government "takings" (compensation for property taken for public uses). Throughout this chapter, the key normative issue concerns the appropriate weight to be afforded to economic liberty. How important are contract and property rights compared with political and civil liberties? When government acts for the public's health, how concerned should we be about impeding commercial opportunities?

A BRIEF HISTORY OF COMMERCIAL REGULATION

A distinctive and powerful governmental tradition
devoted in theory and practice to the vision of a well-
regulated society dominated United States social and
economic policymaking from 1787 to 1877. . . . At

the heart of the well-regulated society was a plethora
of bylaws, ordinances, statutes, and common law
restrictions regulating nearly every aspect of early
American economy and society. . . . Taken together
they explode tenacious myths about nineteenth-century
government (or its absence) and demonstrate the
pervasiveness of regulation in early American versions
of the good society: regulations for public safety and
security . . . and the open-ended regulatory powers
granted to public officials to guarantee public health
(securing the population's well-being, longevity, and
productivity). Public regulation—the power of the
state to restrict individual liberty and property for the
common welfare—colored all facets of early American
development. It was the central component of a
reigning theory and practice of governance committed
to the pursuit of the people's welfare and happiness in
a well-ordered society and polity.
                                        William J. Novak (1996)

Much public health regulation of commercial activities takes place at
the local level and involves the status of cities.[5] Cities in colonial
America had the primary governmental responsibility for public health.
Early legislative activities were organized around reducing filth and regulating dangerous trades.[6] As to the reduction of filth, perhaps the oldest sanitary law, in 1634, prohibited residents of Boston from depositing fish or garbage near the common landing.[7] Beginning in 1652, a
series of ordinances were enacted to control the sanitary condition and
location of privies, prohibit the dumping of rubbish onto public thor-
oughfares and waterways, and impound stray animals from the streets
and remove dead animals and offal.[8]

As to the regulation of hazardous trades and businesses, regulations
limited the location and methods of operation of butchers, blubber-
boilers, slaughterhouses, tanners, and other enterprises. For example,
the first Massachusetts general assembly, in 1692, empowered selectmen in market towns to prohibit slaughterhouses, the trying out of tallow, and the currying of leather, except in assigned locations.[9] At the
same time, legislatures were also overseeing the production of food
(principally bread and meat) by requiring inspections and enforcing
standards.[10]

By the mid-nineteenth century, the industrial revolution was transforming societies in Western Europe and the United States, making possible substantial advances in economic prosperity. Laissez-faire political economics reinforced beliefs in free markets, expansion of industry, and consequent migration to the city to secure jobs and livelihood.[11] The United States was becoming one of the most successful industrial economies in the world.

The sheer success of industrialization and urbanization posed such momentous hazards to community health and well-being that it made possible a political shift in favor of extensive commercial regulation. Public health advocates—a progressive coalition of sanitary engineers, physicians, and public spirited citizens known as "Sanitarians"[12]— observed and documented the profound health and safety risks that arose from the new industrial civilization.[13] The engine of industrial growth, the factory, was causing injury to workers and harm to communities. The migration to the cities for work resulted in overcrowding, slum conditions, homelessness, squalor, and violence. There existed a growing realization that disease caused by garbage, sewage, pollution, and contaminated food and drinking water affected the entire community and was within the proper sphere of government control. By the end of the century, the Sanitarians were pressing for an ambitious regulatory agenda to control noxious substances and unsanitary conditions, as well as to promote town planning.[14] The most important public health report of the time, written by Lemuel Shattuck, commenced with a call for sanitary legislation:[15]

> The condition of perfect public health requires such laws and regulations as will secure to man associated in society the same sanitary enjoyments that he would have as an isolated individual; and as will protect him from injury from any influences connected with his locality, his dwelling house, his occupation, . . . or from any other causes. It is under the control of public authority, and public administration; and life and health may be saved or lost, as this authority is wisely or unwisely exercised.

A pervasive regulatory system evolved in state and local governments to ameliorate the health effects of industrialization and urbanization. Even the most casual perusal of treatises on city government in the late nineteenth century reveals the extensive regulatory system that was then in place, controlling every aspect of civil society.[16] Public health regulations extended to dangerous buildings, public conveyances, corporations, use of travel ways (e.g., streets, highways, and navigable waters), objectionable trades, disorderly houses, storage of gunpowder, sale of food, sale and prescription of dangerous drugs, health and safety of workers, and many other commercial activities.[17]

During the latter half of the nineteenth century the criminal law was the preferred method of sanctioning violations of health and safety regulations. Violation of these laws was usually a misdemeanor, but conviction was facilitated by imposing strict liability, and convicted entrepreneurs faced short terms of imprisonment.[18] The criminal method of enforcing health and safety laws (which would substantially, but not completely, give way to civil penalties in the twentieth century) was significant. Criminal penalties were far more stigmatic than civil remedies and undermined the prestige and status of business persons.[19] The transition from criminal to civil penalties also influenced social perceptions of harmful corporate behavior.

In summary, despite the prevalent contemporary belief that the nineteenth century was a time of free markets and undeterred entrepreneurs, in fact, it was a well-regulated society. A range of sanitary legislation had been enacted to ensure that economic activity did not bring with it excessive risks to health and safety. Public health laws were often backed up with criminal penalties imposed on business executives themselves. Finally, as the following discussion suggests, the administrative infrastructure of public health departments was reinforced to cope better with the rising regulatory system. Tighter control by well-organized government was grounded in the belief that commercial activities, while contributing to prosperity, created harms to the commons. Government's raison d'être was to protect the community's interests by curtailing individual economic freedoms.

PUBLIC HEALTH AGENCIES AND THE RISE OF THE ADMINISTRATIVE STATE

The success or failure of any government in the final
analysis must be measured by the well-being of its
citizens. Nothing can be more important to a state
than its public health; the state's paramount concern
should be the health of its people.
        Franklin Delano Roosevelt (1932)

Sanitary regulation commenced even before cities and states had well-organized and effective public health infrastructures that could support regulation. During the early nineteenth century, public health administration was simple in organization and limited in scope. Only a few major cities had established formal boards of health; the first local health departments were established in Baltimore in 1793, Philadelphia in 1794, and in Massachusetts's municipalities in the late 1790s.[20] At this time, public health officials had no qualifications, no career advancement, and no job security.[21] Even in the latter part of the nineteenth century, many large urban areas had no health departments, and expertise among public health officials was only beginning to emerge.[22]

The burgeoning social problems of the industrial cities convinced legislatures to form more elaborate and professional public health administrations within municipal government.[23] For example, a properly constituted health board was first established in the city of New York in 1866 with "An Act to Create a Metropolitan Sanitary District and Board of Health." The Board comprised experts in medicine and public health and was granted extensive power both to create and to administer regulations relating to the preservation of the public health.[24] This public health infrastructure was necessary to ensure careful regulatory scrutiny of the burgeoning industrial civilization. Boards of health, therefore, were established to obtain an effective ministerial agency to supervise and direct the details of the execution of ordinances. To accomplish its tasks, state legislatures granted local boards of health the power to enact detailed administrative regulations, inspect businesses and property owners to ensure compliance, and adjudicate and sanction those who violated regulatory standards.[25]

Public health administrations within the states came even later than those in municipalities.[26] It was not until after the Civil War that states formed boards of health. The first working state health board was formed in Massachusetts in 1869, followed by a number of other states in the 1870s, such as California, Maryland, Minnesota, and Virginia.[27] County and rural health departments did not emerge until the early twentieth century.[28]

Despite the advances in public health administration, campaigners still observed patronage, inefficiency, and unprofessionalism in state and local health authorities into the twentieth century. Charles Chapin, the superintendent of health for the city of Providence, Rhode Island, pressed for a corps of public health officials who were highly qualified and trained with adequate compensation and opportunities for career advancement.[29] These are problems in public health professionalism that exist to this day: the need for leadership in public health, the ability of public health professionals to work constructively with elected officials, and the short tenure of politically appointed public health officials (see chapter 11).

STATE PUBLIC HEALTH AGENCIES

The state's police powers to protect the health and welfare of its inhabitants are inherent aspects of sovereignty and not derived from another source. The state's plenary power to safeguard citizens' health, moreover, includes the authority to create administrative agencies devoted to that task.[30] State legislation determines the administrative organization, mission, and functions of public health agencies.

Contemporary public health agencies take many different forms that defy simple classification.[31] Before 1960, state public health functions were located in health departments with policymaking functions residing in boards of health (e.g., issuing and enforcing regulations).[32] As programs expanded (e.g., increased federal funding for categorical programs and block grants), certain public health functions were assigned to other state agencies (e.g., mental health, medical care financing for the indigent, and environmental protection). Currently, fifty-five state-level health agencies exist (including the District of Columbia, American Samoa, Guam, Puerto Rico, and the U.S. Virgin Islands), each of which may be a freestanding, independent department or a component of a larger state agency. The trend, since the 1960s, has been to merge state health departments with other departments—often social services, Medicaid, mental health, and/or substance abuse—to form superagencies. Under this framework (Model 1), the public health unit is often called a Division of Health or Public Health (see Figure 16). Another common framework is to assign public health functions to a cabinet-level agency. Under Model 2, the public health unit is often called a Department of Health or Public Health (see Figure 17).[33]

The trend has also been to eliminate or reduce the influence of boards of health. These boards, once ubiquitous and highly influential, are now often replaced or supplemented with specialized boards or committees established by state statute to oversee technical or politically controversial programs (e.g., genetics, rural health, and expansion of health care facilities).[34] The chief executive officer of the public health agency—the commissioner, director, or less often, the secretary—is usually politically appointed by the governor, but may be appointed by the head of a superagency or, rarely, the board of health. Qualification standards may include medical and public health expertise, but increasingly, chief executives with political or administrative experience are appointed.[35]

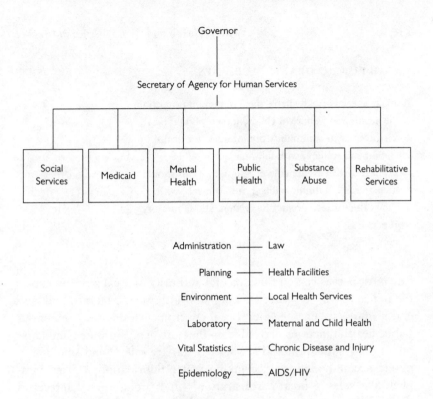

Figure 16.   Model 1: public health as a division of a superagency.

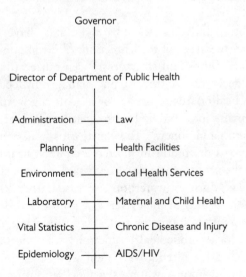

Figure 17.   Model 2: public health as a cabinet agency.

LOCAL PUBLIC HEALTH AGENCIES

To make everywhere available these minimum protections
of the health and welfare of children, there should be a
district, county or community organization for health,
education and welfare, with full-time officials,
coordinating with a statewide program. . . . This should
include: trained, full-time public health officials, with
public health nurses, sanitary inspection, and laboratory
workers.

Herbert Hoover (1931)

The most pervasive and fundamental authority of local governments is the police power to protect the public health, safety, morals, and general welfare (see chapter 2).[36] Local government exercises voluminous public health functions derived from the state (e.g., air, water, and noise pollution;[37] sanitation and sewage;[38] cigarette sales[39] and smoking in public accommodations;[40] drinking water fluoridation;[41] drug paraphernalia sales;[42] firearm registration[43] and prohibition;[44] infectious diseases;[45] rodents and infestations;[46] housing codes;[47] sanitary food and beverages;[48] trash disposal;[49] and animal control[50]). Local government also often regulates (or owns and operates) hospitals[51] or nursing homes.[52]

Municipalities and counties, like the states, have created public health agencies to carry out their functions.[53] Local public health agencies have varied forms and structures:[54] centralized (directly operated by the state), decentralized (formed and managed by local government), or mixed.[55] Local boards of health, or less often government councils, still exist in many local public health agencies, with responsibility for health regulation and policy.[56] The courts usually permit local agencies to exercise broad discretion in matters of public health,[57] sometimes even beyond the geographic area, if necessary, to protect city or county inhabitants (e.g., during a waterborne disease outbreak).[58]

Local public health agencies serve a political subdivision of the state, such as a city (a municipality), town, township, county, or borough.[59] Some local public health functions are undertaken by special districts, which are limited government structures that serve special purposes (e.g., drinking water, sewage, sanitation, or mosquito abatement).[60]

These local government entities are subsidiary and largely subordinate to the state.[61] They have delegated authority and may exercise only those police powers granted by the state. The sources of local government power are the state constitution (which delegates power directly from the people to municipalities), state legislation (which grants additional power), and the municipal or county charter (which is usually approved by local voters and expresses the powers of the corporation).[62] Constitutional and statutory grants of generic authority to cities or counties can create autonomy, or home rule, over local affairs.[63] State constitutions sometimes grant considerable public health power to localities: "to exercise any power and perform any function pertaining to [local government and affairs] including, . . . the power to regulate for the protection of the public health, safety, morals, and welfare."[64] This kind of constitutional authority can insulate cities and counties from state interference with purely local public health functions.

Courts construe state grants of police power to ensure that local governments act within the scope of the delegation. The conventional rule of interpretation of state delegated powers was formulated by Judge Dillon.[65] Dillon's Rule holds that local governments can exercise only those powers expressly conferred, necessarily or fairly implied, or essential to the objects and purposes of the municipality. The strict construction of delegations to local governments during the nineteenth century was often used to block public health measures that judges regarded as unwarranted.[66] The modern judiciary appears split on whether to interpret strictly or liberally state delegations of powers to local government.[67] However, courts often find public health powers quintessentially to be within the local sphere.[68]

Relationships among states and localities are complex and highly political. Each level of government may fervently claim jurisdiction over public health matters, such as smoking or infectious diseases. States may seek to deny cities or counties the power to exercise control by withholding grants of power or economic resources, or by preempting local regulation. Localities, on the other hand, may claim implied authority or assert home rule over public health matters of inherent local importance. Consider the political debate over firearm regulation, with the great majority of states preempting local government regulation of gun sales.[69] In response, cities and counties have adopted innovative methods to regulate firearm violence through traditional zoning and licensing authority (e.g., banning dealers in residential areas and creating strict licensing standards).[70]

In summary, states possess inherent, and localities delegated, police power to regulate for the common good. To achieve this goal, states and localities both have developed elaborate administrative agencies.

Powers and duties of agencies are governed by law but are powerfully influenced by politics. One of the most fundamental issues in law and politics is the appropriate scope of agency power. Since agencies are not directly accountable to the voters, the amount of discretion they exercise is of enduring importance, as the following discussion illustrates.[71]

ADMINISTRATIVE LAW: RULEMAKING, ENFORCEMENT, AND QUASI-JUDICIAL POWERS

Public health agencies are part of the executive branch of government[72] but wield considerable authority to make rules to control private behavior, interpret statutes and regulations, and adjudicate disputes about whether an individual or a company has conformed with health and safety standards. Under the separation of powers doctrine (see chapter 2), the executive branch is supposed to enforce the law but not enact or interpret it. Nevertheless, the lines between law making, enforcement, and adjudication have become blurred with the rise of the administrative state (see Figure 18).[73]

The boundaries among the three branches have changed in response to the demands of modern society. Matters of health and safety are highly complex and technical, requiring extensive planning and expertise. Legislators do not have the scientific skills or time necessary to assemble the facts about health risks and to devise solutions. Moreover, delegations to administrative agencies may be politically expedient.[74] A public health issue may become so socially divisive that elected officials simply declare that a health threat exists and leave to the executive branch the task of solving the problem.[75] Consequently, legislatures may have good reasons, based on efficiency and politics, to delegate policymaking and adjudication functions to specialized agencies.

Politicians may have good reasons to delegate complex public health problems to agencies, but the courts, at least theoretically, can carefully scrutinize these grants of power. Conventionally, representative assemblies may not delegate legislative or judicial functions to the executive branch. Known as "nondelegation," this doctrine holds that policymaking functions should be undertaken by the legislative branch of government (because assemblies are politically accountable) while adjudicative functions should be undertaken by the judicial branch (because courts are independent).

The nondelegation doctrine is rarely used by federal courts to limit agency powers, but this may be changing.[76] In its 2001 term, the

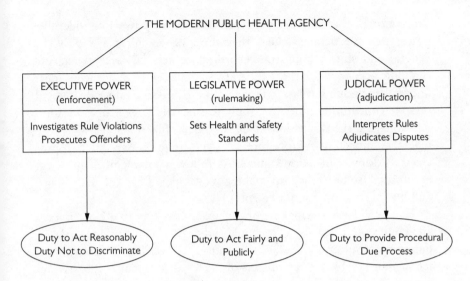

Figure 18.   Powers and duties of the modern public health agency.

Supreme Court agreed to hear *Browner v. American Trucking Associations*, a potentially important case about the allocation of authority in modern adminstrative state.

The nondelegation doctrine has received varying interpretations at the state level[77]—some jurisdictions liberally permit delegations,[78] while others are more restrictive.[79] New York State's highest court, for example, found unconstitutional a health department prohibition on smoking in public places because the legislature, not the health department, should make the "trade-offs" between health and freedom. "Manifestly," the court said, "it is the province of the people's elected representatives, rather than appointed administrators, to resolve difficult social problems by making choices among competing ends."[80]

Even if the courts do not rigidly apply the nondelegation doctrine, they may use it as an aid to statutory construction, interpreting agency authority narrowly if the grant of rulemaking power is vague.[81] For example, the Supreme Court in the *Benzene* case invalidated an OSHA rule that limited benzene in the workplace to no more than one part benzene per million parts of air. The Court reasoned that the broad congressional delegation of power did not permit OSHA to impose health standards for exceptionally low risks with inordinately high economic costs.[82]

Rulemaking. Although public health agencies possess considerable power to issue detailed rules, they must do so fairly and publicly. Federal and state administrative procedure acts (as well as agency-enabling acts) govern the deliberative processes that agencies must undertake in issuing rules.[83] (Procedural due process, under the federal or state constitution, does not apply to rulemaking as it does to adjudication—see the discussion of quasi-judicial functions below.[84]) The federal Administrative Procedure Act (APA) requires two different procedural forms (and many state APAs follow similar paths): informal and formal (some agency rulemaking is exempted from the Act's notice and public procedure requirements).[85]

The APA's basic rulemaking procedure (called "informal" or "notice-and-comment" rulemaking) is simple and flexible, consisting of three requirements:[86] prior notice (e.g., publication in the Federal Register), written comments by interested persons, and a statement of basis and purpose for the rule.[87] The formal rulemaking process ("rulemaking on the record") directs the agency to conduct a hearing and provide interested parties with an opportunity to testify and cross-examine adverse witnesses before issuing a rule.[88] Formal procedures can be costly and futile. For example, the FDA-proposed regulations of vitamin supplements involved eighteen months of hearings; the agency lost on appeal because it had unduly restricted cross-examination of a government expert.[89]

Negotiated rulemaking (sometimes known as "regulatory negotiation," or "reg-neg") emerged in the 1980s as an alternative to traditional procedures.[90] The basic idea is that, in certain situations, the agency can bring together various interest groups to negotiate the text of a proposed rule. The negotiators seek a consensus through a process of evaluating priorities and making trade-offs.[91] The benefits of negotiated rulemaking include reduced time and resources to develop rules, earlier implementation, greater compliance, and more cooperative relationships.[92]

Enforcement. Health departments do not possess only legislative power. They also have the executive power to enforce the regulations they have promulgated. Enforcement of laws and regulations is squarely within the constitutional powers of executive agencies. Legislatures set the penalty for violation of health and safety standards; the executive branch monitors compliance and seeks redress against those who fail to conform. Pursuant to their enforcement power, health departments may inspect premises and businesses, investigate complaints, and generally monitor the activities of those who come within the orbit of health and safety statutes and administrative rules.

Quasi-Judicial. Modern administrative agencies do not simply issue and enforce health and safety standards; they also interpret statutes and rules as well as adjudicate disputes about whether standards are violated. Federal and state administrative procedure acts, and agency-enabling legislation, often enumerate the procedures that agencies must follow in adjudicating disputes. Under the federal APA, formal adjudications ("evidentiary" or "on-the-record" hearings) apply only in the relatively rare cases where the agency's authorizing statute directs the agency to hold an evidentiary hearing.[93] Formal adjudications typically are conducted by an administrative law judge (ALJ), followed by an appeal to the agency head.[94] Formal adjudications usually include notice, the right to present oral and written evidence, cross-examination of hostile witnesses, and agency findings of fact and law as well as reasons for the decision. Even in the absence of statutory requirements, federal and state constitutions require procedural due process if the regulation deprives an individual of "property" or "liberty" interests (see chapter 3).

In summary, modern administrative agencies exercise legislative power to issue rules that carry heavy penalties, executive power to investigate potential violations of health and safety standards and to prosecute offenders, and judicial power to interpret law and adjudicate disputes over violation of governing standards. Agency powers have developed for reasons of expediency (because of agency expertise) and politics (because "specialists" are presumed to act according to disinterested scientific judgments).

While ample agency power is important for achieving public health purposes, it is also troubling and perplexing in a constitutional democracy. Commercial regulation may simply transfer wealth from one private interest group to another rather than promoting a public good. For example, licenses can exclude competitors from the market, or regulation of one industry may benefit another providing comparable services (e.g., coal, electrical, or nuclear energy). A related problem is that agencies may be unduly influenced, or "captured," by powerful constituencies or interest groups. The idea that, over the long term, agencies come to defend the economic interests of regulatory subjects is much discussed in the literature.[95] Finally, agencies may operate in ways that appear unfair or arbitrary, inefficient or bureaucratic, or unacceptable to the public. The very strengths of public health authorities (e.g., neutrality, expertise, and

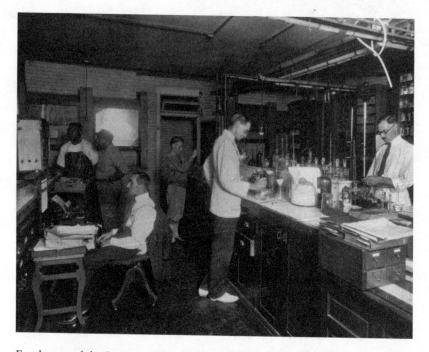

Employees of the Bureau of Chemistry of the U.S. Department of Agriculture at work in a laboratory, circa 1910. The 1906 Pure Food and Drug Acts assigned the Bureau responsibility for enforcing prohibitions against adulterations and misbrandings of food and drugs. The Bureau later evolved into the Food and Drug Administration.

broad powers) can become liabilities if they appear politically unaccountable and aloof from the real concerns and needs of the governed. This is why governors' offices, representative assemblies, and courts struggle over the political and constitutional limits that should be placed on agency action nominally intended for the public's health and safety.

THE REGULATORY TOOLS OF PUBLIC HEALTH AGENCIES

I have discussed the structure, functions, and powers of public health agencies. It is important also to consider the techniques of regulation. Public health authorities possess a number of regulatory tools: licensing trades, professions, and institutions; inspecting for violations of health and safety standards; and abating public nuisances (see Figure 19).

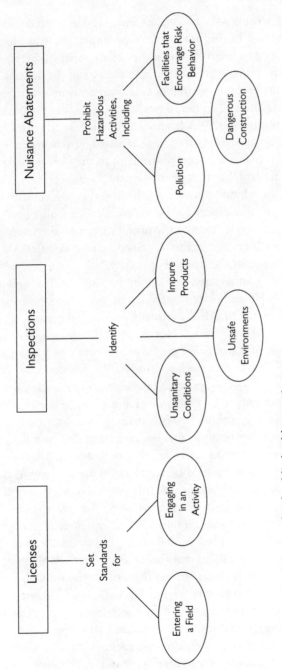

Figure 19. Regulatory tools of public health agencies.

LICENSES AND PERMITS

Licenses and permits have become an integral part of civil society[96] and a staple of public health practice.[97] One important way that government monitors and controls the affairs of persons, businesses, and institutions is to require licenses for the pursuit of an activity.[98] (A related, but different, requirement is registration, which involves recording data such as names, dates, and events for identification and informational purposes.[99]) A license literally is formal permission from the government to perform certain activities. Licenses are required only if the conduct involved is first prohibited; in the absence of a prohibition, governmental permission obviously is unnecessary. A license, therefore, is an administrative act whereby the government sanctions conduct that would otherwise be unlawful. Consequently, legislative language is phrased in terms of a prohibition and then a permission: "No person shall engage in the [specified] activities unless she has obtained a license from the [specified] agency."[100]

Licenses are administered principally by state or local public health agencies or a body authorized by the legislature or agency. Licensing authorities may be the health department, a board of regents, a special licensing agency, or a professional or occupational board. Members of licensing boards, of course, may not have a direct or pecuniary interest in the license.[101] The courts readily allow public health authorities to administer licensing systems, provided the legislature has adequately stated the facts, conditions, or qualifications for issuing the license.[102] The delegation of licensing authority to private entities is constitutionally troublesome,[103] but may be allowable under certain circumstances.[104]

Licenses are part of an active regulatory system that involves setting standards for entering a field or engaging in an activity. Agencies can set any licensing conditions reasonably necessary to protect the public health, safety, morality, or general welfare.[105] First, agencies license a broad range of professions, trades, and occupations. They license and credential health care professionals (e.g., physicians, nurses, pharmacists, dentists, and occupational therapists)[106] as well as other persons engaging in trades or occupations that affect the public's health and safety (e.g., barbers, plumbers, and electricians).[107] (Note that many private professional or occupational specialties, such as medical specialties, nursing specialties, and dietitians, also operate credentialing systems designed to obtain recognition for their members' special qualifications.)[108] Licensing authorities set standards relating to qualifications, experience, and safe practice of professionals and tradespersons.

Second, agencies license various public health institutions (e.g., hospitals, nursing homes, laboratories).[109] Here, they can set standards relating to the security and health of patients or residents. Finally, agencies license businesses (e.g., alcohol beverage retailers, food services, and tatoo parlors).[110] The agency can set standards relating to the safety of workers, purity of goods, and protection of consumers (e.g., from fraud, deception, or unreasonable risks).

A licensing system does not merely sift out the unqualified or unsafe, but also offers continuous monitoring and supervision through inspecting, monitoring, and punishing violators (e.g., withdrawal of licenses as well as civil or criminal penalties). Consequently, licensing systems regulate both prospectively, by limiting entry into the field and imposing operational requirements, and retrospectively, by punishing transgression of standards.

State and local governments have the power to impose reasonable license fees.[111] However, fees must be proportionate to the government's regulatory costs.[112] Thus, if the license has a revenue-raising purpose (e.g., the fee is considerably higher than the administrative and policing costs), then it may be invalidated as an impermissible tax.[113]

Social and Economic Fairness.   Although licensing achieves important public goals in the form of consumer health, safety, and fraud prevention, it presents problems related to social and economic justice. Licensing can be unfair because it parcels out a privilege based upon the discretion of officials. This discretionary authority can be exercised in a discriminatory fashion against disfavored groups such as racial[114] or religious[115] minorities and women.[116] For example, in striking down a licensing system that was hostile to Chinese-Americans, the Supreme Court said, "Though the law be fair on its face and impartial in appearance, yet, if it is applied and administered by public authority with an evil eye and unequal hand . . . [it is] a denial of equal justice."[117] Apart from frank social and cultural discrimination, the legal conditions for issuing a license can operate to exclude the poor and minorities, because they cannot meet educational and qualification standards that may be set artificially high.[118] In many geographic areas authorities historically granted few, if any, licenses to African-Americans for certain professions (e.g., barbers and plumbers).[119] For example, when the American Medical Association co-opted medical licensing in the early twentieth century, it forced the closure of many existing black medical schools, resulting in marked declines in the number of African-American physicians.[120]

The problem of economic and social discrimination is compounded by the fact that members of the regulated profession may dominate, or influence, licensing authorities (e.g., medical licensing boards composed primarily of practicing physicians), creating the appearance, or reality, of exclusionary practices.[121] Licensing grants a certain amount of monopoly power to the profession or occupation.[122] This can enable private actors to exclude classes of people for anticompetitive reasons.[123] Seen in this way, a licensing system, even if it originated in the public interest, can be used by the regulated group to limit new entrants, thus assuring those already in the field of higher incomes and professional status.[124]

Procedural Fairness. A license can be a valuable property interest that triggers a constitutional right to procedural due process (see chapter 3). Proceedings before licensing authorities determining whether to grant or deny applications can be informal, but they must comport with fundamental fairness. In such a proceeding, a citizen should be entitled to legal representation, adequate opportunity to present her case and cross-examine witnesses, a reasonable record of the proceedings, and reasons for the decision.[125]

Constitutionally Troublesome Conditions. Regulations requiring a license for the exercise of a fundamental right or freedom raise important constitutional concerns. For example, licenses may burden the free exercise of religion (e.g., religious processions),[126] expression (e.g., adult cinemas),[127] or assembly (e.g., bathhouses).[128] Courts will not necessarily overturn licensing decisions that burden the exercise of constitutional rights, but they will require neutral health and safety standards as well as the absence of unbridled discretion and arbitrary decision-making.[129]

ADMINISTRATIVE SEARCHES AND INSPECTIONS

An inspection, or administrative search, is perhaps the most important and commonplace method of monitoring and enforcing health and safety standards. It also is among the oldest state powers, being mentioned expressly in the Constitution.[130] An inspection represents a formal and careful examination of a product, business, or premises to ascertain its authenticity (e.g., possession of a valid license), quality (e.g., purity and fitness for use), or condition (e.g., safe and sanitary). Inspection laws authorize and direct public health authorities to conduct administrative searches to assure private conformance with health and safety regulations. Inspection systems operate in many different public health contexts, ensuring the safe construction and maintenance of buildings or residences,[131] purity of food and drugs,[132] sanitary condition of farms[133] or restaurants,[134] safe workplace environments,[135] and control of pesticides[136] and toxic emissions.[137]

Search and Seizure under the Fourth Amendment. Although administrative searches are conducted in the public interest, they invade a sphere of privacy protected explicitly in the Constitution.[138] The Fourth Amendment guarantees the "right of people to be secure in their persons, houses, papers, and effects, against unreasonable searches and seizures." For most of the nation's history, public health inspections were rarely challenged and presumed to be constitutional.[139] However, in 1967, in the companion cases of *Camara v. Municipal Court*[140] and *See v. City of Seattle*,[141] the Supreme Court held that public health inspections are governed by the Fourth Amendment and are presumptively unreasonable if conducted without a warrant.[142]

Administrative search warrants, therefore, are generally required for health or safety inspections of both residential[143] and private commercial property.[144] However, the judiciary permits searches without a warrant in at least three circumstances. First, a legally valid consent justifies an administrative search,[145] and, in practice, most health and safety inspections are conducted with the permission of an authorized person (e.g., the owner or occupier of the property).[146] Second, public health authorities may inspect a premises in an emergency to avert an immediate threat to health or safety.[147] Third, under the so-called open-fields doctrine, inspectors may search a public place[148] (e.g., an eating area of a restaurant)[149] or test pollutants emitted into the open air.[150]

Generally speaking, courts issue warrants in criminal investigations only on evidence of probable cause to believe that a person has committed an offense.[151] However, courts issue warrants for health and safety inspections on grounds that are far less stringent than in criminal investigations.[152] To obtain a warrant for an administrative search, public health agencies need only demonstrate specific evidence of an existing violation of a health and safety standard,[153] or a reasonable plan supported by a valid public interest.[154]

Public health authorities may not use an inspection to investigate a crime.[155] If their primary purpose is to discover evidence of criminal activity, authorities must obtain a search warrant based on probable cause.[156] Agencies, of course, often have both a public health and criminal investigative purpose; after all, violation of a health and safety standard can itself result in criminal penalties. Provided that the public health purpose is dominant, courts will not invalidate an otherwise lawful inspection that combines criminal law and administrative objectives.[157] Similarly, public health authorities may seize criminal evidence if it is discovered during a lawful inspection.[158]

The courts have carved out a major exception to the general rule that agencies must obtain a warrant for an inspection. Courts permit reasonable inspections of pervasively regulated businesses without a warrant.[159] In *New York v. Burger* (1987), the Supreme Court held that an inspection without a warrant of a pervasively regulated industry is reasonable if (1) there is a substantial public interest for the regulatory scheme, (2) the search is necessary to achieve the objective, and (3) the enabling statute gives notice to owners and limits the discretion of inspectors.[160] The courts permit inspections without warrants for a wide range of heavily regulated (and often hazardous) businesses, such as mining,[161] firearms,[162] alcoholic beverages,[163] propane,[164] and transport.[165] They also permit inspections without warrants for licensed businesses with substantial public health significance, such as nursing homes[166] and health care facilities.[167] Finally, the courts allow health inspectors to conduct routine audits of data (e.g., medical or pharmacy records) that, by statute, they have a legal right to search.[168] The judiciary permits administrative searches of pervasively regulated businesses without a warrant because of the importance of routine inspections in enforcing health and safety standards (warrants may afford owners time to conceal hazards)[169] and the reduced expectation of privacy in highly regulated commercial activities.[170]

The courts place certain limits on the time, place, and scope of searches without a warrant.[171] Further, if public health authorities violate the Fourth Amendment (e.g., by not obtaining a warrant when it is required or exceeding the proper scope of the search), the exclusionary rule may apply (i.e., authorities are prohibited from using illegally collected evidence).[172] However, the judiciary often does not apply the exclusionary rule to administrative proceedings if the regulatory subject is facing civil penalties or minimal burdens.[173]

NUISANCE ABATEMENT

Many wrongs are indifferently termed nuisance or
something else, at the convenience or whim of the
writer. Thus, injuries to ways, to private lands, various
injuries through negligence, wrongs harmful to the
physical health, disturbances of the peace . . . are
commonly spoken of as nuisances.

Joel Bishop (1889)

Private and public nuisances have common origins[174] but are distinctly different doctrines. A private nuisance, discussed in the next chapter, is an unreasonable interference with the possessor's use and enjoyment of land (e.g., flooding or contaminating adjoining land). Private nuisances principally are part of the common law and are redressed through the tort system. A public nuisance is an unreasonable interference with the community's use and enjoyment of a public place or harm to common interests in health, safety, and welfare.[175] Public nuisances need not involve interference with interests in land but all activities that harm common pool resources, such as silence, clean air or water, or species diversity.[176] The interest claimed must be common to the public as a class, and not merely applicable to one person or even a small group.[177] Public nuisances were originally part of the common law but are now principally legislative and enforced by public health agencies. Private citizens lack standing to bring public nuisance actions unless they suffer an interference with their enjoyment of land distinct from the general public interest.[178]

Public nuisances are exceptionally difficult to define—a point (as we will see) of major significance, since the Supreme Court resurrected the doctrine in a famous "takings" case in 1992. At common law, a public nuisance was an act or omission "which obstructs or causes inconvenience or damage to the public in the exercise of rights common to all."[179] Early American illustrations of public nuisances included explosives,[180] garbage and offal,[181] decaying animals,[182] improper sewage,[183] and keeping of hogs in a filthy condition.[184]

Today, public nuisances are usually defined by the legislature. Alternatively, the legislature delegates to state and local public health agencies the power and duty "to define, prevent, and abate nuisances."[185] The legislative or administrative definition is often broad and virtually coterminous with the police power (e.g., "anything which is injurious to health, or indecent or offensive to the senses, or to an obstruction to the free use of property, so as to interfere with the comfortable enjoyment of life or property"[186]). Legislatures or agencies also specify particular conditions as public nuisances, such as "a breeding place for flies, rodents, mosquitos,"[187] or a place that is conducive to "high risk sexual activity."[188]

Legislative or administrative definitions of nuisances are presumed constitutional, but courts reserve the right to determine the presence of a nuisance. The standard for judicial review (unless the regulatory action affects a constitutionally protected interest, such as free expression[189]) is whether the nuisance abatement is reasonably necessary to avert a health threat,[190] even if it represents "a derogation of pre-existing private rights of property."[191] Consequently, the modern courts have sustained a wide spectrum of traditional nuisance abatements, including noxious odors,[192] diseased crops,[193] hazardous waste,[194] pollution,[195] unsanitary or dangerous buildings,[196] and fire hazards.[197] Courts have also sustained nuisance abatements in response to public health problems of more recent origin, such as unsafe health care practitioners,[198] public meeting places that increase risks of STDs (e.g., adult entertainment),[199] and violence by abortion protesters.[200] For example, in many cities public health agencies have used nuisance laws to close down bathhouses in response to the HIV epidemic, believing that they create opportunities for anonymous sex. In response, the gay community has argued that closure infringes the freedom of association, while positive measures, such as education and condom distribution would help prevent high-risk sexual behavior.[201] The judiciary has consistently sided with public health authorities in such debates.[202]

Courts possess broad equitable powers to alleviate nuisances. These powers include issuing injunctions to abate nuisances (e.g., ordering cleanup, repair, discontinuance of hazardous activity, or closure), awarding damages to the injured parties, or destruction of property. If abatement is the remedy, public policy suggests that, where there is no emergency, the person should be given reasonable time and opportunity to rectify the hazardous condition.[203] If the public health agency has to intervene, it should avoid unnecessary property damage.[204]

In summary, public health agencies have ample methods to regulate commercial activities, including licenses, inspections, and nui-

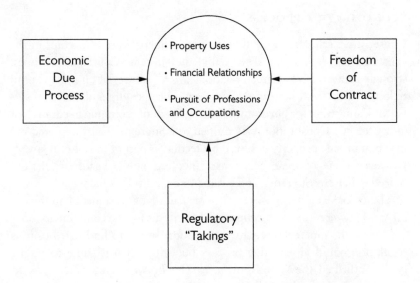

Figure 20.   Economic liberties protected under the U.S. Constitution.

sance abatements. At the same time, these regulatory techniques, if applied in an arbitrary or discriminatory manner, can be unjust and trample constitutional protection of liberty and property interests. One question that has long troubled scholars is the relative importance of economic freedoms. I conclude this chapter by exploring economic rights.

ECONOMIC LIBERTY AND THE PURSUIT OF PUBLIC HEALTH: CONTRACTS, PROPERTY USES, AND "TAKINGS"

The regulatory techniques used by public health authorities (e.g., licensing, inspection, and nuisance abatement), while protecting the public's health and safety, undoubtedly interfere with economic liberties. The Framers clearly intended to protect economic liberties, as evidenced by several constitutional provisions. Notably, the Constitution forbids the state from depriving persons of property (or life or liberty) without due process of law (economic due process),[205] impairing the obligations of contracts (freedom of contract),[206] and taking private property for public use without just compensation ("takings") (see Figure 20).[207] In this section, I examine the normative and constitutional justifications for economic liberties.

ECONOMIC DUE PROCESS

Conservative scholars argue that economic liberties are important in the constitutional design and observe that the Supreme Court has, at times, strongly protected commercial relationships.[208] However, on more careful reflection, the Court has more often seen public health regulation as a sufficient justification for government infringement of economic freedom. Not long after the Constitution was ratified, the Supreme Court explored the idea that private property deserved protection as part of the natural law.[209] However, none of these early cases involved public health regulation. Indeed, when the Supreme Court came to examine a challenge to sanitary regulation of slaughterhouses in 1873, it said that government had the undoubted power to restrict occupational freedoms for the common good.[210]

During the nineteenth century, the Court began to find that business regulation could violate due process but still, when it came to public health, affirmed the state's power.[211] The *Lochner* era, from 1905 to 1937, was a time when the Court most prized economic freedoms and aggressively invalidated numerous attempts at social and economic regulation. Certainly, the Court struck down a great deal of legislation designed to protect the public's health and security, such as minimum wages, consumer protection, and licensing (see chapter 3). Nevertheless, as evidenced by its decision in *Jacobson v. Massachusetts* (1905), the Court conceded, at least nominally, that the state could exercise its police power even if it interfered with liberty.[212] Since Franklin Delano Roosevelt's New Deal, the Court has granted police power regulation a strong presumption of validity even if it interferes with economic and commercial life.[213]

FREEDOM OF CONTRACT

Some scholars espouse a belief in free economic relationships; nevertheless, the Contracts Clause has become a relatively unimportant limitation on public health powers. The clause applies only to the states; challenges to federal restrictions on contractual freedom must be brought under the Due Process Clause. Moreover, the clause applies only to existing contracts; states are free to limit the terms of future contracts.[214] Although most public health regulation affects future economic relationships, it sometimes can affect existing contracts. The Supreme Court, however, has emphasized that the police power "is an exercise of the sovereign right of the Government to protect the lives, health, morals, comfort, and general welfare of the people, and is paramount to any rights under contracts between individuals."[215]

The modern Court uses a three-part test to assess government regulation that interferes with private contracts:[216] (1) Is there a substantial impairment of a contractual relationship? (2) If so, does it serve a significant and legitimate public purpose? (3) Is it reasonably related to achieving the goal?[217] Like substantive due process, this is a highly permissive standard that generally affirms governmental power to regulate contractual relationships reasonably in the public interest.

REGULATORY TAKINGS

Attorney General Meese . . . had a specific, aggressive,
and it seemed to me, quite radical project in mind: to
use the takings clause of the Fifth Amendment as a
severe brake on federal and state regulation of business
and property.

Charles Fried (1991)

Many of the changes in takings law . . . correspond quite
closely to a blueprint for the takings doctrine proposed
by Professor Richard Epstein. . . . This observation [is]
both remarkable and troubling. After all, Epstein's work
was almost universally criticized . . . [and its] proposed
end result—the overturning of a century's worth of
health, safety, and economic regulation—would sink this
country in a constitutional crisis. . . . What we have
found is a large and increasingly successful campaign by
conservatives and libertarians to use the federal judiciary
to achieve an anti-regulatory, anti-environmental agenda.

Douglas T. Kendall and Charles P. Lord (1998)

The federal government and the states have the power of eminent domain, which is the authority to confiscate private property for a governmental activity. However, the Fifth Amendment imposes a significant constraint on this power by requiring "just compensation" for private property taken for a public use.[218] The theory behind the "Takings" Clause is that individuals should not have to bear public burdens, which should be borne by the community as a whole. Consequently, the Takings Clause is about government spreading loss when pursuing the public interest.[219]

Despite its just purposes, an expansive interpretation of the Takings Clause would shackle public health agencies by requiring them to provide compensation whenever regulation significantly reduced the value of private property. Since public health regulation, by definition, restricts commercial uses of property, it has become a focal point for a sustained conservative critique of social action itself.[220]

Government confiscation or physical occupation of property is a "possessory" taking that certainly requires compensation. During the early twentieth century, however, the Supreme Court held that government regulation that "reaches a certain magnitude" also is a taking requiring compensation.[221] Initially, this idea of "regulatory" takings was not highly problematic for public health agencies because the Court suggested that government need not compensate property owners when regulating within the police power.[222] However, regulatory takings took on public health significance in the 1992 case of *Lucas v. South Carolina Coastal Council.*[223] In *Lucas,* Justice Antonin Scalia, the most intellectually powerful conservative voice on the Court, said that a person suffers a taking if regulation denies all economically beneficial or productive use of real property[224] and there were no similar restrictions "that background principles of the State's law of property and nuisance already place upon land ownership."[225] Justice Scalia suggested that common law nuisance was the key to resolving the question of when regulation amounted to an uncompensated taking; an owner who lost the value of her land would suffer a taking if the public health regulation was not considered a nuisance under the common law.

The Court's reasoning in *Lucas* is problematic because it forces public health authorities to define and abate public hazards according to vague and outdated common law understandings of nuisance. Even the most astute legal scholars perceive common law nuisance as confusing and indecipherable.[226] Consequently, when democratically elected government, according to modern standards, regulates to avert a serious public harm, it cannot be certain whether it will be compelled to compensate property owners. This narrowing of what may be considered a nuisance, and expansion of property interests, effectively constrains police power regulation. The Court, in effect, has simultaneously frozen the understanding of public health that existed in earlier times, while allowing the normative value of property to expand to meet modern libertarian expectations.

Since *Lucas,* state and lower federal courts often have resisted expansion of the takings doctrine, ruling against compensation resulting from environmental regulation.[227] However, other courts have used the "property rights" tenor of Justice Scalia's opinion to strike down important public health and environmental regulation.[228] The Court of Appeals for the Federal Circuit established a rule that government may have to compensate an owner for any regulation that causes a diminution in value, unless there is a "reciprocity of advantage" by which the owner receives "direct compensating benefits."[229] This kind of balancing appears to place private property interests on a par with the state's sovereign interests in community well-being. Takings litigation can penetrate deeply into core public health concerns. Consider the decision of the First Circuit Court of Appeals holding that Philip Morris was likely to succeed in its claim that a state law requiring manufacturers to disclose the ingredients in cigarettes was a regulatory taking.[230]

If Charles Fried was correct in describing a conservative plan to use the Takings Clause as a severe constraint on public health regulation, then the outcome remains uncertain. Much depends on the direction of the Supreme Court which, at present, has four members apparently committed to expansion of the regulatory takings doctrine.[231] This split among the justices was manifested in a 1998 case when a bitterly divided Court said that some public programs allocating benefits and burdens of economic life to promote the common good effect a taking. The plurality, representing the four-member conservative bloc on this issue, supported a balancing test (i.e., "the economic impact of the regulation, its interference with reasonable, investment backed expectations, and the character of the governmental action") that elevates economic justice to a new level in our constitutional democracy.[232]

THE NORMATIVE VALUE OF ECONOMIC LIBERTY

When health is absent
Wisdom cannot reveal itself,
Art cannot become manifest
Strength cannot fight,
Wealth becomes useless
and intelligence cannot be applied.
     Herophilus (325 B.C.)

Government regulation for the public's health, as we have seen throughout this book, inevitably interferes with personal or economic liberties. The Court usually grants the legislature deference in the exercise of police powers. A permissive approach to government regulation is justified, in part, by democratic values; citizens elect representatives to enable them to make complex policy choices.[233] A legislative choice to prefer collective health and well-being over individual interests deserves respect and insulation from aggressive judicial scrutiny. This is broadly the judicial approach to public health regulation affecting personal autonomy. Heightened scrutiny is reserved for those rare instances where public health interventions intrude on fundamental rights and interests, such as total deprivation of liberty (see chapter 3).

The normative issue is whether there is something in the nature of economic liberty that warrants a departure from the normal deference to public health regulation. Put another way, how important is unbridled freedom in property uses, financial relationships, and the pursuit of occupations? I see no reason why the diminution of economic liberties should be taken more seriously than the many deprivations of personal autonomy and privacy that routinely occur with public health regulation (e.g., vaccination, reporting, and contact tracing). Courts generally understand that some loss of individual freedom is necessary for the common welfare. Regulation that interferes with civil liberties does not cause conservative thinkers undue concern; nor is there any discussion of compensation to those who must forgo liberty for the collective good.

The same logic ought to apply to economic regulation for the common welfare. The reason for the governmental intervention is to prevent owners from using their private property in ways that are harmful to the public interest. Thus, the state's aim is not to deny economic opportunity per se, but only to foreclose commercial activities that are detrimental to public health and safety. The creation of private wealth, moreover, hardly can be regarded as a fundamental interest akin to total loss of personal freedom, for private wealth creation is not essential to the achievement of a healthy and fulfilling life. Rarely does economic regulation affect an individual's basic ability to obtain the necessities of life, such as food, shelter, and medical care.

The conservative claim, of course, is not only that economic liberties have intrinsic value, but that they have instrumental value as well. They claim that preserving economic liberty will help create wealth for the community at large. Even assuming that economic freedom reliably leads to greater overall prosperity, it is still reasonable for a legislature to make a social choice that favors immediate health and safety benefits over future wealth creation. A community cannot benefit from increased prosperity if it experiences excess morbidity and mortality from hazardous commercial activity.

Government, to be sure, ought not carelessly or gratuitously interfere with economic freedoms. If government has a reason, however, based on averting a significant risk to the public's health, then there appears nothing in the nature of economic liberty that should prevent the state from intervening, nor is there any reason why the state should provide compensation for regulating private commercial activities deemed detrimental to the communal good.

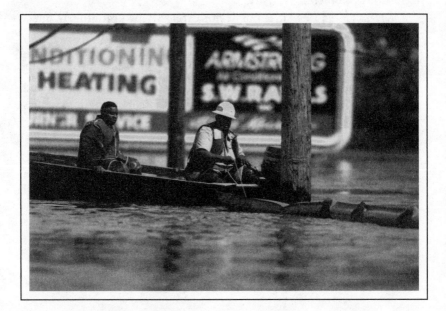

Contractors with the Hazardous Materials Emergency Response team pull oil-absorbing containment booms through flood waters in Franklin, Virginia, after Hurricane Floyd in September, 1999. A wide area was contaminated by petroleum products from motor vehicles and heating-oil tanks leaking into the water. (AP/Wide World Photos)

10 Tort Law and the Public's Health

Indirect Regulation

Both tort and statutory law have regulatory effects. Tort law can regulate behavior not only directly through providing injunctive relief, but indirectly—and more commonly—through the award of damages. Similarly, statutes can regulate behavior directly through standard setting and indirectly through fees [and] subsidies. . . . The line between common law tort actions and regulatory interventions has blurred in recent years as courts look for design defects, agencies propose incentive schemes, and statutes permit private rights of action.

Susan Rose-Ackerman (1991)

Thus far, I have considered regulation principally as the actions taken by legislatures and administrative agencies to prevent injury or disease and to promote the public's health. The creation of private rights of action in the courts can also be an effective means of public health regulation.[1] This chapter concerns one important form of civil litigation: the role of tort law in public health to redress harms to people and the environment they inhabit.[2]

A tort, derived from the Latin *torquere,* "to twist," is a civil, noncontractual wrong for which an injured person or group of persons seeks a remedy in the form of monetary damages.[3] Tort law, then, characteristically is a private, rather than public, right of action, and a civil, rather than a criminal, proceeding. It remedies a wrong by awarding monetary damages, rather than an injunction or civil or criminal penalties. Tort law is composed of a series of related doctrines that impose civil liability upon persons or businesses whose (usually) substandard conduct causes injury or disease.

The functions, or goals, of tort law—although highly controversial and imperfectly achieved[4]—are the (1) assignment of *responsibility* to individuals or businesses that impose unreasonable risks causing injury or disease; (2) *compensation* of persons for loss caused by the conduct of individuals or businesses; (3) *deterrence* of unreasonably hazardous conduct; and (4) encouragement of *innovation* in product design, packaging, labeling, and advertising to reduce the risk of injury or disease. In thinking about tort law as a tool of public health, it is important to emphasize the role of litigation in preventing risk behavior and providing incentives for safer product design.

A vast potential for using tort litigation as an effective tool to reduce the burden of injury and disease exists.[5] Attorneys general, public health authorities, and private citizens resort to civil litigation to redress many different kinds of public health harms: environmental damage (e.g., air pollution[6] or groundwater contamination[7]); exposure to toxic substances (e.g., pesticides,[8] radiation,[9] or chemicals[10]); unsafe pharmaceuticals, vaccines, or medical devices (e.g., diethylstilbestrol [DES],[11] live polio vaccines,[12] or contraceptive devices[13]); hazardous products (e.g., tobacco, firearms, or alcoholic beverages[14]); and defective consumer products (e.g., children's toys,[15] recreational equipment,[16] or household goods[17]).

While tort law can be an extremely effective method of advancing the public's health, like any form of regulation, it is not an unmitigated good. The tort system imposes economic costs and personal burdens on individuals and businesses that warrant careful consideration. The costs entailed in adjudication—transaction expenses (e.g., the court system and attorney fees) and liability—can discourage businesses from entering markets, render it economically burdensome to stay in markets, and/or increase consumer prices. Litigation as a form of regulation, then, holds enormous potential for improving public health, but also entails economic costs and diminution of autonomy. Like any form of regulation, we trade off the public goods from civil litigation against the burdens.

The tort system is full of detail and complexity well beyond the scope of a text on public health law. Nevertheless, to understand tort actions designed to achieve a public good, I first explain the major theories of liability. Next, I examine the complicated problems of scientific proof and uncertainty in bringing tort litigation. After examining the doctrine and scientific evidence, I demonstrate the value of tort law as a tool of public health. Two paradigmatic case studies are presented: one relating to chronic disease (tobacco lawsuits) and one relating to accidental and intentional injury (firearm lawsuits). Finally, I look at some of the limitations of traditional tort doctrine in addressing major public health problems, including the economic costs and burdens as well as the indirect regulatory effects.

MAJOR THEORIES OF TORT LIABILITY

As explained above, the tort system is composed of a series of related doctrines that impose liability on persons, businesses, or governments whose conduct causes injury or disease. Tort law classifies cases according to the degree of culpability inherent in the risk-taking behavior—negligent, intentional, and no fault. Plaintiffs may adopt multiple theories of recovery but must prove each element in a cause of action by a preponderance of evidence.

NEGLIGENCE

The rule that you are to love your neighbor becomes in
law, you must not injure your neighbor; and the
lawyer's question, Who is my neighbor? receives a
restricted reply. You must take reasonable care to avoid
acts or omissions which you can reasonably foresee
would be likely to injure your neighbor. Who, then, in
law is my neighbor? The answer seems to be—persons
who are so closely and directly affected by my act that
I ought reasonably to have them in contemplation.

James R. Atkin (1932)

The use of fault as a basis of civil liability is so much a part of the American experience with tort law that a New York judge, in 1873, was able to assert: "[T]he rule is, at least in this century, a universal one, which, so far as I can discern, has no exceptions or limitations, that no one can be made liable for injuries to the person or property of another without some fault or negligence on his part."[18] It was not always this way, though. While negligence has remained the dominant standard in tort law, prior to the nineteenth century persons were held liable for harm caused by accidents irrespective of fault.[19] The transition from strict liability to fault is often attributed to private enterprise values designed to protect youthful industries from inordinate liability during the industrial revolution.[20] The modern elements of a cause of action based on negligence are duty of care, breach of duty, causation, and loss or damage (see Table 11).[21]

TABLE 11

NEGLIGENCE: THE ELEMENTS

Duty of Care	Legal obligation to protect others against unreasonable risks of harm
Breach of Duty	Defendant fails to conform to the legally recognized standard of safe behavior *Reasonable person standard:* Would a "reasonable person of ordinary prudence" have engaged in that risk behavior? *Rule of custom:* What is the usual and customary practice adopted in the industry or among fellow professionals? *Rule of law:* Did the person or business meet existing regulatory standards?
Causation	Reasonably close causal connection between unreasonably risky conduct and resulting injury *Causation "in fact":* Harm would not have occurred but for the defendant's conduct. *Proximate cause:* Was the injury a foreseeable consequence of the defendant's behavior?
Loss or Damage	Plaintiff must have suffered actual loss or damage and not mere insult to dignity

Duty of Care. A duty of care is an obligation recognized in law to conform to a standard of conduct to protect others against unreasonable risks of harm. Philosophically, the difference between an act ("misfeasance" or active misconduct) and an omission ("nonfeasance" or passive inaction) is far from clear, but the law traditionally draws a distinction. Generally, with respect to affirmative acts, we all owe a duty to every other person in the community to conduct our activities in reasonably safe ways to avoid foreseeable harm. On the other hand, a person usually is not liable for failing to take steps to protect others—that is, no general duty to rescue exists.[22] However, a person does have an affirmative duty to protect another from harm if—by custom, sentiment, and public policy—they share a special relationship, particularly where one person has expert knowledge and the other is vulnerable, such as in a physician-patient relationship.[23]

Breach of Duty. A breach of duty—that is, the person is "negligent"—occurs when a person fails to conform to the legally recognized standard of safe behavior. The standard of care is often characterized as the behavior that would be undertaken by a "reasonable person" or a person of "ordinary prudence."[24] The standard is intentionally vague, relying on the jury to make a normative judgment about the reasonableness of the activity—a legal fiction that randomly selected lay persons will act as the informed conscience of the community.

The "reasonable person" is informed by two concepts—objectivity and foreseeability.[25] Under the "objective" standard, the jury inquires whether a person of ordinary care and skill would have acted the same way under the circumstances. (Some professionals, such as physicians, are held to a higher standard relating to the skill that would be exercised by similarly situated professionals.) The law of negligence is not concerned with the particular actor's actual intent to do good or to cause harm, nor does the law take account of the actor's individual characteristics or capacity for safe behavior. While allowance is made for physical disabilities (e.g., acts of the blind are compared with reasonable conduct of others who cannot see), no allowance is made for the actor's intelligence, character, or mental faculties. If a person exercises his judgment to the best of his ability, he will not necessarily avoid liability in negligence. The logic of reasonable care, however, does require that the harm be reasonably foreseeable. Thus, a person must know, or reasonably should know, that the behavior poses a risk of harm; failing to reduce a risk about which an individual does not, and reasonably could not, know is not negligence.[26]

Courts define negligence by reference to rules of custom and law. Since negligence is a community standard, evidence of the usual and customary conduct of others under similar circumstances is highly probative. Thus, courts examine the practices adopted in the industry or among fellow professionals. For example, medical malpractice law follows a strict rule of custom so that physician behavior is measured against a national standard of how similar generalists or specialists practice in the country. In addition to custom, courts look to standards set by statutes, regulations, and guidelines. Breach of statutory or regulatory standards may be negligence per se or, at least, highly suggestive of negligence. If OSHA requires employers to reduce lead exposure to a specified level, failure to achieve that level may be conclusive evidence of negligence. Even the issuance of nonbinding guidelines by government agencies (e.g., the CDC) or professional organizations (e.g., the AMA) strongly influences legal standards of care in a negligence action. Compliance with lax regulatory standards, of course, can also be used as a shield against liability; for example, environmental tort litigation sometimes flounders because polluters successfully argue that their conduct met low regulatory standards.[27]

Causation. Liability for negligence requires a reasonably close causal connection between the unreasonably risky conduct and the resulting injury. Causality is often examined in terms of "proximate" (or legal) cause, including "causation in fact." Philosophically, causal relationships can be traced to innumerable antecedent events, but legal responsibility is limited to actions that actually cause harm and to sequences of events that are foreseeable. Courts often adopt a "but for" rule to explain causation in fact—that is, the harm would not have occurred but for the defendant's conduct; or, conversely, the harm would still have occurred without the defendant's conduct.[28] A clear definition of proximate cause is difficult to enunciate, because the term is meant to convey the circumstances when, as a matter of law, it is fair to impose liability. Some courts hold that a defendant is liable if her conduct is the direct, rather than a remote, cause of the injury; others say that the harm must be a natural and probable consequence of the act. Most definitions of proximate cause, however, turn on whether the injury was a foreseeable consequence of the defendant's behavior—that is, whether the defendant reasonably could have anticipated the harm at the time she engaged in the risk behavior.

Loss or Damage. Finally, liability for negligence requires actual loss or damage, and not a mere insult to dignity. (This separates negligence from "intentional torts," such as battery, where plaintiffs may recover nominal damages even if no tangible harm has occurred.) For example, a needle-stick injury caused by a hospital's negligence will not result in liability unless the plaintiff actually contracted a bloodborne infection or, at least, was exposed and genuinely fears infection.[29]

In summary, negligence is a measure of legally acceptable risk; a person must exercise due care to avoid unreasonable risks of harm to others. Notice that the law of negligence does not require avoidance of all possibilities of harm; nearly all human activity carries risk, and it is only "unreasonable" risks that are deemed to be negligent. There is much imprecision, of course, in separating "reasonable" from "unreasonable" risks. Some jurists and scholars propose a "negligence calculus" that assesses risk, benefit, and cost: the probability that the conduct may cause harm; the severity of the harm should the risk materialize; the social utility and economic costs of the activity; and the benefits, risks, and costs of the alternatives available to the actor.[30] Judge Learned Hand famously stated the negligence calculus as an algebraic formula: "[I]f the probability [of harm] be called P; the [gravity of the resulting] injury, L; and the burden [of adequate precautions

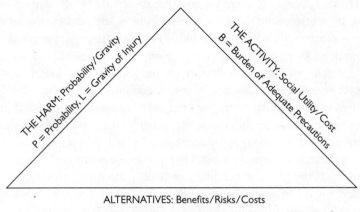

ALTERNATIVES: Benefits/Risks/Costs

LIABILITY occurs when B < PL

Figure 21.   The "negligence calculus": balancing risks, benefits, and costs.

to avert the harm], B; liability depends upon whether B is less than L multiplied by P: i.e., whether B is less than PL" (see Figure 21).[31]

Suppose a manufacturer foresees that a live vaccine will cause death in 1 in 10,000 cases. Should the manufacturer be liable to the person who contracts a vaccine-induced disease? The level of risk is mixed: probability is very low, but severity of harm (death) is high. Balanced against the risk is the social utility, which, in the case of vaccines, is high. Perhaps the conclusive factors would be the costs and benefits of alternative vaccines. If a dead vaccine achieves the same protection and causes disease only in one case in a million, it may be unreasonable to use the live vaccine. However, if the live vaccine costs $1 per dose and the dead vaccine $25 per dose, should the manufacturer be liable? From a population-based perspective, the answer may be "no," but the parent of a child that contracts a vaccine-induced disease may think differently.

PRIVATE NUISANCE

Chapter 9 discussed public nuisances, which are principally legislative and enforced by public health agencies. This chapter discusses private nuisances, which are principally part of the common law and redressed through the tort system. A private nuisance is an unreasonable interference with the possessor's use and enjoyment of land (e.g., contaminating adjoining land[32]).

The components of a private nuisance theory are (1) the defendant intends to interfere with the use and enjoyment of land and (2) the interference is substantial and unreasonable.[33] The intent requirement refers only to the defendant's knowledge of the nuisance—if he knows that his activity creates an interference with property use and still continues, he has the requisite intent. For example, if a person continues the activity after he is notified that his emissions are polluting an adjoining stream, he is deemed to intend the result. It does not matter whether the person's motivation is to pollute or if it is the by-product of socially desirable activity.

The interference must be substantial, not minor or ethereal. An invasion that affects the physical condition of land is almost always substantial, particularly if it results in measurable economic loss. For example, knowledge that pollution of soil or underground water affects natural resources has considerable weight in judicial thinking. It is more difficult to demonstrate that physical or psychological discomfort is a substantial interference. Modern society requires landowners to bear many annoyances due to noise, smells, and unsightly conditions. An annoyance of this kind must create an appreciable interference with property interests judged by the standard of an ordinary member of the community with normal sensitivity and temperament. Nuisances are measured in the context in which they occur, including the neighborhood, property uses, and culture.[34]

Closely associated with "substantiality" is the notion that interference with property uses must be unreasonable. The courts assess reasonableness by weighing the parties' interests much as they would in a negligence action: the extent and duration of harm, the social value of the activity, the cost of avoiding or ameliorating the harm, and comparative economic effects (i.e., the relative capacity of the parties to bear the loss).[35]

Economists often reason that in a well-functioning market it is fairer, and more efficient, if companies "internalize" socially harmful activities as a cost of business.[36] Thus, an entrepreneur engaged in a socially useful activity, such as mining coal or refining petroleum, should pay for the harm caused to the surrounding community, even if modern scientific processes are used to reduce environmental harm.[37] Under this economic theory, monetary damages would be preferred over injunctive relief. A nuisance abatement stifles an enterprise rather than requiring it to bear the fair cost of the activity. Yet courts may grant injunctions in nuisance actions if an unreasonable activity is ongoing, particularly if a danger to humans or the environment persists. For example, in United States v. Reserve Mining Company (1974), a

court enjoined a mining operation to prevent the discharge of carcinogenic fibers into the water supply. The court reasoned that "in matters
of public health, by their very nature, monetary damages are usually
incapable of compensating those who are or who will be injured by the
nuisance."[38]

Courts, then, have three choices: social equities may militate in favor
of the plaintiff bearing the burden (no relief), the defendant internaliz-
ing the cost (monetary damages), or the defendant forbearing the harmful enterprise completely (injunction).

STRICT LIABILITY

[My Lords], if the Defendants, not stopping at the
natural use of their close, had desired to use it for any
purpose which I may term a nonnatural use . . . [and
the plaintiff was injured] . . . then for [that evil] the
consequence . . . is that, in my opinion, the
Defendants would be liable.

Hugh McCalmont Cairns (1868)

Torts based on negligence can be difficult to prove due to lack of evidence of substandard care. For certain risk-taking behaviors, however,
the judiciary affixes liability without regard to culpability (e.g., for unduly hazardous activities and for the sale of defective products). The law
holds that even if the defendant exercises reasonable (or even extreme)
care, she has to carry the cost of injuries. Strict, or no-fault, liability may
be thought of as mandatory insurance against designated risks for reasons of social policy; it remains a highly controversial legal doctrine.

Strict liability does not impose absolute liability, but has the following limits: *intention*—the defendant must knowingly engage in the activity; *proximate cause*—liability is confined to the consequences
caused by the activity and to persons foreseeably harmed; *public duty
privilege*—liability is not imposed when the law expressly authorizes or
imposes a duty to conduct the activity; and *sovereign immunity*—the
Federal Tort Claims Act waives sovereign immunity for claims of government negligence, but not strict liability.[39]

Abnormally Dangerous Activities.   Strict liability in the modern era
originated in the English case of *Rylands v. Fletcher* (1868), in which
the House of Lords found that if "a person brings, or accumulates, on

his land anything which, if it should escape, may cause damage to his neighbour, he does so at his peril."[40] Thus, if a nonnatural substance "does escape, and causes damage, he is responsible, however careful he may have been, and whatever precautions he may have taken."[41]

The rule of *Rylands v. Fletcher* found its way into American law through the doctrine of "abnormally dangerous activities," defined by reference to a number of factors:[42] high degree of risk, seriousness of resulting harm, inability to eliminate the risk by the exercise of due care, and the activity's danger compared with its value to the community. Lord Cairns's formulation of a "natural use" is reflected in the modern notion of "common usage." If an unsafe activity is prevalent (e.g., driving automobiles), it is not abnormally dangerous.[43] Common usage depends, in part, on whether the activity is inappropriate to the place where it is conducted. For example, the storage of explosives may be abnormally dangerous in a densely populated area, but not in a rural community.

In summary, strict liability may be imposed where an activity, although lawful, is so dangerous, unusual, and inappropriate (within the context of its place and manner of use) to justify allocating the risk of loss to the enterprise. Strict liability is particularly important in environmental law, where chemical production or disposal may be considered ultrahazardous.[44] Similarly, production of nuclear energy or transport of nuclear materials may be abnormally dangerous activities.[45]

Products Liability.   The emerging market in consumer products at the turn of the twentieth century had enormous benefits for the population, but individuals injured by those products faced insuperable obstacles in gaining compensation. The extant law permitted actions for negligence only against the party with whom an injured person had a contractual relation, that is, "privity."[46] Contractual privity was abandoned in the famous 1916 decision *MacPherson v. Buick Motor Company*, where consumers were permitted to sue automobile manufacturers.[47] While *MacPherson* was a negligence action, no-fault products liability soon followed. Notably, consumers could sue under "implied warranty of merchantability," a contractual theory that did not require negligence.[48] Sellers, however, began to undermine implied warranty litigation by using safety disclaimers in consumer contracts. In response, strict liability for defective products emerged in the middle part of the century[49] and, by the 1970s, most states adopted the theory.[50] The two most important concepts in products liability law are the meaning of "products" and "defects."

A product is broadly understood to be tangible goods.[51] Products liability applies to virtually all goods capable of causing injury, ranging from motor vehicles,[52] household appliances,[53] and work[54] and recreational equipment[55] to pharmaceuticals,[56] vaccines,[57] and medical devices.[58] Activities (e.g., "abnormally dangerous" activities within the meaning of *Rylands v. Fletcher*) and services are not "products" and, therefore, are not covered under products liability law.[59] For example, blood is not a product: statutes in every state provide that blood suppliers are deemed to provide services so that strict liability theory does not apply.[60]

The courts have adopted varied tests of a product "defect," and no single standard is universally accepted. A common standard is whether the product performed "as safely as an ordinary consumer would expect when used in an intended or reasonably foreseeable manner."[61] The reasonable expectation standard works well for many product defects, but not if the consumer lacks the expertise to evaluate a complex or scientific product such as a medical device. As a result, many courts use a risk-utility balancing test to determine if a defective product is "unreasonably dangerous to the consumer": is the cost of making a product safer greater than the danger from the product in its present condition?[62] Product defects generally fall into three categories: manufacturing defects, design defects, and failures to warn.[63] Some courts also use a misrepresentation theory in finding products defective (see Figure 22).

A product contains a *manufacturing defect* when, as produced, it does not conform to the manufacturer's own design.[64] This means that a flaw was not present in the product design, but, despite due care, the defect resulted from the construction process. Manufacturing defects tend to be random and usually do not affect the entire product line.[65] Since it is usually difficult for consumers to detect a manufacturing flaw, courts impose liability on the seller. Thus, injured consumers do not have to demonstrate that the manufacturer used faulty materials, lacked due care in construction, or failed to inspect properly.

A product contains a *design defect* when it is defective although produced as planned by the manufacturer. Consequently, a design defect is usually apparent in an entire product line. Manufacturers are liable for design defects when "the foreseeable risks of harm posed by the product could have been reduced or avoided by the adoption of a reasonable

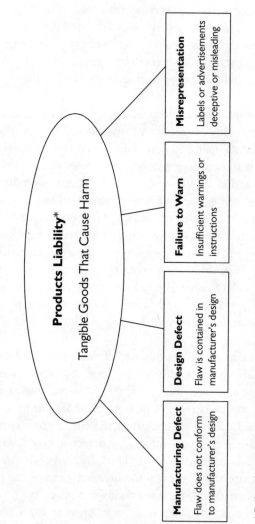

Products Liability*

Tangible Goods That Cause Harm

Manufacturing Defect

Flaw does not conform
to manufacturer's design

Design Defect

Flaw is contained in
manufacturer's design

Failure to Warn

Insufficient warnings or
instructions

Misrepresentation

Labels or advertisements
deceptive or misleading

* **Rules that shield manufacturers from strict liability:**
Unavoidably unsafe products: products that are incapable of being made safe (e.g., pharmaceuticals and vaccines)
Products in common use: common and widely distributed products (e.g., alcoholic beverages and firearms)

Figure 22. Products liability theories.

alternative design . . . and the omission of the alternative design renders the product not reasonably safe."[66] "Reasonable design alternative" is a liability-limiting test because it requires the plaintiff to show that the product could have been made safer.[67] The design defect theory is controversial because the manufacturer intended the "defective" design feature with due consideration of price, attractiveness, and functionality.

A product has a *"failure to warn" defect* when the seller fails to inform consumers adequately about the risks or provide instructions for safe use.[68] The theory underlying this product defect is consumer sovereignty, the notion that customers deserve sufficient data to make informed purchasing choices. Courts use a "reasonableness" test in evaluating failure to warn cases: could the foreseeable risks have been reduced by reasonable instructions or warnings, and did the omission of instructions or warnings render the product unreasonably dangerous?[69] The fact that "failure to warn" cases often turn on the reasonableness of the action suggests a similarity to negligence theory. Some courts, however, unabashedly adopt strict liability for failure to warn even if the dangers were "undiscoverable at the time."[70]

Closely related to "failure to warn" theory is *misrepresentation,* where the seller misinforms consumers orally, in writing, or through other conduct calculated to convey a false impression.[71] Misrepresentation is established through labels, packet inserts, or advertisements that are inaccurate, deceptive, or misleading. Intentional concealment of the truth also can be misrepresentation, such as when a tobacco company fails to disclose internal research of the harmful effects of cigarettes on smokers.[72] Given the pervasive advertising of modern products, misrepresentation claims may become a very important theory of liability for advancing the public's health.[73]

Strict liability is not available for *unavoidably unsafe products.* According to the Restatement (Second) of Torts § 402A, comment k, products that are highly socially beneficial but inherently risky escape strict liability if, "in the present state of human knowledge, they are quite incapable of being made safe for their intended and ordinary use." Pharmaceuticals, vaccines, and medical devices are classic illustrations of unavoidably unsafe products,[74] but courts have applied comment k to other dangerous products such as asbestos[75] and solvents.[76] Comment k "vindicates the public's interest in the availability and affordability" of a desirable consumer product.[77] The doctrine is intended to preserve incentives for socially useful products, but it also has the effect of shifting the risk of loss from manufacturers to injured consumers.

Strict liability is also unavailable for inherently dangerous products that are in *common use* and made according to the manufacturer's design (e.g., "good" whiskey and tobacco[78]). The Restatement of Products Liability says that "common and widely distributed products such as alcoholic beverages, firearms, and above-ground swimming pools" may be held defective only if they are sold without reasonable warning or if reasonable alternative designs could have been adopted.[79] The rationale is that, since these hazardous products have received long-term market acceptance, the legislature is thought to be the appropriate regulatory agency. However, many would find it odd that tobacco and firearms are immunized from strict liability (along with vaccines and prescription drugs) while far safer and socially advantageous products, such as children's toys and food products, must meet rigorous strict liability standards. If the functions of strict liability are to encourage safer product design and to spread the risk of injury and disease, then cigarettes, alcoholic beverages, and firearms would seem to be prime candidates for tort regulation.

SCIENTIFIC CONUNDRUMS IN MASS TORT LITIGATION: EPIDEMIOLOGY IN THE COURTROOM

Thus not only our reason fails us in the discovery of
the ultimate connexion of causes and effects, but even
after experience has inform'd us of their constant
conjunction, 'tis impossible for us to satisfy ourselves
by our reason, why we shou'd extend that experience
beyond those particular instances, which have fallen
under our observation. We suppose, but are never able
to prove, that there must be a resemblance betwixt
those objects, of which we have had experience, and
those which lie beyond the reach of our discovery.
                                        David Hume (1739)

The cultures and purposes of law and science differ markedly, and these differences span centuries of interactions between the two fields.[80] Both fields seek the truth, but each has a different meaning of truth.[81] While law seeks finality and closure, scientific inquiry is continuous; while law in civil litigation makes decisions by the preponderance of evidence (greater than 50 percent), science uses statistical significance (greater than 95 percent, with a confidence limit that does not include 1.0); while law follows an adversarial method, science embraces the experimental design (the "scientific" method); while legal evidence is testimonial, scientific evidence is empirical. These different understandings do not mean that one field discovers truth and the other less than truth.[82] Rather, the two fields have different missions and each operates, at least partly, in the other's environment. Science and law, therefore, must seek to understand the other, and each must accommodate the methods and cognitive processes of the other.

Interactions between law and science center on issues of causality—did an act, event, or exposure produce a certain harm? The law's purpose is to assign responsibility for the harm. Problems of proof in traditional tort actions, such as motor vehicle accidents, are usually surmountable. If X hits Y, who then sustains an immediate injury, causality is readily established by an eyewitness who observes the event and a medical expert who testifies that the harm resulted from the impact. What if a product (P) or activity (A) is associated with an increased rate of harm (H) in the population? How difficult is it to marshal scientific proof that A or P caused H?

This is the kind of scientific conundrum that arises in so-called mass exposure ("toxic tort") litigation. Mass tort actions characteristically involve large populations that are exposed to one or more toxic substances. Toxic substances in mass exposure litigation are as diverse as commercial materials (e.g., lead paint), chemical compounds (e.g., dioxin), personal items (e.g., tampons or silicone breast implants), pharmaceuticals (e.g., Bendectin), vaccines (e.g., swine flu), and low-level radiation. Plaintiffs claim these substances cause a variety of health conditions ranging from carcinogenic (cancer), teratogenic (birth defects), and mutagenic (genetic mutations) effects to autoimmune and nervous system dysfunction. The health effects of exposure to toxic substances usually are not immediately apparent and may take a decade (e.g., asbestosis) or even a generation (e.g., birth defects) to emerge.

Problems of scientific proof in mass exposure litigation relate to the massive scope of the population, the exposure, the health conditions, and the latency period. First, a large number of people are exposed to the same toxic substance, and some of them have the alleged health effect and some do not (e.g., the massive exposure to methyl isocyanate from a Union Carbide plant in Bhopal, India[83]). Second, the population at risk probably has been exposed to many different toxic substances and their levels (or doses) of exposure vary widely. Third, the health conditions from which the population claims to suffer are also present in background levels appearing in groups who were not exposed.[84] Finally, because of the passage of time between the original exposure and the onset of symptoms, plaintiffs find it difficult to gather evidence and to discount the multiple intervening variables that may explain their present health condition. Consider a population that claims a higher prevalence of leukemia and other cancers due to exposure to atomic testing during the 1940s and 1950s. The same diseases occur in the general population with complicated etiologies such as genetics, smoking, and exposure to radon. In such circumstances, it is extraordinarily difficult to prove that the exposure to atomic testing definitively caused the cancers.[85]

Plaintiffs in mass exposure litigation must establish two types of causation: general and specific.[86] General (or generic) causation assesses whether the substance (at the dosage to which the plaintiffs were exposed)[87] is capable of causing the harm found in increased levels in the population. Specific causation assesses whether exposure to the substance in fact caused the plaintiff's harm.[88] Professors Tom Christoffel and Stephen Teret explain that even if plaintiffs can show that factor X is responsible for a significant percentage of all cases of harm Y in a population (general causation), it can rarely be proven that the harm Y suffered by a particular individual was one of the cases caused by factor X (specific causation).[89]

Courts often favor single-cause explanations for injury and seek a traceable causal chain of events.[90] The preferred form of proof is the "eyewitness"—the treating physician who testifies that a specific event caused the patient's harm. Toxic tort plaintiffs, however, use probabilistic evidence to establish a legally cognizable connection between the exposure and the harm (i.e., the likelihood that the exposure that caused the harm was sufficiently high to demonstrate cause and effect).[91] Certainly, as the epigraph by David Hume explains, positive correlations never establish causation; yet epidemiologists use statistical significance to explain positive correlations between two phenomena (i.e., the exposure and the harm) to infer causality[92] (e.g., causality is assumed if there exists more than a 95 percent chance that an exposure resulted in harm[93]).

THE ADMISSIBILITY OF SCIENTIFIC EVIDENCE: "JUNK SCIENCE" IN THE COURTROOM

Issues of causation are often determined by scientific evidence, but the courts have struggled with the vexing question of when scientific testimony may be admitted in a trial. In *Frye v. United States*,[94] decided in 1923, the court set a standard for the admissibility of scientific evidence that lasted for more than seventy years. *Frye*'s "general acceptance" test permitted into evidence only "a well-recognized scientific principle or discovery . . . sufficiently established to have gained general acceptance in the particular field."[95] Thus, establishing a consensus within the scientific community was crucial to the admission of expert testimony. In 1975, Congress enacted the Federal Rules of Evidence, which reflected a more liberal attitude toward the admission of evidence: "[I]f scientific, technical or other specialized knowledge will assist the trier of fact to understand the evidence . . . a witness qualified as an expert . . . may testify."[96] The Federal Rules favor the admission of relevant testimony, relying on the adversarial process to sort out strong from weak evidence.[97]

The Federal Rules' "let it all in" theory, however, permits the introduction of scientifically unfounded evidence (so-called junk science), with the effect that businesses are held liable for harms that they did not create. Peter Huber argues that trial lawyers have an incentive to introduce scientific evidence irrespective of its rigor; medical experts are willing to testify for a fee; and juries are prone to decide against defendants with "deep pockets."[98] Marcia Angell chronicled the systematic use of pseudoscience in the silicone breast implant cases, where Dow Corning was held liable, even though independent scientific reviews showed that implants do not cause autoimmune or connective tissue diseases.[99] Unscientific evidence proffered by "hired guns" representing either industry or consumers remains a serious problem, although the Supreme Court, as the following discussion shows, is moving toward a more scientifically oriented approach to expert evidence (see Figure 23).

After 1975, courts began to divide on whether the restrictive *Frye* test or the permissive Federal Rules test governed admissibility. The Supreme Court resolved the disagreement in *Daubert v. Merrell Dow Pharmaceuticals, Incorporated* (1993),[100] holding that the *Frye* "general acceptance" test was superseded by the Federal Rules.[101] The Court, however, shifted to a more scientific approach,[102] finding that the trial judge must assume a gate-keeping (or screening) role in assessing the admissibility of expert evidence: "[T]he judge must ensure that . . . scientific testimony or evidence admitted is not only relevant, but reliable."[103]

Daubert—part of a long series of cases alleging that the antinausea drug Bendectin caused birth defects in children—established a two-part test to determine reliability of scientific evidence: reliability and relevancy (or "fit"). The Supreme Court suggested four factors to assess the reliability of scientific evidence:[104] (1) *testing*—whether the scientific theory or

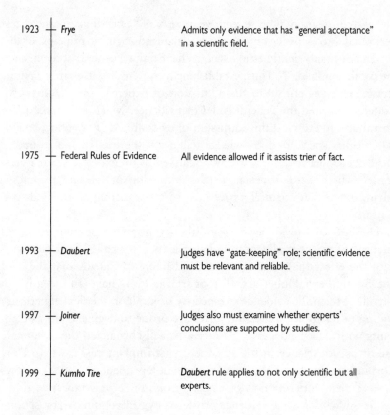

Figure 23.   Admissibility of scientific evidence in the courtroom: a
time line.

technique can be, and has been, tested; (2) *peer review*—whether the theory or technique has been subjected to the strictures of peer review and
publication; (3) *error rate*—whether there is a high known or potential
rate of error; and (4) *general acceptance*—whether the theory or technique enjoys general acceptance within a relevant scientific community.
These four factors are illustrative and nonexclusive, and should be applied flexibly by the trial court.[105]

After considering the reliability of the scientific evidence, the trial
court must consider the relevance of, or "fit" with, the ultimate issue to
be decided: the evidence must "assist the trier of fact to understand the
evidence or to determine a fact in issue."[106] Thus, to be relevant, testimony must "logically advance a material aspect of the case."[107] In mass
exposure cases, plaintiffs often rely on a complex chain of causation beginning with animal studies.[108] Plaintiffs must satisfy the *Daubert* test

of reliability and relevance for each link in the causal chain and, if they fail to do so, courts exclude the expert testimony.[109]

The Supreme Court in *Daubert* left an important issue about inadmissibility unclear—whether the standards of reliability and relevancy apply only to the expert's methodology or whether they apply to her conclusions as well. In other words, must the trial court blindly accept the anomalous conclusions of an expert who relies on valid studies?[110] The Supreme Court in *General Electric Company v. Joiner* (1997)[111] held that the trial court could critically examine whether the expert's conclusions were supported by the studies cited:[112] "[C]onclusions and methodology are not entirely distinct from one another. Trained experts commonly extrapolate from existing data. But . . . a district court [is not required] to admit opinion evidence which is connected to the existing data only by the *ipse dixit* of the expert. A court may conclude that there is simply too great an analytical gap between the data and the opinion proffered."

The Supreme Court, in *Kumho Tire Company v. Carmichael* (1999),[113] held that the *Daubert* factors apply not only to scientific experts, but to all experts, such as engineers. The Court reasoned that no clear line divides scientific knowledge from technical or other specialized knowledge, and no convincing need exists to make such distinctions.

In summary, the Supreme Court has progressively tightened the permissive admissibility standard in the Federal Rules, giving trial judges considerable discretion to exclude both scientific methodologies and expert opinions of all kinds that fail to meet tests of reliability and relevance. The Court itself said that the law must make certain that an expert "employs in the courtroom the same level of intellectual rigor that characterizes the practice of an expert in the relevant field."[114] The major criticism of the *Daubert* framework, however, is that judges do not possess adequate knowledge or scientific background to assess effectively the validity of theories and data offered by expert witnesses.[115]

Although this critique is undoubtedly true, the courts should adopt some reasonable methodology for ensuring that judicial decision-making is scientifically valid or, at least, does not fly in the face of science. The judge's role as gatekeeper to ensure that experts base their opinions on peer-reviewed data and draw reasonable inferences from those data can be helpful. The judiciary has another method at its disposal that would be even better at solving the problem of unscientific evidence, but judges would need to make greater use of it. Trial judges have the power to appoint independent experts to evaluate the evidence for the jury. Independent experts could be chosen from a panel of scientists well regarded in their fields, without conflicts of interest, and independent from the parties to the case. Independent experts could then draw their conclusions from a wide breadth of peer-reviewed materials, applying scientifically sound principles to the facts of the case.

THE PUBLIC HEALTH VALUE OF TORT LITIGATION

Regulation can be as effectively exerted through an
award of damages as through some form of preventive
relief. The obligation to pay compensation can be,
indeed is designed to be, a potent method of governing
conduct and controlling policy.

Felix Frankfurter (1959)

Tort law can be an important tool for advancing the public's health. Many public health issues are politically charged and powerfully affect businesses and consumers. As a result, it may be exceedingly difficult to directly regulate harmful products or activities through legislation or agency rules. Powerful interest groups, such as the tobacco or firearms lobby, can thwart regulation through the political process. Consumers themselves may rise up in revolt against regulation and taxation of the products they desire. Consider the difficulty of imposing strict emission standards for sport utility vehicles, higher taxes on cigarettes, or safety locks on handguns. Where direct regulation through the political process fails, tort law can become an essential tool in the arsenal of public health advocates.

One major critique of tort law is that it is not a particularly effective deterrent. Some scholars assert that legal doctrine rarely controls human behavior:[116] lay persons are not usually aware of legal rules and, even if they are, they are more likely to be influenced by normal human motivation—a sense of adventure, sexual desire, tolerance for risk, or desire for safety. This critique has validity but misses the point. Tort law affects consumer behavior by altering the way that businesses conduct their activities. Industry may react to tort law by making products safer, providing clearer warnings and instructions, or simply discontinuing product lines, all of which powerfully affect consumer choice and action. Alternatively, businesses may absorb the cost of liability, usually passing the cost on to consumers in the form of price increases. Price increases can reduce demand, particularly for young people, as the experience with cigarettes demonstrates.

Businesses are likely to adjust their behavior in response to legal norms, particularly if economic costs are associated with noncompliance. It matters to a business whether it must bear the cost of environmental damage or personal injury; an enterprise will weigh litigation and liability costs in deciding whether to emit a toxin or design a safer product. The tort system, then, can be a potent form of regulation because it imposes costs on individuals and businesses if they engage in risky behavior.

Perhaps the single greatest limitation of traditional tort law in advancing the public's health is the concept of fault under the negligence theory. It is not usually a problem to demonstrate that industry acts unreasonably when selling unsafe products or engaging in high-risk activities. The real difficulty arises from the notion that individuals contribute to their ill health through their own behavior. Two defenses in negligence actions can be fatal to public health.

The first defense, assumption of risk, holds that if individuals are aware of the risk, but nonetheless engage in the activity, they cannot recover. In numerous situations, individuals understand the risks that they face in smoking cigarettes, drinking alcoholic beverages, or purchasing and using a firearm. In these circumstances, it may be easy for industry to point the finger of blame at the consumer herself, suggesting she is responsible for her own condition. In thinking about assumption of risk, government-imposed labeling and disclosure requirements actually may be helpful to industry. For example, alcoholic beverage manufacturers can rely on government health warnings to resist liability. After all, they will argue, the dangers of the product were prominent on the product package and advertising, so the consumer must accept responsibility for her own behavior.

The second defense, contributory or comparative negligence, holds that a damage award can be reduced, or eliminated, if the plaintiff's negligence contributed to a portion of the injury or disease she suffered. The contributory negligence defense allows industry to assert that the plaintiff's ill health was a product of her own lack of due care. A person who continues to smoke after she experiences extreme breathing difficulties, or drinks excessively after experiencing liver damage, may be easily portrayed as acting unreasonably. Similarly, a person who stores her firearm without a lock and within reach of children, will be seen as lacking common sense. In all these cases, and many more, businesses seek to transfer responsibility in the mind of the jury from themselves to consumers. In this way, industry can argue that the harm results not from its own negligence in the design and marketing of a dangerous product, but from the irresponsible behavior of the user of the product.

The skillful use of assumption of risk and comparative negligence by manufacturers sometimes can appear to be ruinous to public health strategies in tort law. However, upon more careful reflection, in a counterintuitive way, these limitations of tort doctrine may help gather support for limiting health threats that appear to be self-imposed.[117] Because of these limitations, plaintiffs must frame their arguments in terms that make the threat seem to be inflicted from without, rather than from within. This is one important reason tobacco, and now firearm, litigation has finally adopted the device of having governments, rather than injured consumers, sue for damages.

In any event, defenses in negligence actions, such as assumption of risk and comparative negligence, give a major incentive to plaintiffs and public health advocates to reframe the debate in a way that makes what once was a quintessentially voluntary risk, such as smoking or drinking alcoholic beverages, seem ambiguous at best, if not outright involuntary. Thus, public health threats that seem to be self-inflicted become more a matter of industry's efforts to mislead, cajole, and reassure the public;[118] sometimes consumers can point to the product's addictive qualities, as with alcoholic beverages or tobacco. This kind of thinking paves the way for public understanding of the true nature of risk and responsibility in tobacco, alcoholic beverages, firearms, and other major health threats. Similarly, it can be helpful in legislative and agency responses that, like tort doctrine itself, have also resisted regulation of perceived self-inflicted harms.

To illustrate the public health value of tort law, I present two case studies—one on tobacco and the other on firearm litigation. In these case studies, it is interesting to see how public health strategies have shifted over time to overcome the nagging problem of personal blame and responsibility.

"THE TOBACCO WARS": A CASE STUDY

Who are these persons who knowingly and secretly
decide to put the buying public at risk solely for the
purpose of making profits and who believe that illness
and death of consumers is an appropriate cost of their

own prosperity? As the following facts disclose,
despite some rising pretenders, the tobacco industry
may be the king of concealment and disinformation.

Dolores K. Sloviter (1992)

In the early 1950s, before the first lawsuit against the tobacco industry
was filed, the cigarette was a cultural icon—tobacco smoking was chic,
promoted ubiquitously, and portrayed by sports and movie stars as an
accouterment of a good life. Epidemiologists, however, were already reporting an association between cigarettes and cancer,[119] and these data
were soon published in the popular media.[120] The first tobacco lawsuit
was filed in 1954,[121] initiating what torts scholar Robert Rabin called
the first wave of tobacco litigation.[122] During this first wave from 1954
to 1973, approximately 100–150 cases were filed; very few of these
cases ever came to trial and in no case did a plaintiff prevail over the
tobacco industry (see Figure 24).[123]

The first wave of cases was filed principally under theories of negligence, breach of warranty, and misrepresentation.[124] In retrospect, it is
surprising that tobacco litigation was so unsuccessful. At that time,
plaintiffs could not voluntarily assume the risks because they began
smoking without knowledge of the harmful effects. The misrepresentation claims, moreover, appeared powerful since industry advertisements
trumpeted product safety: "Play Safe, Smoke Chesterfield. Nose,
throat, and accessory organs not adversely affected" (1952); and
"More doctors smoke Camels than any other cigarette" (1955).
Epidemiologists also were solving the problems of causation, culminat-
ing in Luther Terry's landmark Surgeon General's Report on Smoking
in 1964.[125] Ironically, around the same time the Surgeon General's
Report so influenced science and the public, the American Law Institute
(ALI) all but absolved the tobacco industry from strict products liability. In the Restatement (Second) of Torts, the ALI stated that "[g]ood
tobacco is not unreasonably dangerous merely because the effects of
smoking may be harmful."[126]

By the time of the second wave of litigation from 1983 to 1992, cigarette smoking was beginning to become a hallmark not of elegance,
but of weak character and lower social class. The public had become
far more health conscious, and cigarettes were thought to be a highly
dangerous product. This new health consciousness was both a blessing
and a curse for litigants. While problems of causation were reduced,
plaintiffs could no longer claim ignorance of the health risks. Instead,

1954	Lowe v. R.J. Reynolds	First suit filed by a smoker against cigarette companies for smoking-related injuries.
1963	Lartigue v. R.J. Reynolds	Court finds that "[cigarette] manufacturers are not insurers against unknowable risks." Tobacco industry found not liable.
1967	Pritchard v. Liggett & Meyers	Tobacco industry convinces jury that plaintiffs assume risks of smoking despite misleading advertisements.
1970	Green v. American Tobacco	Court finds that asserting "unwholesomeness of standardized product line" is legally insufficient for breach of warranty claim. Major ruling for tobacco industry.
1992	Cipollone v. Liggett Group	After eight years of litigation, jury awards the plaintiff's estate $400,000 for cigarette-related illness–the first damage award against the industry. On appeal, the U.S. Supreme Court holds that the federal cigarette labeling act preempts negligence, but not fraud, claims against the industry.
1994	Tobacco Papers	Disclosure of evidence that tobacco companies knew of health risks and conspired to conceal information.
1997	Medicaid settlements	Texas, Mississippi, and Florida attorneys general reach settlements for Medicaid medical cost reimbursement.
1998	Master settlement agreement	Forty-six states and tobacco companies reach $206 billion settlement.
1999	Broin v. Philip Morris Co.	Flight attendants sue for exposure to secondhand smoke. Tobacco companies settle.
1999	Individual suits	Several plaintiffs in Oregon, California, and Florida obtain large verdicts against cigarette manufacturers for tobacco-related illnesses.
1999	Federal government lawsuit	Department of Justice files civil action against tobacco companies for Medicare cost reimbursement.
1999	Engle v. R.J. Reynolds	All Florida smokers addicted to cigarettes and suffering from certain conditions allowed to file claims.
2000	Engle v. R.J. Reynolds	First jury verdict for class action against tobacco companies.

Figure 24.   "The tobacco wars": a time line.

defense counsel portrayed plaintiffs as morally responsible for their own illness. Individuals, after all, made their own choice to smoke, fully apprised of the risks. Federal antitobacco regulation, moreover, was used by the industry as a shield against litigation. The Cigarette Labeling and Advertising Act, enacted in 1965, required warning labels on cigarette packages.[127] Defense counsel could point to those warnings as nearly definitive evidence that plaintiffs were informed of the risks.

During this second wave of litigation, nearly 200 cases were filed, many under new theories of failure to warn and strict liability.[128] This was a time when litigants were making stunning advances in mass torts cases ranging from Agent Orange and DES to the Dalkon Shield and Bendectin. One would have thought that if any product would fare badly under the "risk utility" analysis in this era of mass torts, it would be cigarettes—this product caused more illness and death than any other in American history, and its effects were disproportionately borne by young people, ethnic minorities, and the poor. Nevertheless, despite marked changes in science, tort theory, and social attitudes, the results were the same. It was not until 1990 that a New Jersey jury awarded damages of $400,000 to the estate of Rose Cipollone, a smoker who died of cancer at the age of 58. The jury verdict (which was overturned on appeal) was the first in the history of the extensive tobacco litigation in which a plaintiff was awarded damages.[129] To understand why the industry was so successful, it is important to examine its tactics.

"KING OF THE MOUNTAIN": INDUSTRY TACTICS IN THE TOBACCO WARS

[The industry has prevailed] by resisting all discovery, thus requiring a court hearing before plaintiffs can obtain even the most rudimentary discovery . . . by getting confidentiality orders attached to the discovery materials they finally produce, thus preventing plain- tiffs' counsel from sharing the fruits of discovery and forcing each plaintiff to reinvent the wheel . . . by taking exceedingly lengthy depositions and naming multiple experts of their own for each specialty, thereby putting plaintiffs' counsel [to inordinate expense] . . . [and] by taking dozens and dozens of oral depositions, all across the country, of trivial fact witnesses.

  William E. Townsley and Dale K. Hanks (1989)

The aggressive posture we [the tobacco companies] have taken regarding depositions and discovery in general continues to make these cases extremely burdensome and expensive for plaintiffs' lawyers. . . . To

paraphrase General Patton, the way we won these cases
was not by spending all of [R.J. Reynold's] money, but
by making that other son of a bitch spend all his.

                                        J. Michael Jordan (1993)

The tobacco industry resorted to an unusual but highly effective strategy
during the first two waves of tobacco litigation—aggressive and uncom-
promising litigation.[130] First, the industry was relentless in pretrial maneu-
vering, intending to deplete plaintiffs' resources and to delay the trial end-
lessly. Since plaintiffs' lawyers were characteristically situated in small firms
and practiced on a contingency basis, they could not cope with the large
up-front expenses preceding a trial. The industry adopted a conscious policy of devoting inexhaustible resources, never settling a case, and always
fighting to the bitter end. For example, the *Cipollone* case produced twelve
federal opinions and cost the plaintiff's attorneys roughly $4 million; the at-
torneys withdrew from the case before it went to trial a second time.[131]
Second, the industry adopted a "no-holds-barred" defense in which it
would probe the moral habits of the plaintiff, urging juries to find personal
blameworthiness. Since risks of cancer and heart disease unfold over
decades, it was easy for defense counsel to examine every possible behavioral risk factor. What was intended to be a sober adjudication of corporate responsibility became a searching examination of the plaintiff's morality. Finally, the industry consistently disputed the health risks. A 1972
memorandum outlined the industry's strategy of "creating doubt about the
health charge without actually denying it; and advocating the public's right
to smoke without actually urging them to take up the practice."[132]

THE PREEMPTION BATTLE: THE CIGARETTE
LABELING ACT AND ROSE CIPOLLONE

The Cigarette Labeling and Advertising Act of 1965,[133] as amended in
1969,[134] preempts state regulation based on "smoking and health."
Following Rose Cipollone's jury verdict, the Supreme Court granted
certiorari, setting the stage for the landmark decision in *Cipollone v.
Liggett Group, Incorporated* (1992).[135] Justice John Paul Stevens, in a
plurality decision, held that the 1969 Act preempts tort claims based on
"failure to warn and the neutralization of federally mandated warnings
to the extent that those claims rely on omissions or inclusions in the
[manufacturers'] advertising or promotions." However, the act does
not preempt tort claims based on express warranty, intentional fraud

and misrepresentation, or conspiracy.[136] The Supreme Court's decision left ample room for tobacco litigation based on theories of misinformation and deceit. During the third wave, plaintiffs succeeded in ways that scarcely could have been imagined.

MEDICAL COST REIMBURSEMENT AND CLASS ACTIONS: THE "THIRD WAVE" OF TOBACCO LITIGATION

The third wave did not begin quietly. On May 12, 1994, a paralegal at the law firm representing Brown and Williamson Tobacco delivered over 10,000 pages of internal industry documents to Professor Stanton Glantz at the University of California, San Francisco. The "Tobacco Papers" contained damaging evidence about the tobacco industry's actual knowledge and intent.[137] Despite the industry's public claims, the Tobacco Papers demonstrated that executives understood the health effects of smoking, the addictive quality of nicotine, and the toxicity of pesticides contained in cigarettes. The industry, moreover, manipulated the nicotine content of cigarettes and marketed their products to young persons. These documents, and others obtained through press reports[138] and discovery,[139] would be used with great effect in the ensuing litigation—notably medical cost reimbursement, class actions, and individual smoker lawsuits.

Medical cost reimbursement became a dominant theme in the third wave. State attorneys general filed direct claims against the tobacco industry for reimbursement of public money that had been spent to pay for tobacco-related illness. Following the original Medicaid reimbursement suit filed in Mississippi in 1994,[140] most states joined the litigation. On June 20, 1997, the tobacco industry and the attorneys general ended their negotiations and presented a settlement that required Congress to grant the industry immunity from certain forms of litigation. In exchange, the states would receive $368 billion over twenty-five years. However, federal attempts to codify the settlement ultimately failed. For example, a bill sponsored by Senator John McCain would have increased the tax on cigarettes, raised the settlement amount, and altered the civil immunity provisions.[141] As a result, RJR-Nabisco withdrew support for federal tobacco legislation, and the bill died in committee.

In the wake of federal failure, four states (Florida, Minnesota, Mississippi, and Texas) settled with the tobacco industry for a total of $40 billion.[142] As the cost of individual settlements mounted, the industry negotiated a Master Settlement Agreement with forty-six states and six U.S. territories. The agreement, concluded on November 16, 1998, requires industry to compensate states in perpetuity, with payments totaling $206 billion through the year 2025; creates a charitable foundation to reduce adolescent smoking; disbands the Council for Tobacco Research; provides public access to documents through the Internet; and restricts outdoor advertising, the use of cartoon characters, tobacco merchandising, and sponsorship of sporting events. The industry received civil immunity for future state claims, but not for individual or class action lawsuits.[143]

The success of state attorneys general has encouraged other groups to seek medical expense reimbursement, notably the federal government for recoupment of Medicare costs,[144] union health funds to recover money spent to treat smoking-related disease,[145] and even foreign countries to obtain costs expended by their public health care systems.[146] Perhaps the most unusual plaintiffs are bankrupt asbestos companies, which had been found liable for causing lung cancer in workers. These companies are suing the tobacco industry for contributions to the lung cancer burden that juries attributed solely to asbestos.[147]

Tobacco litigants have adopted a strategy of class action litigation. In 1994, nonsmoking flight attendants filed a class action against tobacco manufacturers alleging that they suffered injuries caused by inhalation of secondhand smoke in airplane cabins. The judiciary certified the class,[148] and the parties reached a settlement for a $300 million medical foundation; the settlement permits individual lawsuits.[149] On April 7, 2000, a jury awarded compensatory damages to three Florida smokers in the first class action verdict.[150]

The judiciary, however, has thus far thwarted the most ambitious class actions. For example, in *Castano v. American Tobacco Company* (1996),[151] the court decertified a class of all nicotine-dependent smokers in the United States because variations in state law would render the class impracticable. Plaintiffs' attorneys promised to bring state-by-state class actions,[152] but some courts have refused to certify state classes.[153]

The tobacco industry also faces litigation from individual smokers in the third wave. Plaintiffs in Florida,[154] Oregon,[155] and California[156] have won substantial verdicts, and numerous individual suits are pending.[157] With the formation of the Tobacco Trial Lawyers Association (a network that shares information, expert witnesses, and tactics), stricter judicial case management, and new rules regarding work-product discovery,[158] individual lawsuits may emerge as a force in the tobacco wars.[159]

The tobacco wars have been a stunning, and highly unexpected, public health success. Considering that numerous tobacco suits over several decades failed to clear the obstacle of smoker responsibility, the global settlement is a remarkable achievement. The result of the cash settlement will certainly increase the price of cigarettes, thus decreasing consumer demand. Additionally, the voluntary ban on outdoor advertisements, cartoon characters, merchandising, and sports sponsorship will reduce the omnipresent images of tobacco in American culture.

Despite the undeniable benefits of the litigation, the victory is tarnished in several respects. First, the financial settlement offered a missed opportunity for investment in smoking prevention; experience with the fairness doctrine shows that counter-advertising is a highly effective technique.[160] Unfortunately, the states have used the discretionary funds primarily for general education, social programs, tax relief, and other political priorities.[161] Second, disbanding the Council for Tobacco Research actually may be advantageous to the industry. The Council had become a vehicle for discovering harms from tobacco use and, eventually, industry concealment of those harms, which rebounded to its disadvantage. Thirdly, advertising restrictions still permit ample scope for creative industry promotion of its product in multiple fora accessible to young people.

Perhaps the most important effect of tobacco litigation was to transform public and political perceptions about risk and responsibility in smoking, making clear what manufacturers knew, how they concealed this knowledge, and how they manipulated consumers. Far-reaching tobacco legislation in the aftermath of the settlement seemed achievable, but ultimately failed. Here we have a case where tort law reframed the debate from personal to corporate responsibility; yet the industry managed, at least in the political realm, to alter the discourse to one involving freedom of choice for the smoker, evils of "big government" regulation, and unfair taxation.

TORT LITIGATION TO PREVENT FIREARM INJURIES: A CASE STUDY

A gun is an article that is typically and characteristically
dangerous; the use for which it is manufactured and
sold is a dangerous one, and the law reasonably may

presume that such an article is always dangerous. . . .
In addition, the display of a gun instills fear in the
average citizen; as a consequence, it creates an
immediate danger that a violent response will ensue.

John Paul Stevens (1986)

Firearms are pervasive in the United States and are a major cause of
morbidity and mortality.[162] Private citizens own approximately 200
million firearms, and 41 percent of all households contain a firearm.[163]
In 1997, over 32,000 deaths were associated with firearms in the
United States, with twice as many nonfatal injuries requiring emergency
care.[164] Firearm injuries particularly affect young persons (mainly
homicides) and the elderly (mainly suicides).[165] Firearm injuries are
also borne disproportionately by African-American males, who incur
such injuries at four times the rate of the U.S. population.[166] The public health burden of firearms is much greater in the United States than
in comparable societies. For example, the firearm death rate for U.S.
children is nearly twelve times higher than in twenty-five industrialized
countries combined.[167]

Tort law provides a tool to help prevent many of the injuries and
deaths due to firearms. Tort theorists might ask two related questions.
From a public health perspective, which party could most effectively
prevent these injuries and deaths? From a justice perspective, which
party is best able to suffer the loss—manufacturer, retailer, owner,
shooter, or victim? (See Figure 25.)

The shooter could reduce harm by exercising greater care, but many
shooters are children and/or suffer self-inflicted wounds. In any case,
courts already impose liability in negligence on adults for the unintentional discharge of a firearm causing injury—a very high degree of care
is required because a firearm is a dangerous instrument.[168] Victims usually are not in a position to avoid harm and are perhaps least able to
absorb the loss.

Firearm manufacturers, retailers, and owners are in the best position to
prevent harm and should be held accountable in civil litigation for gun-
related morbidity and mortality.[169] Firearm sellers can reduce risks by taking care to sell only to lawful and responsible customers. The law holds
firearm sellers liable under a theory of "negligent entrustment."[170] Thus,
retailers have been found liable for the sale of a weapon to a person who
is, or reasonably should be, known to be mentally ill, intoxicated, or underage.[171] This doctrine could be usefully extended to sales to "straw"

1971	Reida v. Lund	Father negligent for keeping gun locked in case, when child knew location of key.
1983	Mavilia v. Stoeger Industries	Risk-utility analysis could not be applied to firearms.
1985	Perkins v. F. I. E. Corp.	Strict liability theory is not applicable because dangers of guns are obvious and well known.
1985	Kelley v. R.G. Industries Inc.	Manufacturer strictly liable for injuries from a Saturday Night Special (ruling later overturned by legislation).
1996	Hamilton v. ACCU-Tek	First jury finds manufacturers liable for negligently creating market that foreseeably put handguns into hands of criminals.
1997	Kitchen v. K-Mart Corp.	K-Mart, the seller of the firearm, is liable to an injured party for selling a gun to an intoxicated buyer.
1998	Morial v. Smith & Wesson	New Orleans becomes first city to sue gun industry to recover costs of gun-related violence.
1998	Chicago v. Beretta U.S.A. Corp.	Chicago sues gun industry, claiming that the industry marketed guns illegally to criminals.
1999	NAACP v. American Arms Inc.	NAACP files suit against manufacturers, claiming negligent marketing to persons of color and negligent distribution to criminals.
1999	Cincinnati v. American Arms Inc.	Court dismisses Cincinnati suit against the gun industry, holding that "public nuisance does not apply to the design, manufacture, and distribution of a lawful product."
1999	City lawsuits increase	As of October 1999, twenty-eight cities and counties have filed suit against the gun industry under products liability, public nuisance, and negligent marketing theories.

Figure 25. Firearms in the courts: a time line.

purchasers who buy guns for disqualified persons such as juveniles or felons or for mass distribution to supply the criminal market.[172]

Gun owners can reduce risks by taking care to store guns safely[173]— unloaded and in a locked area separate from ammunition so that they cannot be accessed by children or other unauthorized users.[174] Yet, many owners—even those with children[175]—store guns loaded and/or unlocked.[176] Several states have enacted child access prevention statutes that render gun owners criminally responsible for unsafe storage.[177] Other states, under the same theory of "negligent entrustment" applied to retailers,[178] impose liability if a child gains access to, and uses, a carelessly stored firearm.[179] The one party that has effectively escaped tort liability is the entity best able to abate harm and absorb loss—the manufacturer.

TORT LIABILITY FOR FIREARM MANUFACTURERS:
"DANGEROUS BY DESIGN"

Injury prevention programs often achieve the greatest success when they focus on safer product design rather than on safer operation. While human behavior is difficult to control, manufacturers can create products that reduce injuries.[180] The design of firearms contributes significantly to unintentional injuries and deaths.[181] Injury control experts regard at least three design features to be unsafe:[182] (1) trigger devices sufficiently easy to pull so that young children can operate them, (2) no reliable indication of whether a round of ammunition is in the firing chamber, and (3) the universal ability of unauthorized users to operate the firearm. Readily achievable alternative designs could make firearms safer, including stiffer trigger devices, trigger locks, loaded-chamber indicators, and personalized guns that can be discharged only by an authorized user.[183] Additionally, certain weapons appear to be designed to deliver mass injuries, such as those that permit fully automatic firing.[184]

Despite the public health benefits of better design (apart from manufacturing defects, such as an exploding gun barrel,[185] and manufacturer mistakes, such as shipping a loaded gun[186]), the judiciary has strongly resisted indirect regulation of firearm producers through the tort system. Plaintiffs have sought liability under theories of design defect, failure to warn, and ultra-hazardous activities. While it will be difficult to prevail on these legal theories, I will show that good reasons exist for holding manufacturers liable.

Most firearm design defect cases fail.[187] Courts often find that consumers have a "reasonable expectation" that firearms will be dangerous.[188] Courts have concluded that firearm risks, for the most part, are open and obvious, and consumers do not require expert knowledge to assess the risks.[189] Firearms, moreover, are in "common use"—if they are functioning properly, they may be exempt from strict liability based on the theory that they are "good" (well-made) guns.[190] In addition, the courts have not found that the "risk-utility" theory affords a basis for strict liability.[191] Finally, problems of causation exist but are not insurmountable. Although violence through firearm use is foreseeable,[192] the chain of causation may be broken by an intervening intentional or criminal act. (However a California appellate court was the first to find that a manufacturer had a duty of care to persons injured by the criminal misuse of its product.[193])

Despite judicial reluctance, firearm manufacturers should be vulnerable to design defect claims that "reasonable alternatives" exist.[194] As discussed above, firearms present inherent risks of serious injury, and existing technology can reduce those risks without undue costs or interference with product performance. If they chose to look, courts could find ample evidence of an unfavorable risk-utility balance: certain firearms have little usefulness for recreation or self-defense and pose inordinate risks, and alternative firearms exist to serve acceptable societal purposes. Judges may believe that, due to the contentious nature of the firearms debate in America, legislative rather than judicial resolution is preferable. However, theories of democracy did not stop courts from imposing liability on manufacturers of other potentially dangerous products. Tort liability, therefore, can become part of a comprehensive strategy for reducing firearm violence.[195]

Most firearm marketing defect cases fail as well.[196] Nevertheless, "failure to warn," "misrepresentation," and "oversupplying the market" theories are intriguing and could potentially succeed. Advertising campaigns encourage consumers to purchase guns to protect their person and property,[197] despite evidence that handguns possessed in homes result in increased risk of homicide and suicide.[198] Further, some advertising appears to be directed toward criminal activity (e.g., promoting small size, easy concealment, and "resistance to fingerprints"). Finally, marketing and distribution practices may be calculated to saturate the lawful market, creating a reservoir of handguns for criminals. For example, a Brooklyn jury found manufacturers liable for negligently oversupplying the market, rendering it easier to obtain guns in New York City.[199]

Commentators have argued effectively that firearm manufacturers should be held strictly liable because they are engaged in an "ultrahazardous" activity.[200] The courts, however, have rejected this doctrine because firearms are products rather than activities; their use, rather than manufacture, is dangerous; and firearm manufacture and distribution are prevalent, which implicates the "common usage" principle.[201] Despite the judicial reticence, many of the arguments supporting the "abnormally dangerous activity" doctrine apply to firearms: they pose a high risk of serious harm, the risk cannot be eliminated by the exercise of due care, and the activity's danger is great compared with its value to the community.

MUNICIPAL TORT ACTIONS AGAINST THE FIREARM INDUSTRY

The burdens imposed by firearms are not borne solely by individuals and families, but also by the body politic. Government incurs billions of dollars in costs annually from firearm violence, including medical care, emergency systems, public health services, law enforcement, the court system, and prisons.[202] Much of these costs are borne by urban communities.[203] As a result, more than thirty cities have filed, or intend to file, tort actions against the gun industry.[204]

The city lawsuits proceed on different theories of recovery. In *Morial v. Smith & Wesson*,[205] New Orleans is suing the gun industry under a products liability theory: design defects (i.e., failure to produce guns with safety devices) and marketing defects (i.e., failure to warn about risks and failure to issue adequate safety instructions).

In *Chicago v. Beretta U.S.A. Corporation*,[206] the city is suing under a public nuisance theory,[207] claiming that industry marketing practices are calculated to move firearms from the legal marketplace into the possession of criminals:[208] manufacturers circumvent Chicago's gun control ordinance by oversupplying handguns in surrounding jurisdictions, failing to set standards for retailers to prevent unlawful sales, and designing and marketing guns that are attractive to criminals.

Firearm litigation, like that for tobacco, is premised on the theory that the industry has made conscious choices that increase injury and death, particularly among children: design innovation focused on firepower rather than safety, distribution that indirectly supplies criminal markets, production of rapid-fire weapons with no legitimate use in recreation or self-defense, and promotion of guns in homes without disclosure of risks to families.[209]

In 2000, Smith & Wesson, the largest gun manufacturer in the United States, agreed to a settlement in the municipal lawsuits. The company agreed, inter alia, to include child safety locks, ensure background checks at retail stores and gun shows, and take so-called ballistic fingerprints of its guns. [210]

Private and public lawsuits could create incentive systems to encourage safer practice. Tort liability would render it less expensive to redesign firearms than to defend personal injury and wrongful-death cases. Gun producers would carry insurance to cover tort costs, to spread the loss, and to add a third party interested in prevention. Tort liability would also raise prices, which would reduce demand for firearms. Finally, tort actions would raise public attention to the relationship between industry practices and personal safety.[211]

Whether tort law can achieve all of these public health goals is uncertain. Firearm litigation is still languishing in the terrain of personal responsibility—the pernicious idea that it is not the manufacturer of the gun that kills, but rather the shooter. It is in this regard that the emerging tort strategy of municipal lawsuits against the firearm industry has advantages over individual tort actions.[212] Cities have the resources to engage in mass litigation and seek damages incurred collectively by taxpayers. Furthermore, a manufacturer cannot attribute blame for firearm violence to cities the way it can to those who purchase and use guns. Finally, discovery powers in civil litigation may provide needed evidence about the industry's intentions in design, promotion, and distribution.

Tort law appears to offer the best, and perhaps only, hope of serious safety regulation of firearms. Despite the benefits of safer firearm design and public support for innovative programs,[213] Congress has expressly removed firearms from the jurisdiction of the Consumer Products Safety Commission.[214] The resistance to change by the political organs of government is also apparent in the failure to enact major gun control legislation in the aftermath of mass shootings in schools and other communities (although at least one attorney general has used the state's unfair and deceptive trade practices statute to regulate the safety and performance of handguns[215]). State legislatures have even tried to thwart tort litigation by forbidding localities from bringing suit against firearm manufacturers, trade associations, or dealers.[216]

Like tobacco companies, the firearms industry has managed to frame the debate as one involving personal freedom and the burdens of governmental regulation. If there is fault, according to the industry, it lies in a violent society and purposeful, or at least negligent, mishandling of firearms. However, this attribution of risk to personal behavior can go only so far. In countless other areas, such as motor vehicles and consumer products, public health research has demonstrated that injuries are best prevented by safer product design. In the end, tort law offers at least the possibility that industry behavior can be shifted in the direction of safer design, marketing, and sale of firearms.

THE LIMITATIONS OF TORT LAW: SOCIAL AND ECONOMIC COSTS

I have devoted the entire chapter to the idea that tort law is an important vehicle for advancing the public's health. However, I do not want to leave the impression that the tort system achieves only socially desirable results. Tort costs (liability and litigation expenses) have potentially detrimental effects that warrant consideration.

Economic Burdens. Tort costs, as explained earlier, must be absorbed by the enterprise, which will often pass the costs onto its employees or consumers through loss of employment (or loss of benefits of employment, such as wages and health insurance) and/or higher prices. Since socioeconomic status has important health effects,[217] lower employment or wages and higher consumer prices are important from a public health perspective. The advantages of deterrence, therefore, have to be weighed against the adverse effects on employment and prices. Imposing costs on a polluter or the supplier of an unsafe product may appear to be an unmitigated public good, but it does entail social cost.

Penalizing Business Judgment. Suppose that the enterprise does not pass on tort costs, but rather redesigns its products to avoid potential hazards. I have depicted this kind of redesign as clearly beneficial, but this is not inevitably the case. Businesses may forgo product features that are attractive, convenient, and offer better value for consumers in exchange for relatively small safety advantages. Certainly, safety is a fundamental public good, but it is not the only good.

Overdeterrence and Stifled Innovation. Tort costs may be, or may be perceived to be,[218] so high that businesses do not enter the market, leave the market, or curtail research and development. Society, it may be argued, would not be any poorer if tort costs made it difficult for dangerous, socially unproductive enterprises (e.g., tobacco and firearms) to operate within the market. Tort costs, however, appear to be just as high for socially advantageous goods and services. While it is in society's interest to encourage safety in the production of health-related products and services, overdeterrence may result in less investment. It matters to society if industry cuts back on the research or marketing of childhood vaccines[219] or prescription drugs.[220] The same may be true of certain medical specialties, such as obstetrics, neurosurgery, and orthopedics, where malpractice insurance costs have potent deterrent effects.[221]

Wrong Incentives. Sometimes the tort system sends the wrong deterrent signal, with the result that behaviors are changed in unintended ways. Consider the effects of medical malpractice litigation. Ideally, the tort system wants to send a signal that physicians should exercise due care to avoid medically induced injury. Physicians, however, sometimes understand the law to be encouraging the practice of defensive medicine (e.g., ordering intrusive diagnostic tests that are not clinically indicated). As a result, patients may have to undergo unnecessary procedures and the health care system incurs unnecessary cost.

These potential adverse consequences do not militate against tort litigation to achieve important public health objectives. However, I do want to make a point that recurs throughout this text and that applies with equal force to tort law: Regulation intended to promote the public interest has personal and economic consequences. Regulation may help solve a particular public health problem, but it can create or exacerbate another problem for individuals or for society at large. The resulting dilemmas—legal, scientific, and ethical—are perplexing but exceedingly important to the study of public health law.[222]

PART THREE

The Future of Public Health Law

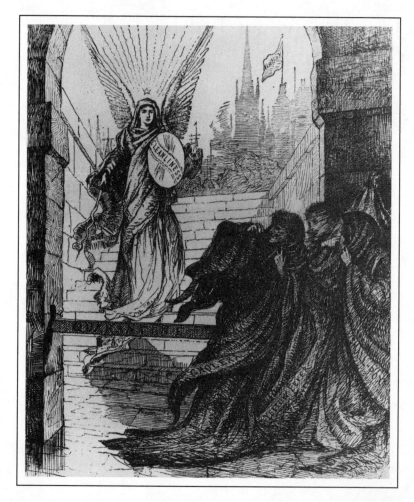

This print, entitled "At the gates—our safety depends on official vigilance," comes from an 1885 issue of Harper's Weekly. The angel holds a shield at the port of New York defending the city against cholera, yellow fever, and smallpox.

11 Public Health Law Reform

> Public health is the science and the art of preventing disease,
> prolonging life, and promoting physical health and efficiency
> through organized community efforts for the sanitation of
> the environment, the control of community infections, the
> education of the individual in principles of personal hygiene,
> the organization of medical and nursing service for the early
> diagnosis and preventive treatment of disease, and . . .
> organizing these benefits in such fashion as to enable every
> citizen to realize his birthright of health and longevity.
>
> *Charles-Edward Winslow (1920)*

Public health typically is regarded as a scientific pursuit and, undoubtedly, our understanding of the etiology and response to disease is heavily influenced by scientific inquiry. Nonetheless, this book has been devoted to the core idea that law is essential for creating the conditions for people to lead healthier lives. Law creates a mission for public health authorities, assigns their functions, and specifies the manner in which they may exercise their authority. The law is a tool in public health work, which is used to influence norms for healthy behavior, identify and respond to health threats, and set and enforce health and safety standards. The most important social debates about public health take place in legal fora—legislatures, courts, and administrative agencies—and in the law's language of rights, duties, and justice. It is no exaggeration to say that "the field of public health . . . could not long exist in the manner in which we know it today except for its sound legal basis."[1]

The Institute of Medicine (IOM), in its foundational 1988 report, *The Future of Public Health,* acknowledged that law was essential to public health, but cast serious doubt on the soundness of public health's legal basis. Concluding that "this nation has lost sight of its public health goals and has allowed the system of public health activities to fall into disarray," the IOM placed some of the blame on an obsolete and inadequate body of enabling laws and regulations.[2] The IOM recommended that "states review their public health statutes and make revisions necessary to accomplish the following two objectives: [i] clearly delineate the basic authority and responsibility entrusted to public health agencies, boards, and officials at the state and local levels and the relationship between them; and [ii] support a set of modern disease control measures that address contemporary health problems such as AIDS, cancer, and heart disease, and incorporate due process safeguards (notice, hearings, administrative review, right to counsel, standards of evidence)."[3]

This chapter responds to the IOM's critique of public health law and offers guidelines for law reform.[4] The frankly utilitarian premise adopted is that public health law ought to be as effective as possible in helping agencies to create the conditions necessary for the health of the populace. To do this, the law should reflect our best understanding of how agencies work to promote health, as well as the political and financial constraints under which they operate. Public health laws should also be consistent with prevailing legal standards and social norms.

This final chapter, therefore, provides a subjective account of the field of public health and makes proposals for the future. First, I explore the inherent problems in public health practice: politics and money, leadership and jurisdiction, and legitimacy and trust. Next, I discuss three concepts of public health and liberty: the power to regulate, limits on regulatory power, and positive promotion of health and social status. Finally, I propose guidelines for law reform: consistency and uniformity of approach, mission and essential functions, powers, substantive limits, procedural limits, and protection against discrimination and invasion of privacy.

It is important to emphasize that no single model of law reform is likely to fit the entire spectrum of public health ranging from the regulation of food, drugs, and the water supply to the workplace, environment, and infectious diseases. The proposed guidelines, therefore, represent general themes important to good governance of public health agencies engaged in a variety of public health activities.

THE INHERENT PROBLEMS OF PUBLIC HEALTH

The essential job of public health authorities is to identify what makes people healthy and what makes them sick, and then to take the steps necessary to make sure that the population encounters a maximum of the former and a minimum of the latter. At first glance, this would seem to be uncontroversial, but the pursuit of public health creates fundamental social and political disputes almost by definition. Public health is rooted in the biomedical and social sciences, but from the moment of asserting some collective responsibility for the population's health, authorities have to manage a complex political process and operate with finite resources. Public health authorities, in particular, confront inherent problems concerning politics and money, leadership and jurisdiction, and legitimacy and trust. These are not barriers to good public health that somehow can be overcome by law reform. They are, rather, unavoidable conditions of public health, conditions with which authorities must find ways to cope to achieve the gains in health that are possible in an imperfect political, social, and economic environment.

PUBLIC HEALTH, POLITICS, AND MONEY

From my perspective, as a White House official watching
the budgetary process, and subsequently as head first of
a health care financing agency and then of a public
health agency, I was continually amazed to watch as
billions of dollars were allocated to financing medical
care with little discussion, whereas endless arguments
ensued over a few millions for community prevention
programs. The sums that were the basis for prolonged,
and often futile, budget fights in public health were
treated as rounding errors in the Medicare budget.

William Roper (1994)

The ability of public health authorities to attract support is essential to their success, for, as its daily practice reminds us, public health operates in a world of choices in the allocation of limited resources. The great health officer Hermann Biggs famously remarked that "public health is purchasable,"[5] but because there will always be limits on how much we are willing to buy, public health will turn on allocational decisions. Thus, the field of public health is as inherently political (i.e., concerned with the allocation of resources in society) as it is technological (i.e., concerned with the deployment of professional knowledge of injury and disease).[6]

If the field of public health is essentially political, then one might assume that attracting public and financial support would not be difficult given the undoubted communal benefits of health. However, as William Roper's epigraph illustrates, the condition of public health is one of paradox. Most people support a high level of public health, fewer are eager to pay for it, and many are positively opposed to changing their own activities to promote it. Public health authorities have enormous legal power, yet they often cannot exercise it for political, cultural, or resource reasons. The public cares passionately about health threats, but often in inverse relation to the quantitative magnitude of the risk.[7] The measures that will provide the most societal benefit often provide little or no discernible benefit to any one person, and vice versa.[8] Although there is a virtually bottomless purse for treating illness, it appears there is little in the budget to prevent it or, more generally, to ensure the conditions in which people can be healthy. Overall, the proportion of national health expenditures allocated to population-based public health initiatives is approximately 1 percent.[9]

Even within the relatively modest budgets devoted to public health, hard choices remain. Public health authorities are inevitably faced with the need to divide a small pie among many worthy competitors for resources. Injuries, HIV, emerging infectious diseases, bioterrorism, chronic diseases, and many other health threats are, in some sense, in competition for prevention resources. Difficult decisions must be made about the most effective allocation of funds. Thus, rationing—a controversial notion in medicine—is, in public health, a "moral imperative . . . in the face of scarce resources."[10]

LEADERSHIP AND JURISDICTION

Agencies devoted to improving the public's health face the challenge of explaining why injury, disease prevention and health promotion are important and deserving of policymakers, and the public's support.[11] Effective public health work requires leaders who can win battles in the halls of government. Programs have to be approved by executives and funded by legislators in an environment of scarcity and, often, political polarization. Effective leaders appreciate the process of developing public health initiatives, including the legislative process, as an opportunity to define important health issues and take the lead in solving them. Drafting legislation or regulations provides a chance to gather and build relationships among important stakeholders. Any interaction with legislators is an occasion to get their attention and educate them about public health needs and methods.

Despite its importance, public health scholars and practitioners perceive a crisis in leadership.[12] Although some health department leaders are astute politically and have established their credibility in government and the community, many others view politicians and legislators as unwelcome impediments to effective public health action.[13]

Public health leadership requires planning, collaboration with each of the branches of government, building of popular support, and the capacity to exercise political skill. Public health policy development requires setting priorities for health problems, identifying solutions, and determining who can best implement them. Ideally, public health policy should include long-range planning that forecasts resource needs, maintains the public health infrastructure, and anticipates new health threats.[14] Without long-range planning, health departments may find crises—such as an environmental accident, a disease outbreak, or a new or perceived health risk—driving their priority setting and policymaking. From the leadership point of view, a planning process that includes communities in identifying priorities and fashioning responses is an excellent way to create political support for health programs, quite apart from its benefits in making better programs in the first place.[15] Unfortunately, only a minority of states consistently engage in community planning for public health, and only a handful of health departments are required to do so by law.[16]

Even the most powerful and best-led public health agency could not exercise direct authority over the full range of activities that affect health. Occupational safety, environmental protection, the purity of food and drinking water, and the prevention of violence and injuries are normally the province of other agencies, and much of the behavior that public health authorities try to change (e.g., eating a diet high in fat) is not subject to direct legal regulation at all. Since many of the determinants of health are outside the jurisdiction of health departments, public health authorities, in developing policy, should collaborate with other state agencies (e.g., environmental, agricultural, highway safety, housing, welfare, social services, and law enforcement), community-based organizations (e.g., nongovernmental entities, activists, and persons with disease), the private sector (e.g., business and labor), and academic institutions (e.g., schools of public health, nursing, dentistry, and medicine).

Public health agencies can often accomplish their goals only by instigating and coordinating health-enhancing activities in these spheres.[17] Thus, every health agency faces the challenge of using its expertise and persuasive power to encourage and facilitate others to take actions that are consistent with the goals of public health. The jurisdictional problem, therefore, casts the health agency in the roles of educator and persuader. It also requires the health department to act as an expert for other agencies and to coordinate government policy affecting the population's health.

LEGITIMACY AND TRUST

Public health agencies rely on voluntary cooperation by those at risk and the support of the population at large. Consequently, they must appear credible in the advice they render and trustworthy in their practices. Despite its importance, agencies face a considerable challenge in maintaining public confidence because they are organs of government and because, by necessity, they are engaged in a highly political process.

Public health agencies are fixtures of public administration, part of the structure of government since the earliest times of the Republic.[18] As such, they possess the trappings of government: generalized mistrust, doubts about efficiency, and fear of oppression. If the public perceives health officials as simply the tool of an overreaching government, captured by special interests, their ability to win compliance and support is compromised. Likewise, public health measures become subject to general legal limitations on governmental activity and to prevailing attitudes about the sorts of things government ought to do. Many disputes turn less on public health's goal, which everyone professes to support, and more on the proper scope of government intervention to achieve it.

To maintain legitimacy and trust, public health authorities rely on expert knowledge derived from the sciences of public health. Scientific decisions are thought to be more objective and systematic, and less captive to political ideology. Health officials know that this expertise gives them the authority and the ability to convince. At the same time, health authorities, to be effective, must be willing to embrace and excel in the political process. It is precisely this political involvement that risks weakening the impression of professional neutrality and expertise from which public health officials draw their public credibility.

Winning and maintaining the trust of those at risk of disease and the general public is a precondition for effective public health programs. This helps explain the importance of finding a way to maintain scientific rigor while still engaging effectively in the political process.

THREE CONCEPTS OF PUBLIC HEALTH AND LIBERTY

There is a distinction between negative liberty, that
which the individual must be allowed to enjoy without
state interference, and positive liberty, that which the
state permits by imposing regulations that, by necessity, limit some freedoms in the name of greater liberty
for all. Both kinds of liberty are required for a just
society.

Isaiah Berlin (1959)

A model public health statute should reflect at least three principles—each
is important but, to some extent, conflicts with the others. First, the law
should afford public health authorities ample power to regulate individuals and businesses to achieve the communal benefits of health and security.
This idea of regulatory power is counterintuitive to a civil libertarian, but
natural and instinctive to a sanitarian. The power to regulate is the power
to make people secure in the most important aspect of their lives—health
and well-being. As detailed in chapter 1, individuals cannot exercise civil
or political rights, or enjoy a life full of contentment, without a certain
measure of health. One important way of assuring the health of the community is by giving government adequate powers to regulate. Individuals
acting independently, without organized community activity, cannot assure many of the essential conditions of health. Sound and effective public health statutes, therefore, should afford agencies ample authority to set
standards of health and safety and to assure compliance.

Second, the law should restrain government in the exercise of regulatory
power to achieve the benefits of liberty and freedom in a democracy. This
idea of regulatory restraints is found in most liberal formulations of a good
society. As explained in chapter 4, government must refrain from interference with individual liberty and autonomy unless it has a sound justification. The liberal position holds that doing harm and causing offense to others exhaust the class of adequate reasons for the exercise of governmental
power.[19] Although liberals exclude harm to the person himself (paternalism) as a sufficient justification for regulation, I will assume (for the reasons
given in chapter 4) that certain forms of paternalism that impose minimal
burdens and high benefits can also be justified (e.g., compulsory seat belts,
motorcycle helmets, and water fluoridation). Sound and effective public
health statutes, therefore, should set clear substantive and procedural limits on public health powers to ensure objective and fair decision-making.

Finally, the law should impose duties on government to promote health and social status within the population.[20] Affirmative duties, as explained in chapter 2, are highly controversial and not generally part of the constitutional design. However, there is nothing to stop legislatures from imposing statutory obligations on agencies to perform essential public health functions, nor is there anything to stop legislatures from protecting individuals against threats to their dignity and social status, such as by enacting adequate privacy and antidiscrimination protection. Public health statutes can create expectations that agencies (within reasonable resource limitations) will assure the conditions for public health, while at the same time creating safeguards of privacy and fair treatment.

Sound public health statutes, therefore, should be based on three concepts of health and liberty: (1) adequate regulatory power, (2) appropriate restraints on power, and (3) positive duties to promote the health and social status of the population. As to the first, public health statutes should provide ample authority to regulate for the public's health. This means that public health authorities should have all the power they need, and the flexibility to exercise their professional judgment to prevent injury and disease and promote health. As to the second, public health statutes should set objective standards and ensure fair procedures for the exercise of power. This means that public health regulation should, *inter alia,* be based on a significant risk to the public and that persons subject to regulation should be entitled to procedural due process. As to the third, statutes should set a clear mission for public health agencies, ensure that they perform essential functions, and provide adequate safeguards of privacy and against discrimination. By doing so, public health statutes will recognize and balance effectively each of the three important concepts of public health and liberty.

GUIDELINES FOR PUBLIC HEALTH LAW REFORM

Effective public health protection is technically and politically difficult. Law cannot solve all, or even most, of the challenges facing public health authorities, yet law can become an important part of the ongoing work of creating the conditions necessary for people to live healthier lives. A public health law that contributes to health will, of course, be up to date in the methods of assessment and intervention it authorizes. It will also conform to modern standards of law and prevailing social norms. It should be designed to enhance the reality and the public perception of the health department's rationality, fairness, and responsibility. It should help health agencies overcome the defects of their limited jurisdiction over health threats facing the population. Finally, both a new law and the process of its enactment should provide an opportunity for the health department to challenge the apathy about public health that is all too common both within the government and the population at large.

CREATE MODERN, CONSISTENT, AND UNIFORM PUBLIC HEALTH LAWS

The law relating to public health is scattered across countless statutes and regulations at the state and local level. Problems of antiquity, inconsistency, redundancy, and ambiguity render these laws ineffective, or even counterproductive, in advancing the population's health. In particular, health codes frequently are outdated, built up in layers over different periods of time, and highly fragmented among the fifty states and territories.

Problem of Antiquity. The most striking characteristic of state public health law, and the one that underlies many of its defects, is its overall antiquity. Certainly, some statutes are relatively recent in origin, such as those relating to health threats that became salient in the latter part of the twentieth century (e.g., environmental law). However, a great deal of public health law was framed in the late nineteenth and early to mid-twentieth century and contains elements that are 40 to 100 years old, such as infectious disease law. Old laws are not necessarily bad laws. A well-written statute may remain useful, effective, and constitutional for many decades.

Nevertheless, old public health statutes that have not been substantially altered since their enactment are often outmoded in ways that directly reduce both their effectiveness and their conformity with modern standards. These laws often do not reflect contemporary scientific understandings of injury and disease (e.g., surveillance, prevention, and response) or legal norms for protection of individual rights. Rather, public health laws utilize scientific and legal standards that prevailed at the time they were enacted. Society faces different sorts of risks today and deploys different methods of assessment and intervention. When many of these statutes were written, public health (e.g., epidemiology and biostatistics) and behavioral (e.g., client-centered counseling) sciences were in their infancy. Modern prevention and treatment methods did not exist.

At the same time, many public health laws predate the vast changes in constitutional (e.g., tighter scrutiny and procedural safeguards) and statutory (e.g., disability discrimination) law that have transformed social and legal conceptions of individual rights. Failure to reform these laws may leave public health authorities vulnerable to legal challenge on grounds that they are unconstitutional or that they are preempted by modern federal statutes, such as the Americans with Disabilities Act. Even if state public health law is not challenged in court, public health authorities may feel unsure about applying old legal remedies to new health problems within a very different social milieu.

Problem of Multiple Layers of Law. Related to the problem of antiquity is the problem of multiple layers of law. The law in most states consists of successive layers of statutes and amendments, built up in some cases over 100 years or more in response to existing or perceived health threats. This is particularly troublesome in the area of infectious diseases, which forms a substantial part of state health codes. Because communicable disease laws have been passed piecemeal in response to specific epidemics, they tell the story of the history of disease control in the United States (e.g., smallpox, yellow fever, cholera, tuberculosis, venereal diseases, polio, and AIDS).

Through a process of accretion, the majority of states have come to have several classes of communicable disease law, each with different powers and protections of individual rights: those aimed at traditional STDs (or venereal diseases), including gonorrhea, syphilis, chlamydia, and herpes; those targeted at specific currently or historically pressing diseases, such as tuberculosis and HIV; and those applicable to "communicable" or "contagious" diseases, a residual class of conditions ranging from measles to malaria whose control does not usually seem to raise problematic political or social issues.[21] There are, of course, legitimate reasons to treat some diseases separately. Nevertheless, affording health officials substantially different powers, under different criteria and procedures for different diseases, is more an accident of history than a rational approach to prevention and control.

The disparate legal structure of state public health laws can significantly undermine their effectiveness. Laws enacted piecemeal over time are inconsistent, redundant, and ambiguous. Even the most astute lawyers in public health agencies or offices of the attorney general have difficulty understanding these arcane laws and applying them to contemporary health threats.

Problem of Inconsistency among the States and Territories. Public health laws remain fragmented not only within states but among them. Health codes within the fifty states and territories have evolved independently, leading to profound variation in the structure, substance, and procedures for detecting, controlling, and preventing injury and disease. In fact, statutes and regulations among American jurisdictions vary so significantly in definitions, methods, age, and scope that they defy orderly categorization. Ordinarily a different approach among the states is not a problem and is often perceived as a virtue; an important value of federalism is that states can become laboratories for innovative solutions to challenging health problems. Nevertheless, there may be good reason for greater uniformity among the states in matters of public health. Health threats are rarely confined to single jurisdictions, but pose risks within whole regions or the nation itself. For example, geographic boundaries are largely irrelevant to issues of air or water pollution, disposal of toxic waste, or the spread of infectious diseases. Similarly, a bioterrorism event threatens the nation and is not confined to a single location.

Public health law, therefore, should be reformed so that it conforms with modern scientific and legal standards, is more consistent within and among states, and is more uniform in its approach to different health threats. Rather than making artificial distinctions among diseases, public health interventions should be based primarily on the degree of risk, the cost and efficacy of the response, and the burdens on human rights. A single set of standards and procedures would add needed clarity and coherence to legal regulation, and would reduce the opportunity for politically motivated disputes about how to classify newly emergent health threats.

DEFINE A MISSION AND ESSENTIAL PUBLIC HEALTH FUNCTIONS

State public health statutes should define a cogent mission for the health department and identify a full set of essential public health functions that it should, or must, perform.[22] Broad and well-considered mission statements in state public health statutes are important for organizational, political, and legal reasons. From an organizational perspective, they establish the purposes or goals of public health agencies.[23] By doing so, they inform and influence the activities of government and, perhaps ultimately, the expectations of society about the scope of public health. From a political perspective, mission statements demonstrate a legislative commitment to public health. They also provide a measure of the kinds of activities that are politically sanctioned. When it is acting under a broad mission statement, a public health agency can better justify its decisions to legislators, the governor, and the public. Further, legislative language that explains that public health agencies exist to assure the conditions for population health can provide a mandate for the health department to take the lead within the executive branch in devising strategies for reducing injury and disease. From a legal perspective, courts pay deference to statements of legislative intent, and may permit a broad range of activities consistent with mission statements.[24] Thus, even if the aspirational qualities of mission statements do not produce the desired results, they can help support agency action in courts of law.

Public health statutes that hold agencies responsible for providing essential public health functions support good practice for many of the same reasons. By creating agency duties, the legislature can ensure that the full range of public health services will be available to the population in a given geopolitical area. Researchers, and the agency itself, can also use these essential functions as a way to monitor and evaluate agency performance.[25]

Despite the importance of a defined mission and functions, a Columbia University study found that few state public health statutes define a cogent mission for the health department or identify a full set of essential public health functions.[26] Public health law, therefore, should provide a clear statement of mission and essential public health functions. Figure 26, taken from the Public Health Functions Project (a collaborative effort of the U.S. Public Health Service and national public health organizations), specifies both a proposed mission statement and ten essential public health functions.

PROVIDE A FULL RANGE OF PUBLIC HEALTH POWERS

Voluntary cooperation is the primary way to obtain compliance with public health measures. However, where voluntary strategies fail, public health officials need a full range of powers to assure compliance with health and safety standards. At present, public health officials in many states have the sterile choice of either exercising draconian authority, such as deprivation of liberty, or refraining from any coercion at all. The temptation is either to

Vision:
Healthy People in Healthy Communities

Mission:
Promote Physical and Mental Health and Prevent Disease, Injury, and Disability

Public Health
- Prevents epidemics and the spread of disease
- Protects against environmental hazards
- Prevents injuries
- Promotes and encourages healthy behaviors
- Responds to disasters and assists communities in recovery
- Assures the quality and accessibility of health services

Essential Public Health Services
- Monitor health status to identify community health problems
- Diagnose and investigate health problems and hazards in the community
- Inform, educate, and empower people about health issues
- Mobilize community partnerships to identify and solve health problems
- Develop policies and plans that support individual and community health efforts
- Enforce laws and regulations that protect health and ensure safety
- Link people to needed personal health services and assure the provision of health care when otherwise unavailable
- Assure a competent public health and personal health care workforce
- Evaluate effectiveness, accessibility, and quality of personal and population-based health services
- Research for new insights and innovative solutions to health problems

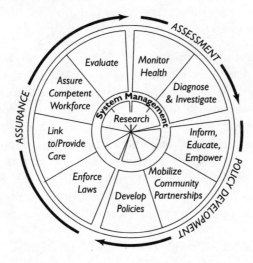

Adopted: Fall 1994, Source: Public Health Functions Steering Committee, Members (July 1995): American Public Health Association, Association of Schools of Public Health, Association of State and Territorial Health Officials, Environmental Council of the States, National Association of County and City Health Officials, National Association of State Alcohol and Drug Abuse Directors, National Association of State Mental Health Program Directors, Public Health Foundation, U.S. Public Health Service—Agency for Health Care Policy and Research, Centers for Disease Control and Prevention, Food and Drug Administration, Health Resources and Services Administration, Indian Health Services, National Institutes of Health, Office of the Assistant Secretary for Health, Substance Abuse and Mental Health Services Administration

Figure 26.   Mission and essential functions of public health.

exercise no statutory power or to reach for measures that are too restrictive of individual liberty to be acceptable in a modern democratic society. As a result, authorities may make wrong choices in two opposite directions: failing to react in the face of a real threat to health or overreacting by exercising powers more intrusive than necessary.

Public health authorities need a more flexible set of tools, ranging from incentives and minimally coercive interventions to highly restrictive measures. Reformed public health statutes should expressly grant agencies the authority to employ a broad variety of measures to encourage and, if necessary to ensure, safer behaviors: traditional prevention strategies (e.g., counseling, education, and health communication campaigns); incentives for behavioral change (e.g., tax breaks, cash allowances, food, transportation, or child care); means for behavioral change (e.g., condoms or sterile drug injection equipment); mandatory attendance for counseling, education, testing, or treatment; directly observed therapy; and outpatient care or treatment in a clinic for STDs, TB, or drug dependency. These less restrictive powers would enable public health authorities to encourage, supervise, and/or control persons who pose a significant health risk without full deprivation of liberty.

IMPOSE SUBSTANTIVE LIMITS ON POWERS: A DEMONSTRATED THREAT OF SIGNIFICANT RISK

While public health authorities should have all the powers they need to safeguard the public's health, statutes should place substantive limits on the exercise of those powers. The legislature should state clearly the circumstances under which authorities may curtail autonomy, privacy, liberty, and property interests. At present, only a few state statutes articulate clear criteria for the exercise of public health powers; others provide vague or incomplete standards; still others leave their use partly or wholly within the discretion of public health officials. Public health authorities may prefer an unfettered decision-making process, but the lack of criteria does not serve their interests or the interests of regulatory subjects.

Statutes that fail to provide clear criteria hamper public health work in a variety of ways. Paradoxically, a lack of statutory guidance may lead public health officials either to overuse or to underuse coercive powers. Without clear criteria, public health officials may restrict an individual's liberty without valid public health grounds or may be so unsure of their authority to act that they do not use these measures to respond to actual threats. Broad discretion and the absence of criteria also invite abuse of compulsory powers and their discriminatory use against stigmatized or marginalized groups, or create the perception of such abuse against the vulnerable even when health officials have no malevolent intentions.

Effective and constitutionally sound public health statutes should set out a rational and reliable way to assess risk to ensure that the health measure is necessary for public protection. In chapter 4, I proposed and defended criteria to govern the regulation of public health threats. Most important, public health authorities should be empowered to utilize a compulsory intervention only to avert a significant risk (not speculative, theoretical, or remote). Risk assessments in public health statutes should be based on objective and reliable scientific evidence and made on an individualized (case-by-case) basis. Public health authorities should consider the nature of the risk, the duration of the risk, the probability that harm will occur, and the severity of the harm if the risk were to materialize.

In addition to incorporating the significant risk standard, statutes should also require health officials to choose the least restrictive alternative that will accomplish the public health goal. This does not require authorities to adopt a less effective measure, but only to choose the least intrusive measure that would achieve the public health end. This would help align public health statutes with evolving standards of both antidiscrimination law and constitutional law, by allowing only those measures that are reasonably necessary to contain a serious health threat without unduly interfering with personal liberty.

IMPOSE PROCEDURAL LIMITS ON POWERS:
PROCEDURAL DUE PROCESS

There are good reasons, both constitutional and normative, for legislatures to require health authorities to use a fair process whenever their decisions seriously infringe upon autonomy, liberty, proprietary, or other important interests (see chapter 3). For example, if health authorities seek to close a restaurant, withdraw a professional (e.g., physician) or institutional (e.g., restaurant) license, or restrict personal freedom (e.g., civil confinement), they should provide procedural due process. Procedural protections help to ensure that health officials make fair and impartial decisions and reduce community perceptions that public health agencies arbitrarily employ coercive measures. Where few formal

procedures exist, public health officials risk rendering biased or inconsistent decisions and erroneously depriving persons and businesses of
their rights and freedoms. Although public health authorities may feel
that procedural due process is burdensome and an impediment to expe-
ditious action, it can actually facilitate deliberative and accurate decision-making.

Because of the importance of a fair process, public health statutes
should require due process prior to serious interference with personal and
property interests. The procedures required in any given case depend on
the nature, severity, and duration of the public health power. If authorities are exercising powers that are minimally invasive, statutes may have
few, if any, procedural requirements. However, if authorities intend to exercise highly coercive powers (e.g., civil confinement), due process may
require the full panoply of procedures: written notice of the threat the
person is alleged to pose and the behavior required of him by the agency,
appointment of counsel, discovery, presentation of evidence at an impartial hearing, cross-examination, a written decision, and an appeal.

Public health authorities, of course, should not have to provide procedural due process if they need to act urgently to prevent an imminent
health threat. For example, if a person is actively infectious or food
products are contaminated, health authorities need not delay effective
action to comply with procedural requirements. In cases of urgency,
procedural due process can be afforded after the fact to ensure that the
agency has not overreached its authority.

PROVIDE STRONG PROTECTION AGAINST DISCRIMINATION

Throughout the modern history of disease control, the stigma associated with serious diseases and the social hostility that is often directed
at those with, or at risk of, disease have interfered with the effective operation of public health programs.[27] The field of public health has always had to grapple with issues of race, gender, sexual orientation, disability, and socioeconomic status. Persons who fear social repercussions
may resist testing or fail to seek needed services. As part of any effort
to safeguard the public's health, legislators must find ways to address
both the reality and perception of social risk.

A great deal of protection against discrimination is already found in
disability discrimination law and, to a lesser extent, in disease-specific
statutes (see chapter 7).[28] These laws apply to persons with a wide
range of injury and disease, typically those with substantial physical or

mental impairments or those perceived as having such impairments. Disability statutes usually proscribe discrimination in a variety of different contexts, such as employment, public services, and public accommodations. Public health statutes should have nondiscrimination provisions that are as strong as those in disability discrimination law. At the very least, public health statutes should not have provisions that are inconsistent with, or undercut, the safeguards afforded in disability discrimination and disease-specific statutes.

Strong reasons exist, moreover, for public health statutes to have antidiscrimination provisions that are even stronger than those found in many disability laws. As explained in chapter 7, the Supreme Court has narrowed the definition of disability, excluding large numbers of persons from the protection of the ADA.[29] Moreover, federal courts have held that Title II of the ADA, which proscribes discrimination by public entities such as state health departments, is unconstitutional because it authorizes lawsuits against agencies without the state's permission; some courts see this as an unconstitutional abrogation of the state's sovereign immunity (see chapter 2).[30]

State public health statutes could remedy these, and other, problems of scope and effectiveness that exist under disability discrimination law. Since the ADA expressly does not preempt stronger safeguards against discrimination[31] and, particularly, does not preempt certain public health efforts,[32] state public health laws could provide much needed protection against discrimination.

PROVIDE STRONG PROTECTION FOR PRIVACY AND SECURITY OF PUBLIC HEALTH INFORMATION

Privacy and security of public health data are highly important both from the perspective of the individual and the public at large. Individuals seek the protection of privacy so that they can control intimate health information. They have an interest in avoiding the embarrassment and stigma of unauthorized disclosures to family or friends. They similarly have an interest in avoiding discrimination that could result from unauthorized disclosures to employers, insurers, or landlords. At the same time, privacy and security protection can advance the public's health. Privacy assurances can facilitate individual participation in public health programs and promote trust between health authorities and the community. Public health laws, therefore, should have strong safeguards of privacy to protect these individual and societal interests.

Public health legislation, however, should not grant individuals absolute privacy. Authorities need reasonable access to data and the power to use those data for important public health purposes, such as surveillance and response to health threats. If privacy rules become overly strict, legislatures risk impeding important public health functions and harming the public interest.

Legislation, therefore, cannot provide absolute privacy protection while still affording reasonable access to data to achieve important public health purposes. What legislation can do is create fair, comprehensive rules to ensure that data are acquired, used, and disseminated according to unambiguous criteria and procedures, under mandated security arrangements, with strict penalties for breaches of privacy. I have already made detailed proposals for safeguarding public health information privacy and security in chapter 5, and elsewhere I have offered a model public health privacy statute endorsed by the CDC.[33]

State legislatures should enact the following standards for collection, use, storage, and disclosure of personally identifiable information: require agencies to justify collection of data for an important public health purpose, provide information for persons and populations about the legitimate uses of personal information, proscribe secret data systems, ensure access by individuals to their personal records, mandate the technology necessary to secure health data, and institute an independent review of privacy and security arrangements within health agencies.

THE PROCESS OF LAW REFORM
AS A PUBLIC HEALTH ACTIVITY

The methods and goals of public health are often misunderstood and undervalued within government and society.[34] Health departments receive modest funding, particularly in comparison with resources allocated to health care services. The fact that public health often polices the commons and champions population-based risk reduction through behavioral change (e.g., smoking cessation, designated drivers, exercise, and diet modification) deprives it of specific beneficiaries who are motivated to form political constituencies. The prevalence of an individualistic, market ideology in political circles makes it difficult even to speak of public health in the vocabulary of contemporary politics.[35] Public health needs opportunities to draw attention to its resource requirements and achievements, and to develop constituencies for programs.

The lawmaking process provides just such an opportunity. A bill is the first step toward a coalition. It is an occasion for contact with interest groups and affected communities, some of whom may be motivated to act in support. Contact and cooperative effort also help to establish long-term ties and to identify important sources of support for other programs. Moreover, the process of negotiating for support can be a useful and concrete way for health agencies to incorporate the views of persons who receive public health services or are subject to regulation.

Legal reform also has the potential to enhance the agency's relationship with the legislature. Positive lawmaking offers a different sort of contact with legislators than tends to occur in the appropriations process. Public health law reform may offer an occasion to deal with a far greater range of legislators outside the context of contentious budget discussions. The drafting, negotiating, and hearing process provides a variety of fora for educating lawmakers and their staffs about public health needs and methods, and also provides health planners with better information about legislative views and priorities.

Law reform, of course, cannot guarantee better public health. However, by crafting a consistent and uniform approach, carefully delineating the mission and functions of public health agencies, designating a range of flexible powers, specifying the criteria and procedures for using those powers, and protecting against discrimination and invasion of privacy, the law can become a catalyst, rather than an impediment, to reinvigorating the public health system.

THE FUTURE OF PUBLIC HEALTH LAW

In this book, I have sought to provide a fuller understanding of the varied roles of law in advancing the public's health. The field of public health is purposive and interventionist. It does not settle for existing conditions of health, but actively seeks effective techniques for identifying and reducing health threats. Law is a very important, but perennially neglected, tool in furthering the public's health. Public health law should not be seen as an arcane, indecipherable set of technical rules buried deep within state health codes. Rather, public health law should be seen broadly as the authority and responsibility of government to assure the conditions for the population's health. As such, public health law has transcending importance in how we think about government, politics, and policy in America.

Although government has the responsibility to assure the conditions for health, it cannot overreach in a democratic society. This leads to one of the most complicated problems in the field: how to balance the collective good achieved by public health regulation with the resulting infringements of individual rights and freedoms. The difficult trade-offs between collective goods and individual rights form a major part of the study of public health law.

Finally, it is important to recall that public health, and the law itself, is highly political, influenced by strong social, cultural, and economic forces. As these forces shift over the years, as different political ideologies and economic conditions take hold, the field of public health will change and adapt. It has always been that way in public health, and it is likely to remain that way for the future, providing intellectually enticing, and socially important, terrain for scholars and practitioners to explore.

Notes

1. A THEORY AND DEFINITION OF PUBLIC HEALTH LAW

SOURCES FOR CHAPTER EPIGRAPHS: Page 3: JAMES A. TOBEY, PUBLIC HEALTH LAW: A MANUAL OF LAW FOR SANITARIANS 6–7 (1926). Page 16: C.-E.A. WINSLOW, THE LIFE OF HERMANN BIGGS 149, 246 (1929). Page 16: *Vital Statistics or the Statistics of Health, Sickness, Disease and Death, in* MCCULLOCH'S STATISTICAL ACCOUNT OF THE BRITISH EMPIRE 567 (1837), *reprinted in* MORTALITY IN MID 19TH CENTURY BRITAIN (Richard Wall ed., 1974); *see* MAJOR GREENWOOD, MEDICAL STATISTICS FROM GRAUNT TO FARR 71 (1948).

1. Elsewhere, my colleague and I make the case for closer public-private partnerships, and we propose economic incentives for managed care organizations to assume traditional public health functions. René Bowser & Lawrence O. Gostin, *Managed Care and the Health of the Nation, 72* S. CAL. L. REV. 1209 (1999). *See* Mark Wolfson et al., *Managed Care, Population Health, and Public Health,* 15 RES. SOC. HEALTH CARE 229 (1998).

2. A government in the republican form is a government of the people; a government by representatives chosen by the people. *See* Duncan v. McCall, 139 U.S. 449, 461 (1891) ("By the Constitution, a republican form of government is guarantied [sic] to every State in the Union, and the distinguishing feature of that form is the right of the people to choose their own officers for governmental administration.").

3. Wendy E. Parmet, *Health Care and the Constitution: Public Health and the Role of the State in the Framing Era,* 20 HASTINGS CONST. L.Q. 267, 312 (1992); *see also* § 3 of the Virginia Constitution of 1776: "That government is, or ought to be, instituted for the common benefit, protection, and security of the people. . . ."

4. U.S. CONST. art. I, § 1 ("All legislative Powers herein granted shall be vested in a Congress of the United States. . . .").

5. *Id.* at § 8, cl. 1 ("The Congress shall have Power To lay and collect Taxes . . . and provide for the common Defence and general Welfare of the United States. . . .").

6. *Id.* at art. II, § 3 (The President "shall take Care that the Laws be faithfully executed. . . .").

7. As to the powers and contemporary functions of the federal executive branch in matters of public health, see chapter 2.

8. U.S. CONST. art. III, § 2, cl. 1 ("The judicial Power shall extend to all Cases, in Law and Equity, arising under this Constitution, the Laws of the United States, and Treaties made. . . .").

9. A public nuisance was thought of as any activity which risked the health or safety of the citizenry. See chapters 9 and 10.

10. MICHAEL WALZER, SPHERES OF JUSTICE: A DEFENSE OF PLURALISM AND EQUALITY 64 (1983).

11. *Id.* at 65–66.

12. DAN E. BEAUCHAMP, THE HEALTH OF THE REPUBLIC: EPIDEMICS, MEDICINE, AND MORALISM AS CHALLENGES TO DEMOCRACY 15 (1988).

13. WALZER, *supra* note 10, at 68. *See also* NEW ETHICS FOR THE PUBLIC'S HEALTH (Bonnie Steinbock & Dan E. Beauchamp eds., 1999).

14. NORMAN DANIELS, JUST HEALTH CARE (1985); Dan W. Brock & Norman Daniels, *Ethical Foundations of the Clinton Administration's Proposed Health Care System,* 271 JAMA 1189 (1994).

15. BEAUCHAMP, *supra* note 12, at 4.

16. *Id.*

17. Daniel Fox, *The Politics of Physician's Responsibility in Epidemics: A Note on History,* 18 HASTINGS CTR. REP. 5 (1988).

18. JOHN B. BLAKE, PUBLIC HEALTH IN THE TOWN OF BOSTON 1630–1822 (1959); JOHN DUFFY, EPIDEMICS IN COLONIAL AMERICA (1953); JOHN DUFFY, A HISTORY OF PUBLIC HEALTH IN NEW YORK CITY 1625–1866 (1968); JOHN DUFFY, THE SANITARIANS: A HISTORY OF AMERICAN PUBLIC HEALTH (1990) [hereinafter THE SANITARIANS]; CHARLES E. ROSENBERG, THE CHOLERA YEARS: THE UNITED STATES IN 1832, 1849, AND 1866 (1964); Elizabeth Fee, *The Origins and Development of Public Health in the United States, in* THE OXFORD TEXTBOOK OF PUBLIC HEALTH 35 (Roger Detels et al. eds., 3d ed. 1997).

19. Parmet, *supra* note 3, at 285–302.

20. THE SANITARIANS, *supra* note 18, at 35–50.

21. JOHN J. HANLON & GEORGE E. PICKETT, PUBLIC HEALTH: ADMINISTRATION AND PRACTICE (9th ed. 1990).

22. C.-E.A. WINSLOW, THE EVOLUTION AND SIGNIFICANCE OF THE MODERN PUBLIC HEALTH CAMPAIGN (1923).

23. LEMUEL SHATTUCK, REPORT OF THE MASSACHUSETTS SANITARY COMMISSION (1850).

24. BARBARA G. ROSENKRANTZ, PUBLIC HEALTH AND THE STATE (1972).

25. THE SANITARIANS, *supra* note 18, at 66–125; WILSON SMILLIE, PUBLIC HEALTH: ITS PROMISE FOR THE FUTURE 167–74, 228–34 (1955). For a selection of public health essays and speeches from the early nineteenth century, *see* ORIGINS OF PUBLIC HEALTH IN AMERICA (Charles E. Rosenberg ed., 1972).

26. INSTITUTE OF MEDICINE, THE FUTURE OF PUBLIC HEALTH 58 (1988).

27. Elizabeth Fee, *Public Health and the State: The United States, in* THE HISTORY OF PUBLIC HEALTH AND THE MODERN STATE 231–33 (Dorothy Porter ed., 1994).

28. ELIZABETH FEE, DISEASE AND DISCOVERY: A HISTORY OF THE JOHNS HOPKINS SCHOOL OF HYGIENE AND PUBLIC HEALTH 1916–1939 (1987).

29. THE SANITARIANS, *supra* note 18, at 138–56, 175–92; *see also* ROSENBERG, *supra* note 18.

30. Stephen Smith, *The History of Public Health, 1871–1921, in* A HALF CENTURY OF PUBLIC HEALTH 1 (Mazych Porche Ravenel ed., 1921).

31. INSTITUTE OF MEDICINE, *supra* note 26, at 66.

32. FITZHUGH MULLAN, PLAGUES AND POLITICS: THE STORY OF THE UNITED STATES PUBLIC HEALTH SERVICE (1989); John K. Iglehart, *Politics and Public Health,* 334 NEW ENG. J. MED. 203 (1996).

33. FEE, *supra* note 27, at 232, 239–42.

34. *Id.* at 246–48; *see also* THE SANITARIANS, *supra* note 18, at 239–73; R.C. WILLIAMS, THE UNITED STATES PUBLIC HEALTH SERVICE, 1798–1950 (1951).

35. Federal Food, Drug, and Cosmetic Act, 21 U.S.C. §§ 301, 395(c)(1994).

36. Lawrence O. Gostin et al., *Water Quality Laws and Waterborne Diseases: Cryptosporidium and Other Emerging Pathogens,* 90 AM. J. PUB. HEALTH 847 (2000).

37. Lawrence O. Gostin & James G. Hodge, Jr., *Piercing the Veil of Secrecy in HIV/AIDS and Other Sexually Transmitted Diseases: Theories of Privacy and Disclosure in Partner Notification,* 5 DUKE J. OF GENDER LAW & POL'Y 9 (1998).

38. Social Security Act, 42 U.S.C. §§ 301–1397 (1994).

39. *See generally* HARRY MUSTARD, GOVERNMENT IN PUBLIC HEALTH 140–82 (1945).

40. James A. Tobey, *Public Health and the Police Power,* 4 N.Y.U. L. REV. 126 (1927).

41. *See generally* PAUL STARR, THE SOCIAL TRANSFORMATION OF AMERICAN MEDICINE (1982).

42. FEE, *supra* note 28, at 2 (1987).

43. BLACK'S LAW DICTIONARY 721 (6th ed. 1990).

44. Roger Detels, *Epidemiology: The Foundation of Public Health, in* OXFORD TEXTBOOK OF PUBLIC HEALTH, *supra* note 18, at 501.

45. JUDITH S. MAUSER & SHIRA KRAMER, MAUSER & BAHN EPIDEMIOLOGY: AN INTRODUCTORY TEXT 1 (2d ed. 1985).

46. Geoffrey Rose, *Sick Individuals and Sick Populations,* 14 INT'L J. EPIDEMIOLOGY 32, 37 (1985).

47. *Id.* at 32.

48. ERIC J. CASSELL, THE NATURE OF SUFFERING AND THE GOALS OF MEDICINE 7 (1991).

49. The preamble of the World Health Organization's constitution (1946) states, "The enjoyment of the highest attainable standard of health is one of the fundamental rights of every human being. . . ." *See generally* LAWRENCE O. GOSTIN & ZITA LAZZARINI, HUMAN RIGHTS AND PUBLIC HEALTH IN THE AIDS PANDEMIC 27–30 (1997).

50. "Public health is the science and the art of preventing disease, prolonging life, and promoting physical health and efficiency through organized community efforts." C.-E.A. Winslow, *The Untilled Fields of Public Health,* 51 SCIENCE 23, 30 (1920).

51. INSTITUTE OF MEDICINE, *supra* note 26, at 19, 37–40.

52. J. Michael McGinnis & William H. Foege, *Actual Causes of Death in the United States,* 270 JAMA 2207 (1993).

53. William M. Sage, *Enterprise Liability and the Emerging Managed Health Care System,* 60 LAW & CONTEMP. PROBS. 159 (1997).

54. J. Michael McGinnis et al., *Objectives-Based Strategies for Disease Prevention, in* OXFORD TEXTBOOK OF PUBLIC HEALTH, *supra* note 18, at 1621–31.

55. Roger Detels & Lester Breslow, *Current Scope and Concerns in Public Health, in* OXFORD TEXTBOOK OF PUBLIC HEALTH, *supra* note 18, at 3–17; Lester Breslow, *From Disease Prevention to Health Promotion,* 281 JAMA 1030 (1999).

56. PUBLIC HEALTH FUNCTIONS PROJECT, PUBLIC HEALTH IN AMERICA (1994) (a collaborative project of the U.S. Public Health Service and national public health organizations).

57. *See* INSTITUTE OF MEDICINE, *supra* note 26 at 7–8, 43–47.

58. Public Health Functions Project, *Public Health in America* (visited April 19, 2000), <http://www.health.gov/phfunctions/public.html>; Dept. of Health and Human Servs., *Healthy People 2010* (visited April 19, 2000), <http://www.health.gov/healthypeople>; INSTITUTE OF MEDICINE, IMPROVING HEALTH IN THE COMMUNITY: A ROLE FOR PERFORMANCE MONITORING 1–2 (Jane S. Durch et al. eds., 1997).

59. INSTITUTE OF MEDICINE, LEADING HEALTH INDICATORS FOR HEALTHY PEOPLE 2010: FINAL REPORT (1999); *see* KRISTINE M. GEBBIE, IDENTIFICATION OF HEALTH PARADIGMS IN USE IN STATE PUBLIC HEALTH AGENCIES (1997); *see also* Kristine M. Gebbie, *Community Based Health Care: An Introduction, in* COMMUNITY HEALTH INFORMATION NETWORKS 3–14 (Patricia Brennan et al. eds., 1997).

60. KEN MCKONNELL & PAUL FRONSTIN, EBRI HEALTH BENEFITS DATABOOK 1 (1999).

61. WALZER, *supra* note 10, at 81–82.

62. Charles V. Chapin, *Foreword, in* JAMES A. TOBEY, PUBLIC HEALTH LAW: A MANUAL OF LAW FOR SANITARIANS XV (1926).

63. ALLAN M. BRANDT, NO MAGIC BULLET: A SOCIAL HISTORY OF VENEREAL DISEASE SINCE 1880 (1985); Parmet, *supra* note 3.

64. Jonathan Mann et al., *Health and Human Rights,* 1 J. HEALTH & HUM. RTS. 6 (1994).

65. GOSTIN & LAZZARINI, *supra* note 49.

66. *See generally* AIDS LAW TODAY: A NEW GUIDE FOR THE PUBLIC (Scott Burris et al. eds., 1993).

2. PUBLIC HEALTH IN THE CONSTITUTIONAL DESIGN

SOURCES FOR CHAPTER EPIGRAPHS: Page 32: DeShaney v. Winnebago County Dep't of Soc. Servs., 489 U.S. 189, 195 (1989). Page 35: THOMAS M. COOLEY,

CONSTITUTIONAL LIMITATIONS 587 (6th ed. 1890). Page 47: WILLIAM BLACKSTONE, COMMENTARIES ON THE LAWS OF ENGLAND, vol. IV OF PUBLIC WRONGS (reprint, Univ. of Chicago Press 1979)(1769). Page 51: Mormon Church v. United States, 136 U.S. 1, 57 (1890).

1. As long ago as Martin v. Hunter's Lessee, 14 U.S. (1 Wheat.) 304, 324 (1816), the Supreme Court has puzzled over questions "of great importance and delicacy" in determining whether particular sovereign powers have been granted to the federal government or retained by the states. See New York v. United States, 505 U.S. 144, 155 (1992).

2. ERWIN CHEMERINSKY, CONSTITUTIONAL LAW: PRINCIPLES AND POLICIES 1–6 (1997).

3. JUDITH C. AREEN ET AL., LAW, SCIENCE AND MEDICINE 520 (2d ed. 1996).

4. James G. Hodge, Jr., *Implementing Modern Public Health Goals Through Government: An Examination of New Federalism and Public Health Law,* 14 J. CONTEMP. HEALTH L. & POL'Y 93, 97 (1997).

5. McCulloch v. Maryland, 17 U.S. (4 Wheat.) 316 (1819) (holding that the "necessary and proper" clause of the Constitution permits Congress to incorporate a bank).

6. Gibbons v. Ogden, 22 U.S. (9 Wheat.) 1, 87 (1824) ("[T]he constitution gives nothing to the States or to the people. Their rights existed before it was formed, and are derived from the nature of sovereignty and the principles of freedom.").

7. The Supreme Court recognizes two forms of preemption. In an *express* preemption, the federal statute explicitly declares that it supersedes state or local law. In an *implied* preemption, the language of the statute and the legislative history make clear Congress's intent to supersede state or local law. Two forms of implied preemption exist: field preemption and conflict preemption. In field preemption, the scheme of federal regulation is so pervasive as to make reasonable the inference that Congress left no room for the states to supplement it. In conflict preemption, compliance with both federal and state regulations is a physical impossibility, or state law stands as an obstacle to the accomplishment and execution of the full Congressional objectives. Gade v. National Solid Waste Management Ass'n, 505 U.S. 88, 98 (1992).

8. The Cigarette Labeling and Advertising Act, Pub. L. No. 80-92 § 2, 79 Stat. 282, 283 (1965), Pub. L. No. 91-222 § 2, 84 Stat. 87, 88 (1970) (codified as amended at 15 U.S.C. Ch. 36 (1994)), bars states from imposing requirements or prohibitions on tobacco manufacturers based on "smoking and health." *In re* Lorillard, 80 F.T.C. 455 (1972). The act preempts state tobacco regulation and certain tort claims. Cipollone v. Liggett Group, 505 U.S. 504 (1991); Lindsey v. Tacoma-Pierce County Health Department, 195 F.3d 1065 (9th Cir. 1999) (invalidating a ban on outdoor tobacco advertising on grounds of preemption); *see* Lawrence O. Gostin & Allan M. Brandt, *Tobacco Liability and Public Health Policy,* 266 JAMA 3178 (1991).

9. The Employee Retirement Income Security Act (ERISA), 29 U.S.C. § 1001 (1994), preempts state regulation of risk retention plans. *See* Lawrence O. Gostin & Alan I. Widiss, *What's Wrong with the ERISA Vacuum? Employers' Freedom to Limit Health Care Coverage Provided by Risk Retention Plans,* 269 JAMA 2527 (1993).

10. The Occupational Safety and Health Act of 1970, 29 U.S.C. Ch. 15 (2000) preempts states from establishing an occupational health and safety standard on an issue for which OSHA has already promulgated a standard, unless the state has obtained the Secretary's approval for the state's plan. *See* Gade, 505 U.S. at 88.

11. However, the judiciary, due to its respect for principles of federalism, is sometimes reluctant to infer federal preemption in the absence of clearly expressed Congressional intent. Consequently, courts have sustained state and local public health regulation, despite federal preemption claims, in areas ranging from licensing of nuclear power plants and state tort actions for radiation exposure to smoking abatement and permits for pesticide application to private land. *See, e.g.,* Wisconsin Public Intervenor v. Mortier, 501 U.S. 597 (1991) (holding that express preemption of state labeling requirements in the Federal Insecticide, Fungicide, and Rodenticide Act did not supersede other types of state or local regulation); Silkwood v. Kerr-McGee Corp., 464 U.S. 238 (1984) (holding that an award of punitive damages under state law for exposure to nuclear material was not preempted by the Atomic Energy Act).

12. While all federal judges are appointed to lifetime tenures, many state judges are periodically elected.

13. Although public health commentators sometimes complain about judicial emphasis on the rights of individuals, much of this text demonstrates that, more often than not, the courts are highly deferential to public health decision-making.

14. *See* Lawrence O. Gostin, *The Formulation of Health Policy by the Three Branches of Government, in* SOCIETY'S CHOICES: SOCIAL AND ETHICAL DECISION MAKING IN BIOMEDICINE 335 (Ruth Ellen Bulger et al. eds., 1995).

15. *See* LAWRENCE O. GOSTIN ET AL., IMPROVING STATE LAW TO PREVENT AND TREAT INFECTIOUS DISEASE 1 (1998); Lawrence O. Gostin et al., *The Law and the Public's Health: A Study of Infectious Disease Law in the United States,* 99 COLUM. L. REV. 59 (1999).

16. See chapter 3.

17. Susan Bandes, *The Negative Constitution: A Critique,* 88 MICH. L. REV. 2271 (1990); Mark Tushnet, *An Essay on Rights,* 62 TEX. L. REV. 1363 (1984).

18. DeShaney v. Winnebago County Dep't of Soc. Servs. 489 U.S. 189 (1989).

19. *Id.* at 195.

20. Webster v. Reproductive Health Servs., 492 U.S. 490 (1989).

21. Laurence Tribe, *The Abortion Funding Conundrum: Inalienable Rights, Affirmative Duties, and the Dilemma of Dependence,* 99 HARV. L. REV. 330 (1985).

22. *Webster,* 492 U.S. at 507.

23. *Id.* at 510.

24. Johnson v. Dallas Indep. Sch. Dist., 38 F.3d 198 (5th Cir. 1994), *cert. denied,* 514 U.S. 1017 (1995) (finding students have no constitutional right to affirmative protection from violence at school); Archie v. City of Racine, 847 F.2d 1211 (7th Cir. 1988), *cert. denied,* 489 U.S. 1065 (1989) (denying liability when a 911 dispatcher gave incorrect advice and failed to dispatch an am-

bulance for a caller who then died); Gilmore v. Buckley, 787 F.2d 714 (1st Cir.), *cert. denied*, 479 U.S. 882 (1986) (finding no liability when state officials released a dangerous mental patient they knew had threatened a particular person, leading to her murder).

25. DeShaney v. Winnebago County Dep't of Soc. Services, 489 U.S. 189, 213 (1989) (Blackmun, J., dissenting).

26. Bandes, *supra* note 17, at 2278.

27. Seth F. Kreimer, *Allocational Sanctions: The Problem of Negative Rights in a Positive State*, 132 U. PA. L. REV. 1293, 1295–96 (1984).

28. LOUIS M. SEIDMAN & MARK V. TUSHNET, REMNANTS OF BELIEF: CONTEMPORARY CONSTITUTIONAL ISSUES 52 (1996).

29. *Id.* at 54.

30. McCulloch v. Maryland, 17 U.S. (4 Wheat.) 316, 421 (1819).

31. The enumerated powers of Congress include the power to tax, borrow money, regulate interstate commerce, establish rules for naturalization and bankruptcies, coin money, punish counterfeiting, establish Post Offices, promote the progress of science and art by securing rights in intellectual property, constitute the judiciary, punish piracy and felony on the high seas, declare war, provide for and maintain (in various ways) the military of the United States, and exclusively legislate in the District of Columbia. Congress, moreover, may enact all laws that are "necessary and proper" to carry out its enumerated powers. U.S. CONST. art. I, § 8. Apart from Article I, § 8, the provisions of the Constitution delegating power to Congress include Article IV (the manner in which full faith and credit shall be given to the acts of every state); Article V (ratification of constitutional amendments); the Sixteenth Amendment (national income tax); and various amendments that recognize individual rights that authorize Congress to enforce their provisions by "appropriate legislation."

32. U.S. CONST. art. I, § 9 ("[n]o Capitation, or other direct, Tax shall be laid, unless in Proportion to the Census."). This "apportionment" requirement made it burdensome for the federal government whenever the Supreme Court ruled that a tax, for constitutional purposes, was "direct."

33. Pollock v. Farmers' Loan & Trust Co., 157 U.S. 429 (1895) (holding that income tax, because the source of income is, in part, property, is unconstitutional unless apportioned).

34. Consider excise taxes that have a trust fund with a related public health purpose; for example, the tax on the sale or use of domestic mined coal goes to the Black Lung Disease Trust Fund for Miners. 30 U.S.C. § 901 (1994).

35. OFFICE OF MANAGEMENT AND BUDGET, THE BUDGET OF THE UNITED STATES GOVERNMENT: FISCAL YEAR 1999, at 218 (1998); *see also* HENRY J. AARON, SERIOUS AND UNSTABLE CONDITION: FINANCING AMERICA'S HEALTH CARE 67–68 (1991).

36. *See, e.g.*, R. ALTON LEE, A HISTORY OF REGULATORY TAXATION 1–11 (1973) (discussing the relationship between police power and taxing power).

37. Daniel M. Fox & Daniel C. Schaffer, *Tax Policy as Social Policy: Cafeteria Plans, 1978–1985*, 12 J. HEALTH POL., POL'Y & L. 609, 610 (1987); *see* Daniel M. Fox & Daniel C. Schaffer, *Tax Administration as Health Policy:*

Hospitals, the Internal Revenue Service, and the Courts, 16 J. HEALTH POL., POL'Y & L. 251 (1991).

38. Employer-Sponsored Health Care Plans, 26 U.S.C. § 162 (1989).

39. Fox & Schaffer, *supra* note 37, at 610.

40. M. Gregg Bloche, *Health Policy Below the Waterline: Medical Care and the Charitable Exemption*, 80 MINN. L. REV. 299 (1995).

41. Child and Dependent Care Tax Credit, I.R.C. § 21(a) (1996) (allowing taxpayers to subtract a percentage of money spent on child care from overall tax liability); 26 U.S.C. § 21 (1989).

42. Low Income Housing Credit, 26 U.S.C. § 42 (1989).

43. Clinical Testing Expenses for Certain Drugs for Rare Diseases or Conditions, *id.* at § 45C.

44. Charitable Contributions, *id.* at § 170.

45. *See generally* Jendi B. Reiter, *Citizens or Sinners? The Economic and Political Inequity of "Sin Taxes" on Tobacco and Alcohol Products*, 29 COLUM. J. L. & SOC. PROBS. 443 (1996).

46. Tobacco Tax, 26 U.S.C. § 5701 (1989).

47. Alcohol Tax (Beer), *id.* at § 5051; Alcohol Tax (Distilled Spirits) *id.* at § 5001; Alcohol Tax (Wines) *id.* at § 5041.

48. Firearm Making Tax, *id.* at § 5821.

49. Taxes on Wagering, *id.* at § 4401.

50. Federal Gas Tax, *id.* at § 4081.

51. Ozone-Depleting Chemical Tax, *id.* at § 4681.

52. *See, e.g.*, United States v. Constantine, 296 U.S. 287, 295 (1935) (holding that federal tax that punishes liquor dealers who violate state liquor laws is unconstitutional); Bailey v. Drexel Furniture Co., 259 U.S. 20, 37 (1922) (holding that federal tax imposed on violators of federal child labor regulations has a "prohibitory and regulatory effect and purpose [that is] palpable").

53. United States v. Sanchez, 340 U.S. 42, 44 (1950) (upholding federal tax on distribution or prescription of marijuana), *citing* Sonzinsky v. United States, 300 U.S. 506, 513–14 (1937) (upholding federal tax on firearms capable of concealment).

54. United States v. Kahriger, 345 U.S. 22 (1953).

55. United States v. Butler, 297 U.S. 1, 66 (1936) (holding that Congress's power to tax is expressly conferred by the General Welfare Clause of the Constitution).

56. Helvering v. Davis, 301 U.S. 619, 641 (1937).

57. LAURENCE TRIBE, AMERICAN CONSTITUTIONAL LAW 323 (2d ed. 1988).

58. Pennhurst State Sch. & Hosp. v. Halderman, 451 U.S. 1, 17 (1981).

59. *Id.*

60. South Dakota v. Dole, 483 U.S. 203, 211 (1987).

61. *Halderman*, 451 U.S. at 17.

62. Steward Machine Co. v. Davis, 301 U.S. 548, 590 (1937).

63. *Dole*, 483 U.S. at 203.

64. *See* Albert J. Rosenthal, *Conditional Federal Spending and the Constitution*, 39 STAN. L. REV. 1103, 1104 (1987).

65. 42 U.S.C. § 3756(f) (1994); see Lawrence O. Gostin et al., *HIV Testing, Counseling, and Prophylaxis After Sexual Assault*, 271 JAMA 1436 (1994).

66. Act of Oct. 28, 1991, Pub. L. No. 102-141, Title VI, § 633, 1991 U.S.C.C.A.N. (105 Stat.) 834, 876–77, *reprinted in* note to 42 U.S.C. § 300ee-2 (1994); *see* Lawrence O. Gostin, *The HIV-Infected Health Care Professional: Public Policy, Discrimination and Patient Safety*, 151 ARCHIVES OF INTERNAL MED. 663 (1991).

67. Pub. L. No. 104-146, § 7, 1996 U.S.C.C.A.N. (110 Stat.) 1346, 1369 (codified at 42 U.S.C. § 300 ff (1994)).

68. Ronald O. Valdiserri et al., *Determining Allocations for HIV-Prevention Interventions: Assessing a Change in Federal Funding Policy*, 12 AIDS & PUB. POL'Y J. 138 (1997).

69. 42 U.S.C. §1396a (1994) (Medicaid requirements for establishment of state plans); 42 U.S.C. § 1395i-4 (Medicare requires state grants for planning and implementation of rural health care networks to be based on eligibility as defined in the statute).

70. Rust v. Sullivan, 500 U.S. 173 (1991) (permitting federal regulations prohibiting use of Title X funds in programs where abortion is used as a means of family planning).

71. Coastal Zone Management Act of 1972, 16 U.S.C. §§ 1451–1465 (1994); Federal Water Pollution Control Act, 33 U.S.C. §§ 1251–1387 (1994); Resource Conservation and Recovery Act, 42 U.S.C. § 6901 (1994).

72. New York v. United States, 505 U.S. 144, 159 (1992).

73. NLRB v. Jones & Laughlin Steel Corp., 301 U.S. 1, 37 (1937).

74. United States v. Darby, 312 U.S. 100, 115 (1941).

75. *New York*, 505 U.S. at 159–60 (upholding monetary and access incentive, but invalidating commandeering provisions of the Low-Level Radioactive Waste Policy Act).

76. United States v. Sullivan, 332 U.S. 689 (1948) (upholding Congress's commerce power to regulate the labeling of medicine shipped interstate and being held for future sales in purely local or intrastate commerce); *see* McDermott v. Wisconsin, 228 U.S. 115 (1913) (upholding the Pure Food and Drugs Act of 1906 against a challenge under the Commerce Clause).

77. Hillsborough County v. Automated Med. Labs., 471 U.S. 707 (1985) (upholding federal regulation of blood plasma collection from paid donors).

78. Hodel v. Virginia Surface Mining & Reclamation Ass'n, 452 U.S. 264, 277 (1981).

79. *See* Arkansas v. Oklahoma, 503 U.S. 91, 101 (1992) (holding that the EPA was authorized to issue water quality regulations in Arkansas that affected Oklahoma).

80. Gade v. National Solid Waste Management Ass'n, 505 U.S. 88, 97 (1992) (holding that the Occupational Health and Safety Act implicitly preempts unapproved state regulations).

81. United States Dep't of Energy v. Ohio, 503 U.S. 607, 611–12 (1992) (holding that the national government's immunity from liability for civil fines imposed by a state for past violations of the Clean Water Act is not waived); Kenaitze Indian Tribe v. Alaska, 860 F.2d 312, 314 (9th Cir. 1988), *cert. denied*, 491 U.S. 905 (1989) (finding that a state's definition of "rural area" was in conflict with the federal definition under the Alaska National Interest Land Conservation Act).

82. One rationale for national minimum standards is to prevent states from relaxing environmental protection to attract industry. This "race-to-the-bottom" rationale is thought to help states resist local economic pressures, but it has been criticized. See Richard L. Revesz, *Rehabilitating Interstate Competition: Rethinking the "Race-to-the-Bottom" Rationale for Federal Environmental Regulation,* 67 N.Y.U. L. REV. 1210 (1992).

83. West Lynn Creamery v. Healy, 512 U.S. 186 (1994) (holding that a Massachusetts milk pricing order that subjected all milk sold to Massachusetts retailers to assessment, with entire assessment distributed to Massachusetts dairy farmers, violated the Commerce Clause); Dean Milk Co. v. City of Madison, 340 U.S. 349 (1951) (holding that a local ordinance prohibiting sale of milk unless bottled within five miles from Madison violated the Commerce Clause).

84. Bacchus Imports, Ltd. v. Dias, 468 U.S. 263 (1984) (holding that a Hawaii local liquor tax exemption violated the Commerce Clause).

85. Sporhase v. Nebraska *ex rel.* Douglas, 458 U.S. 941, 958–60 (1981) (invalidating state regulation of ground water because it posed an unreasonable burden on interstate commerce).

86. C & A Carbone, Inc. v. Town of Clarkstown, 511 U.S. 383 (1994) (invalidating a local requirement that solid waste be processed at the town's transfer station because it deprived out-of-state firms access to the local market); Fort Gratiot Sanitary Landfill, Inc. v. Michigan Dep't of Natural Resources, 504 U.S. 353 (1992) (holding that a state prohibition on private landfill operators from accepting solid waste that originated outside the county in which their facilities are located violated the Commerce Clause).

87. City of Philadelphia v. New Jersey, 437 U.S. 617 (1978) (invalidating a New Jersey statute prohibiting the importation of most solid or liquid waste that originated outside the state, because it attempted to regulate out-of-state commercial interests in violation of the Commerce Clause).

88. Chemical Waste Management v. Hunt, 504 U.S. 334 (1992) (Alabama statute imposing added fee on hazardous waste generated outside state).

89. Elizabeth Fee, *Public Health and the State: The United States, in* THE HISTORY OF PUBLIC HEALTH AND THE MODERN STATE 224, 233 (Dorothy Porter ed., 1994).

90. Congress's first significant enactment in the field of public health was the Food and Drug Act of 1906, a broad prohibition against the manufacture or shipment of any adulterated or misbranded food or drug in interstate commerce. Medtronic, Inc. v. Lohr, 518 U.S. 470, 475 (1996). *See* C.C. Regier, *The Struggle for Federal Food and Drugs Legislation,* 1 LAW & CONTEMP. PROBS. 3 (1933).

91. *see generally* R.C. WILLIAMS, THE UNITED STATES PUBLIC HEALTH SERVICE, 1798 1950 (1951).

92. JOHN M. LAST, PUBLIC HEALTH AND HUMAN ECOLOGY 311 (1998).

93. Fee, *supra* note 89, at 246.

94. *Id.* at 249.

95. An early treatise on public health law posted the maxim on its cover page. LEROY PARKER & ROBERT H. WORTHINGTON, THE LAW OF PUBLIC HEALTH

AND SAFETY, AND THE POWERS AND DUTIES OF BOARDS OF HEALTH (1892). *Salus populi* was often used by the courts to uphold police regulations during the nineteenth century. *See* William J. Novak, *Public Economy and the Well-Ordered Market: Law and Economic Regulation in 19th-Century America*, L. & SOC. INQUIRY 1, 7 (1993).

96. WEBSTER'S THIRD NEW INTERNATIONAL DICTIONARY, UNABRIDGED 1753 (1986).

97. OXFORD ENGLISH DICTIONARY 22–25 (2d ed. 1989). For related meanings, see "polity" and "policy."

98. THE FEDERALIST Nos. 17, 34 (Alexander Hamilton), *quoted in* Wendy E. Parmet, *From Slaughter-House to Lochner: The Rise and Fall of the Constitutionalization of Public Health*, 40 AM. J. LEGAL HIST. 476, 478 (1996).

99. Pasquale Pasquino, *Theatrum Politicum: The Genealogy of Capital—Police and the State of Prosperity, in* THE FOUCAULT EFFECT: STUDIES IN GOVERNMENTALITY 105, 108–111 (Graham Burchell et al. eds., 1991) ("police" as "the science of happiness" and the "science of government").

100. RUTH LOCK ROETTINGER, THE SUPREME COURT AND STATE POLICE POWER: A STUDY IN FEDERALISM 10–22 (1957) (cataloguing Supreme Court statements on police power).

101. Gibbons v. Ogden, 22 U.S. (9 Wheat.) 1 (1824).

102. FRANK P. GRAD, THE PUBLIC HEALTH LAW MANUAL 10–15 (2d ed. 1990).

103. Commonwealth v. Alger, 61 Mass. (7 Cush.) 53, 96 (1851).

104. WILLIAM J. NOVAK, THE PEOPLE'S WELFARE: LAW AND REGULATION IN NINETEENTH-CENTURY AMERICA 14 (1996).

105. *Id.*

106. *See, e.g.,* ERNST FREUND, THE POLICE POWER: PUBLIC POLICY AND CONSTITUTIONAL RIGHTS (1904); W.P. PRENTICE, POLICE POWERS ARISING UNDER THE LAW OF OVERRULING NECESSITY 38–41(2d ed. 1939).

107. Gibbons v. Ogden, 22 U.S. (9 Wheat.) 1 (1824).

108. TOM CHRISTOFFEL & STEPHEN P. TERET, PROTECTING THE PUBLIC: LEGAL ISSUES IN INJURY PREVENTION 25–28 (1993).

109. 39 AM. JUR. 2D *Health* § 22 *et seq.* (1968) (state citations omitted).

110. Zucht v. King, 260 U.S. 174 (1922) (holding that a municipality may constitutionally vest in its officials broad discretion in matters affecting the enforcement of health law, specifically vaccinations).

111. Leisy v. Hardin, 135 U.S. 100 (1890) (upholding state confiscation of alcohol).

112. Givner v. State, 124 A.2d 764, 774 (Md. 1956); *see also* See v. Seattle, 387 U.S. 541, 550–52 (1967) (listing historical examples of state inspection) (Clark, J., dissenting).

113. Jones v. Indiana Livestock Sanitary Bd., 163 N.E.2d 605, 606 (Ind. 1960) (finding that in the exercise of police powers, states may take the legislative steps necessary to eliminate nuisances); Francis v. Louisiana State Livestock Sanitary Bd., 184 So. 2d 247, 253 (La. Ct. App. 1966) (upholding statute giving State Livestock Sanitary Board plenary power to deal with contagious and infectious diseases of animals).

114. State *ex rel.* Corp. Comm'n v. Texas County Irrigation & Water Res. Ass'n, 818 P.2d 449 (Okla. 1991) (upholding state's police power to protect fresh groundwater from pollution).

115. Strandwitz v. Board of Dietetics, 614 N.E.2d 817, 824 (Ohio Ct. App. 1992) (finding that in the interest of protecting the health and safety of its citizens, a state may, pursuant to its police powers, regulate businesses regarding food and nutrition).

116. Kaul v. Chehalis, 277 P.2d 352, 354 (Wash. 1955) (en banc) (upholding state law to control dental caries).

117. Safe Water Ass'n v. City of Fond du Lac, 516 N.W.2d 13, 15 (Wis. Ct. App. 1994) (upholding city council's adoption of a water fluoridation program as a valid exercise of state police power). *See, e.g.,* Douglas A. Balog, *Fluoridation of Public Water Systems: Valid Exercise of State Police Power or Constitutional Violation?,* 14 PACE ENVTL. L. REV. 645 (1997).

118. State v. Otterholt, 15 N.W.2d 529, 531 (Iowa 1944) (upholding state licensing requirements for chiropractors).

119. Kassel v. Consolidated Freightways Corp., 450 U.S. 662, 670 (1981).

120. The Slaughter-House Cases, 83 U.S. 36, 62 (1873) (holding that regulation of the slaughter of meat "is, in its essential nature, one which has been . . . in the constitutional history of this country, always conceded to belong to the States").

121. Pacific States Box & Basket Co. v. White, 296 U.S. 176, 181 (1935) (holding that food regulation "is a part of the inspection laws; [and] was among the earliest exertions of the police power in America").

122. Hillsborough County v. Automated Med. Labs., 471 U.S. 707, 719 (1985).

123. Rice v. Santa Fe Elevator Corp., 331 U.S. 218, 230 (1947), *quoted with approval in* Medtronic, Inc. v. Lohr, 518 U.S. 470, 471 (1996).

124. West Virginia v. Chas. Pfizer & Co., 440 F.2d 1079, 1089 (2d Cir. 1971); *see* Daniel B. Griffith, *The Best Interests Standards: A Comparison of the State's Parens Patriae Authority and Judicial Oversight in Best Interests Determinations for Children and Incompetent Patients,* 7 ISSUES IN L. & MED. 283 (1991).

125. *See* THE REPORT OF THE ROYAL COMMISSION ON THE LAW RELATING TO MENTAL ILLNESS AND MENTAL DEFICIENCY 1954–57 paras. 146, 255, 776–7, 846–52 (Cmnd. 169, HMSO, London,1957).

126. 17 Edw. II (1339) St. I. cc. 9, 10.

127. Alfred L. Snapp & Son, Inc. v. Puerto Rico, 458 U.S. 592, 600 (1982) (quoting J. CHITTY, PREROGATIVES OF THE CROWN 155 (1820)).

128. *In re* Estate of Longeway, 133 Ill. 2d 33 (Ill. 1989) (holding that the Probate Act implicitly authorizes a guardian to exercise the right to refuse artificial sustenance on ward's behalf); *see* Gibbs v. Titelman, 369 F. Supp. 38, 54 (E.D. Pa. 1973) (allowing the Commonwealth of Pennsylvania to intervene in a challenge to the constitutionality of state automobile repossession laws under the doctrine of *parens patriae*).

129. Hawaii v. Standard Oil Co. of Cal., 405 U.S. 251, 257 (1972).

130. Santosky v. Kramer, 455 U.S. 745, 746 (1982) (requiring due process safeguards before a state could irrevocably sever a natural parent's right in her child).

131. Decision-makers with total authority over the ward's personal and financial matters are commonly called plenary guardians; decision-makers with authority over financial matters solely are called guardians of the estate or conservators; and decision-makers with control over personal (e.g., medical and placement) questions only are guardians of the person. *See* Marshall B. Kapp, *Ethical Aspects of Guardianship*, 10 CLINICS IN GERIATRIC MED. 501, 502 (1994).

132. *Addington v. Texas*, 441 U.S. at 418, 426; *In re* S.L., 94 N.J. 128, 136 (1983) ("The authority of the state to civilly commit citizens is said to be an exercise of its police power to protect the citizenry and its parens patriae authority to act on behalf of those unable to act in their own best interests."); *see* Developments in the Law, *Civil Commitment of the Mentally Ill*, 87 HARV. L. REV. 1201 (1974).

133. O'Connor v. Donaldson, 422 U.S. 563, 583 (1975) (Burger, C.J., concurring).

134. *In re* D.C., 679 A.2d 634, 643 (N.J. 1996); *In re* Raymond S., 623 A.2d 249 (N.J. Super. Ct. App. Div. 1993).

135. Mormon Church v. United States, 136 U.S. 1, 56–58 (1890).

136. Developments in the Law, *supra* note 132, at 1208, 1212.

137. *Addington*, 441 U.S. at 426 (requiring procedural due process requirements for use in commitment of persons with mental illness).

138. Larry W. Yackle, *A Worthy Champion for Fourteenth Amendment Rights: The United States in Parens Patriae*, 92 NW. U. L. REV. 111, 140–44 (1997).

139. *Id.* at 143. The federal government also has claim to *parens patriae* capacity where its interests in national welfare establish standing similar to that of a state.

140. Louisiana v. Texas, 176 U.S. 1, 19 (1900). Louisiana unsuccessfully sought to enjoin a quarantine maintained by Texas. However, Louisiana was granted standing as *parens patriae* because the quarantine affected its citizens at large.

141. *See* Missouri v. Illinois, 180 U.S. 208 (1901) (holding that Missouri was permitted to sue Chicago sanitation district on behalf of Missouri citizens to enjoin the discharge of sewage into the Mississippi).

142. Kansas v. Colorado, 206 U.S. 46 (1907) (holding that Kansas was permitted to sue as *parens patriae* to enjoin the diversion of water from an interstate stream).

143. Georgia v. Tennessee Copper Co., 206 U.S. 230 (1907) (holding that Georgia was entitled to sue to enjoin fumes from a copper plant across the state border from damaging land in five Georgia counties).

144. New York v. New Jersey, 256 U.S. 296 (1921) (holding that New York could sue to enjoin the discharge of sewage from New Jersey into the New York harbor).

145. Alfred L. Snapp & Son, Inc. v. Puerto Rico, 458 U.S. 592, 593 (1982).

146. *See* Oklahoma *ex rel.* Johnson v. Cook, 304 U.S. 387 (1938).

147. *Alfred L. Snapp & Son*, 458 U.S. at 602.

148. Support Ministries for Persons with AIDS, Inc. v. Village of Waterford, New York, 799 F. Supp. 272 (N.D.N.Y. 1992).

149. *See, e.g.,* Morehead v. New York *ex rel.* Tipaldo, 298 U.S. 587 (1936) (invalidating state minimum wage requirements for women as violating due process).

150. CHEMERINSKY, *supra* note 2, at 174.

151. United States v. Lopez, 514 U.S. 549 (1995).

152. James G. Hodge, Jr., *The Role of New Federalism and Public Health Law,* 12 J.L. & HEALTH 309 (1997–98).

153. *Lopez,* 514 U.S. at 549.

154. The Rehnquist Court's federalism jurisprudence includes Printz v. United States, 521 U.S. 898 (1997); Seminole Tribe of Florida v. Florida, 517 U.S. 44 (1996); New York v. United States, 505 U.S. 144 (1992).

155. Terry v. Reno, 101 F.3d 1412 (D.C. Cir. 1996) (finding the Freedom of Access to Clinic Entrances (FACE) Act constitutional), *cert. denied,* 520 U.S. 1264 (1997); United States v. Bird, 124 F.3d 667 (5th Cir. 1997), *cert. denied sub nom.* Bird v. United States, 523 U.S. 1006 (1998)(upholding FACE).

156. United States v. Franklin, 157 F.3d 90 (2d Cir. 1998) (upholding regulation of machine guns); United States v. Hanna, 55 F.3d 1456 (9th Cir. 1995) (upholding prohibition on possession of a firearm by a convicted felon); United States v. Wilks, 58 F.3d 1518 (10th Cir. 1995) (upholding prohibition on possession of a machine gun); Gillespie v. City of Indianapolis, 185 F. 3d 693 (7th Cir. 1999), *cert. denied,* 120 S. Ct. 934 (2000) (upholding prohibition on gun possession by persons convicted of domestic violence).

157. United States v. Olin Corp., 107 F.3d 1506 (11th Cir. 1997) (finding no Commerce Clause violation in the application of the Comprehensive Environmental Response, Compensation, and Liability Act (CERCLA) to a chemical manufacturer).

158. National Ass'n of Home Builders v. Babbitt, 130 F.3d 1041 (D.C. Cir. 1997), *cert. denied,* 524 U.S. 937 (1998) (finding the application of the Endangered Species Act to an endangered species of fly found only in California was a constitutional exercise of the commerce power).

159. Reno v. Condon, 120 S. Ct. 666 (2000).

160. United States v. Morrison, 120 S. Ct. 1578 (2000). *See* Martha Minow, *Violence Against Women: A Challenge to the Supreme Court,* 341 NEW ENG. J. MED. 1927 (1999).

161. United States v. Wilson, 133 F.3d 251, 257 (4th Cir. 1997) (holding that regulation in Clean Water Act exceeded congressional Commerce Clause authority).

162. The only other case in that half century to invalidate a federal statute on Tenth Amendment grounds was later overruled. National League of Cities v. Usery, 426 U.S. 833 (1976), *overruled in* Garcia v. San Antonio Metro. Transit Auth., 469 U.S. 528 (1985).

163. New York v. United States, 505 U.S. 144 (1992).

164. *Id.* at 169.

165. Printz v. United States, 521 U.S. 898 (1997).

166. U.S. CONST. amend. XI ("The judicial power of the United States shall not be construed to extend to any [suit] commenced or prosecuted against one of the United States by Citizens of another State, or by Citizens or Subjects of any Foreign States.").

167. In *Fitzpatrick v. Bitzer*, 427 U.S. 445 (1976), the Supreme Court held that Congress could abrogate the state's sovereign immunity and allow states to be sued directly pursuant to its enforcement power under the Fourteenth Amendment to remedy discrimination.

168. 517 U.S. 44 (1996) (Congress could not authorize Indian tribe to sue the state in dispute over gaming activities).

169. Alden v. Maine, 527 U.S. 706, 709 (1999).

170. *See id.*

171. Florida Prepaid Postsecondary Educ. Expense Bd. v. College Sav. Bank, 119 S. Ct. 2199 (1999).

172. College Sav. Bank v. Florida Prepaid Postsecondary Educ. Expense Bd., 119 S. Ct. 2219 (1999).

173. Kimel v. Florida Bd. of Regents, 120 S. Ct. 631 (2000).

174. *See, e.g.,* Alsbrook v. City of Maumelle, 184 F. 3d 999 (8th Cir. 1999) (Title II of ADA did not validly abrogate Eleventh Amendment immunity from private suit in federal court).

175. *See, e.g.,* Little Rock Sch. Dist. v. Mauney, 183 F. 3d 816 (8th Cir. 1999).

176. Gregory v. Ashcroft, 501 U.S. 452 (1991).

177. Neil A. Lewis, *A Court Becomes a Model of Conservative Pursuits,* N.Y. TIMES, May 24, 1999, at A1 (4th Circuit Court of Appeals has "quietly but steadily become the boldest conservative court in the nation [issuing] remarkable rulings and a striking tone").

3.   CONSTITUTIONAL LIMITS ON THE EXERCISE
     OF PUBLIC HEALTH POWERS: SAFEGUARDING
     INDIVIDUAL RIGHTS AND FREEDOMS

SOURCE FOR CHAPTER EPIGRAPH: Page 61: People v. Budd, 22 N.E. 670, 676 (N.Y. 1889).

1. Early public health law texts are dominated by discussions of compulsory powers. *See, e.g.,* LEROY PARKER & ROBERT H. WORTHINGTON, THE LAW OF PUBLIC HEALTH AND SAFETY AND THE POWERS AND DUTIES OF BOARDS OF HEALTH XXXVIII (1892) ("It needs no argument to prove that the highest welfare of the State is subserved by protecting the life and health of its citizens by laws which will compel the ignorant, the selfish, the careless and the vicious, to so regulate their lives and use their property, as not to be a source of danger to others. If this be so, then the State has the right to enact such laws as shall best accomplish this purpose, even if their effect is to interfere with individual freedom and the untrammeled enjoyment of property.").

2. The first eight amendments prohibit the federal government from invading individual rights; the Ninth Amendment provides that the enumeration of certain rights in the Constitution shall not be construed to deny other rights retained by the people; and the Tenth Amendment reserves to the states, or to the people, those powers not delegated to the federal government.

3. The following constitutional provisions safeguard individual rights. Article I guarantees the availability of habeas corpus (to test the legality of the detention) and prohibits Bills of Attainder (a special legislative act that inflicts

punishment on a particular person), ex post facto laws (allow criminal conviction of a person for an act done that, when it was committed, was not a criminal offense), and impairments in contractual obligations. Article III guarantees trial by jury and establishes the basic elements of the crime of treason. Article IV provides an entitlement to all privileges and immunities of citizens in the several states. Finally, Article VI prohibits the use of religious tests as a qualification for elected office. In its 1999 term, the Supreme Court resurrected the Privileges and Immunities Clause. See Saenz v. Roe, 526 U.S. 489 (1999).

4. Prior to the twentieth century, there was considerable uncertainty as to whether the Bill of Rights constrained states. See The Slaughter-House Cases, 83 U.S. 36 (1873).

5. From a public health perspective, the most important constitutional provision that remains unincorporated is the Second Amendment's guarantee of "the right of the people to keep and bear Arms." Gun control and injury prevention are seen as major public health objectives. See Jon S. Vernick & Stephen P. Teret, *New Courtroom Strategies Regarding Firearms: Tort Litigation against Firearm Manufacturers and Constitutional Challenges to Gun Laws,* 36 HOUS. L. REV. 1713, 1717–20 (1999); Stephen P. Teret et al., *Support for New Policies to Regulate Firearms: Results of Two National Surveys,* 339 NEW ENG. J. MED. 813 (1998); David Hemenway, *Regulation of Firearms,* 339 NEW ENG. J. MED. 843 (1998). Because the Supreme Court has expressly declined to incorporate the Second Amendment (Presser v. Illinois, 116 U.S. 252 (1886)), states and localities possess broad powers to limit access to, and possession of, firearms. United States v. Miller, 307 U.S. 174 (1939) (finding no Second Amendment right to possession of sawed-off shotguns); Hickman v. Black, 81 F.3d 98 (9th Cir. 1996) (declaring that the plaintiff lacked standing to bring an individual claim premised on a violation of the Second Amendment); Love v. Pepersack, 47 F.3d 120 (4th Cir. 1995) (upholding officers' denial of an application for a handgun on grounds of prior arrests); Fresno Rifle & Pistol Club, Inc. v. Van de Kamp, 965 F.2d 723 (9th Cir. 1992) (law proscribing sale and possession of guns does not violate the Second Amendment because it is limited to federal action). Even as applied to the federal government, the Court narrowly construes the Second Amendment to prohibit federal gun regulation that would interfere with effective state militias and police forces. See United States v. Miller, 307 U.S. 174, 178 (1939) (upholding federal regulation of the transfer of firearms).

6. The following provisions of the Bill of Rights have not been incorporated and thus do not apply to state and local government: the Second Amendment's right to bear arms, the Third Amendment's right not to have soldiers quartered in a person's home, the Fifth Amendment's right to a grand jury indictment in criminal cases, the Seventh Amendment's right to a jury trial in civil cases, and the Eighth Amendment's prohibition of excessive fines.

7. Shelley v. Kraemer, 334 U.S. 1, 13 (1948) (holding that judicial enforcement of racially discriminatory restrictive covenants constituted state action). See Civil Rights Cases, 109 U.S. 3, 17 (1883) (Constitutional rights "cannot be impaired by the wrongful acts of individuals, unsupported by State authority in the shape of laws, customs, or judicial or executive proceedings.").

8. Adickes v. S.H. Kress & Co., 398 U.S. 144, 170–171 (1970).

9. While I attempt to impose clarity with respect to public health activities, multiple, complicated relationships exist between health authorities and private entities. As the Supreme Court observed, to "fashion and apply a precise formula for recognition of state responsibility . . . is an impossible task." Burton v. Wilmington Parking Auth., 365 U.S. 715, 722 (1961).

10. Home Tel. & Tel. Co. v. Los Angeles, 227 U.S. 278 (1913) (holding that even if a state officer misuses his power, state action still exists).

11. American Mfrs. Mut. Ins. Co. v. Sullivan, 526 U.S. 40 (1999); Blum v. Yaretsky, 457 U.S. 991 (1982) (holding that a private nursing home decision to transfer patients to other facilities, thereby terminating their Medicaid benefits, did not constitute state action); Jackson v. Metropolitan Edison Co., 419 U.S. 345 (1974) (finding no state action when a privately owned utility company terminated an individual's electric service).

12. Moose Lodge No. 107 v. Irvis, 407 U.S. 163, 176 (1972) (holding that state sanctions to enforce a discriminatory private rule constitutes state action).

13. Id. at 163 (holding that a private club that discriminated on the basis of race did not implicate the state by simply adhering to state liquor laws).

14. Columbia Broadcasting Sys., Inc. v. Democratic Nat'l Committee, 412 U.S. 94 (1973) (finding no state action in the FCC's refusal to require broadcast licensees to accept editorial advertising).

15. Jackson, 419 U.S. at 345.

16. Blum, 457 U.S. at 1004; Burton v. Wilmington Parking Authority, 365 U.S. 715, 725 (1961) (finding that the city was so "entangled" with a restaurant to which it leased space that there was a "symbiotic relationship" sufficient to constitute state action).

17. Rendell-Baker v. Kohn, 457 U.S. 830, 841 (1982) (finding no state action when a private school, receiving over 90 percent of its funds from the state, fired a teacher because of her speech).

18. Jackson, 419 U.S. at 345.

19. Carter v. Carter Coal Co., 298 U.S. 238 (1936) (invalidating a congressional delegation of regulatory power to private parties); see also PARKER & WORTHINGTON, supra note 1, at 12–13 ("The police power is so clearly essential to the well-being of the State, that the legislature cannot, by any act or contract whatever, divest itself of the power.").

20. See generally, René Bowser & Lawrence O. Gostin, Managed Care and the Health of a Nation, 72 S. CAL. L. REV. 1209 (1999).

21. Jackson, 419 U.S. at 352.

22. Rendell-Baker, 457 U.S. at 842.

23. National Collegiate Athletic Ass'n v. Tarkanian, 488 U.S. 179 (1988) (holding that the NCAA, in regulating collegiate athletics, does not perform a traditional or exclusive state function).

24. Jacobson v. Massachusetts, 197 U.S. 11 (1905).

25. PARKER & WORTHINGTON, supra note 1, at 5 ("[T]he legislature has a discretion which will not be reviewed by the courts; for it is not a part of the judicial functions to criticize the propriety of legislative action in matters which are within the authority of the legislative body.").

26. State *ex rel.* Conway, Atty. Gen. v. Southern Pac. Co., 145 P.2d 530 (Ariz. 1943) (*quoting* State *ex rel.* McBride v. Superior Court, 174 P. 973, 976 (Wash. 1918)).

27. Pre-*Jacobson* understandings of constitutional restraints recognized that "a statute, to be upheld as a valid exercise of the police power, must have some relation to those ends; the rights of citizens may not be invaded under the guise of police regulation." PARKER & WORTHINGTON, *supra* note 1, at 6–7. *See* Mugler v. Kansas, 123 U.S. 623, 661 (1887) (upholding prohibition on sale of alcoholic beverages, but emphasizing the duty of the courts to adjudge whether a statute has a "real or substantial relation" to public health); Brimmer v. Rebman, 138 U.S. 78 (1891) (invalidating state prohibition on sale of meat because of overbroad prevention of sale of wholesome, fresh meat).

28. *Jacobson,* 197 U.S. at 26.

29. *Id.* at 26–27 (citing Commonwealth v. Alger, 7 Cush. 53, 84 (Mass. 1851)).

30. *Jacobson,* 197 U.S. at 27.

31. Ironically, the Court during that era is best known for its libertarian position on questions of economic rights; see the discussion of economic due process and the *Lochner* case later in this chapter.

32. Viemeister v. White, 72 N.E. 97 (N.Y. 1904) (holding that laws requiring vaccination of children as a condition of their attendance in public schools are a valid exercise of the state police powers).

33. *Jacobson,* 197 U.S. at 34.

34. Price v. Illinois, 238 U.S. 446 (1915) (upholding state prohibition on sale of certain food preservatives to protect the public health).

35. New York *ex rel.* Lieberman v. Van de Carr, 199 U.S. 552 (1905) (upholding the state prohibition on the sale of milk without a health board permit).

36. California Reduction Co. v. Sanitary Reduction Works, 199 U.S. 306 (1905) (upholding an ordinance requiring refuse to be cremated or destroyed at the owner's expense).

37. *Jacobson,* 197 U.S. at 28.

38. THE CONCISE OXFORD DICTIONARY OF CURRENT ENGLISH 811 (10th ed. 1999).

39. Even though, under *Jacobson,* the government is permitted to act only in the face of a demonstrable threat to health, the Court did not appear to require the state to produce credible scientific, epidemiologic, or medical evidence of that threat. Justice Harlan said that "what the people believe is for the common welfare must be accepted as tending to promote the common welfare, whether it does in fact or not." *Jacobson,* 197 U.S. at 35 (quoting *Viemeister,* 241, 72 N.E. 97, 99 (N.Y. 1904)).

40. *Jacobson,* 197 U.S. at 31; Nebbia v. New York, 291 U.S. 502, 510–511 (1933) (holding that public welfare regulation must not be "unreasonable, arbitrary, or capricious, and the means selected shall have a real and substantial relation to the object sought to be attained").

41. *Jacobson,* 197 U.S. at 38–39.

42. *Id.* at 39.

43. *Id.* ("We are not to be understood as holding that the statute was intended to be applied to such a case [involving an unfit subject], or, if it was so intended, that the judiciary would not be competent to interfere and protect the health and life of the individual concerned."). It is interesting to note that Henning Jacobson did allege that, when a child, a vaccination had caused him "great and extreme suffering." *Id.* at 36. Jacobson's claim of potential harm was not without merit. In Jenner's original publication in the *Inquiry* in 1799, he noted in case IV a severe adverse reaction to vaccination now termed anaphylaxis. Harry Bloch, *Edward Jenner (1749–1823): The History and Effects of Smallpox, Inoculation, and Vaccination*, 147 AM. J. DIS. CHILD. 772, 774 (1993).

44. Jew Ho v. Williamson, 103 F. 10, 22 (C.C.N.D. Cal. 1900) ("It must necessarily follow that, if a large . . . territory is quarantined, intercommunication of the people within that territory will rather tend to spread the disease than to restrict it.").

45. Lochner v. New York, 198 U.S. 45 (1905).

46. HOWARD GILLMAN, THE CONSTITUTION BESIEGED: THE RISE AND DEMISE OF LOCHNER ERA POLICE POWERS JURISPRUDENCE (1993).

47. *Lochner*-era courts did not uniformly strike down health regulations despite their economic effects. *See* New York *ex rel Liberman v. Van de Carr,* 199 U.S. 552 (1905) (upholding Board of Health regulation of milk sales); Adams v. City of Milwaukee, 228 U.S. 572 (1913) (upholding tuberculin testing of cows from outside the city).

48. *Lochner,* 198 U.S. at 58 ("There is . . . no reasonable foundation for holding this to be necessary or appropriate as a health law to safeguard the public health, or the health of the individuals who are following the trade of a baker.").

49. *Id.* at 69 (Harlan J, dissenting).

50. *Id.* at 71 (Harlan J, dissenting).

51. *Id.* at 62.

52. *Id.* at 73 (Harlan J, dissenting). Ironically, the Court's insistence that government demonstrate a close connection between the intervention and the protection of public health led to better public interest lawyering. In *Muller v. Oregon,* 208 U.S. 412 (1908), Louis Brandeis wrote a richly empirical brief demonstrating the relationship between excessive labor and reproductive health. The extensive use of social and medical science in judicial briefs, often called "Brandeis briefs," therefore originated during the Lochner period.

53. Coppage v. Kansas, 236 U.S. 1 (1915) (invalidating federal and state legislation forbidding employers to require employees to agree not to join a union).

54. Adkins v. Children's Hosp., 261 U.S. 525 (1923) (invalidating a law establishing minimum wages for women).

55. Weaver v. Palmer Bros. Co., 270 U.S. 402 (1926) (striking down a law that prohibited use of rags and debris in mattresses enacted to protect the public health).

56. New State Ice Co. v. Liebmann, 285 U.S. 262 (1932) (striking down a statute forbidding a state commission to license the sale of ice except on proof of necessity).

57. West Coast Hotel Co. v. Parrish, 300 U.S. 379, 391 (1937) (upholding a minimum wage law for women).

58. Williamson v. Lee Optical, 348 U.S. 483 (1955) (upholding a statute prohibiting an optician from selling lenses without a prescription); Turner v. Elkhorn Mining Co., 428 U.S. 1 (1976) (upholding a federal statute providing compensation to coal miners who suffered from pneumoconiosis or black lung disease).

59. Thomas B. Stoddard & Walter Rieman, *AIDS and the Rights of the Individual: Toward a More Sophisticated Understanding of Discrimination*, 68 (Supp. 1) MILBANK QUART. 143, 146–49 (1990).

60. *See, e.g.*, Washington v. Glucksberg, 521 U.S. 702, 719 (1997) ("The Due Process Clause guarantees more than fair process, and the 'liberty' it protects includes more than the absence of physical restraint."); Collins v. Harker Heights, 503 U.S. 115, 125 (1992) (due process "protects individual liberty against 'certain government actions regardless of the fairness of the procedures used to implement them'").

61. Stono River Envtl. Protection Ass'n v. South Carolina Dep't of Health & Envtl. Control, 406 S.E.2d 340 (S.C. 1991) (intervenors in a water quality certification were entitled to due process rights of notice and an opportunity to be heard).

62. Board of Regents v. Roth, 408 U.S. 564, 577 (1972) (holding that the plaintiff had no reasonable expectation to a property interest of receiving tenure).

63. Goldberg v. Kelly, 397 U.S. 254 (1970) (finding a property interest in the receipt of welfare and holding that due process is therefore applicable to the termination of such benefits).

64. *Roth*, 408 U.S. at 577.

65. Hutchinson v. City of Valdosta, 227 U.S. 303, 308 (1913) ("It is the commonest exercise of the police power . . . to provide for a system of sewers and to compel property owners to connect therewith.").

66. *See, e.g.*, Ewing v. Mytinger & Casselberry, 339 U.S. 594, 599–600 (1950) ("One of the oldest examples is the summary destruction of property without prior notice or hearing for the protection of public health."); Hodel v. Virginia Surface Mining & Reclamation Ass'n, 452 U.S. 264, 299–300 (1981) (regulating surface mining to protect society and the environment from adverse effects); North American Cold Storage Co. v. Chicago, 211 U.S. 306 (1908) (upholding emergency seizure of contaminated food).

67. Cleveland Bd. of Educ. v. Loudermill, 470 U. S. 532 (1985) (finding that public employees cannot be denied their property right in continued employment without due process).

68. United States v. Cardiff, 344 U.S. 174 (1952) (holding that an industry that processes apples is entitled to written notice of the intention to inspect).

69. A physician enjoys a protected property interest in a license to practice medicine. *See, e.g.*, Lowe v. Scott, 959 F.2d 323, 335 (1st Cir. 1992). However, procedural due process can be accomplished by using a "post-suspension remedy," especially if the physician poses a health risk. Caine v. Hardy, 943 F.2d 1406 (5th Cir. 1991).

70. St. Agnes Hosp., Inc. v. Riddick, 748 F. Supp. 319, 337 (D.Md. 1990) (holding that the procedures utilized in withdrawing the accreditation of a hospital comported with due process and fairness standards).

71. Fair Rest Home v. Commonwealth Dep't of Health, 401 A.2d 872 (Pa. Commw. Ct. 1979) (requiring the health department to hold a hearing before revoking a rest home's license). *But see* O'Bannon v. Town Court Nursing Ctr., 447 U.S. 773 (1980) (finding that residents had no due process right before their nursing home was decertified; but that the nursing home itself may have had a due process right).

72. Contreras v. City of Chicago, 920 F. Supp. 1370, 1392–94 (N.D. Ill. 1996) (finding that a postdeprivation hearing comports with procedural due process because there is a reduced expectation of privacy for closely regulated businesses such as restaurants).

73. *See, e.g.,* Darlak v. Bobear, 814 F.2d 1055, 1061 (5th Cir. 1987) ("It is well-settled . . . that a physician's staff privileges may constitute a property interest protected by the due process clause.").

74. Board of Regents v. Roth, 408 U.S. 564, 572 (1972).

75. In cases where quick action is required, a post deprivation hearing, or even a common law tort remedy for erroneous deprivation, satisfies due process. *See, e.g.,* Logan v. Zimmerman Brush Co., 455 U.S. 422, 436 (1982).

76. Mathews v. Eldridge, 424 U.S. 319, 335 (1976): (1) the nature and extent of the private interest at stake; (2) the risk of an erroneous deprivation of property or liberty, and the probable value of additional or substitute procedures; and (3) the government's interests, including the achievement of the state's objectives and the fiscal and administrative burdens that additional or substitute procedures would entail. *See* Morales v. Turman, 562 F.2d 993, 998 (5th Cir. 1977) ("The interests of the individual and of society in the particular situation determine the standards for due process."); Washington v. Harper, 494 U.S. 210, 229–30 (1990).

77. Lesser deprivations of liberty (e.g., directly observed therapy) may require a more relaxed procedural standard. For interventions that involve minimal bodily invasion (e.g., vaccination), the health department may not be obliged to provide any particular procedures.

78. Lessard v. Schmidt, 413 F. Supp. 1318 (E.D. Wis. 1976) (requiring due process in civil commitment proceedings); *In re* Ballay, 482 F.2d 648 (D.C. Cir. 1973) (same).

79. Greene v. Edwards, 263 S.E.2d 661 (W.Va. 1980) (entitling patient to a new hearing since counsel was not appointed until after commencement of involuntary commitment hearing).

80. Involuntary civil commitment to a mental institution, for example, is a "massive curtailment of liberty." Vitek v. Jones, 445 U.S. 480, 491–92 (1980).

81. Parham v. J.R., 442 U.S. 584, 609 (1979).

82. Romer v. Evans, 517 U.S. 620, 635 (1996). *See* Cleburne v. Cleburne Living Ctr., Inc., 473 U.S. 432 (1985) (invalidating a zoning ordinance that prevented the construction of a group home for the mentally retarded). Even though *Romer* and *Cleburne* were decided on equal protection grounds, they illustrate the Court's insistence on a valid public interest.

83. Collins v. Harker Heights, 503 U.S. 115, 125 (1992).

84. Washington v. Glucksberg, 521 U.S. 702, 712 (1997).

85. *Id.* at 713.

86. Bolling v. Sharpe, 347 U.S. 497 (1954) (holding that equal protection applies to the federal government through the Due Process Clause of the Fifth Amendment).

87. *Romer* 517 U.S. at 631.

88. Shaw v. Hunt, 517 U.S. 899 (1996) (holding that race was the predominant factor motivating a legislative decision to gerrymander a voting district, triggering strict scrutiny).

89. Plyler v. Doe, 457 U.S. 202, 216 (1982) ("The Constitution does not require things which are different in fact or opinion to be treated in law as though they were the same.").

90. Jew Ho v. Williamson, 103 F. 10, 24 (C.C.N.D. Cal. 1900) (finding that the quarantine was made to operate exclusively against the Chinese community); *see* Yick Wo v. Hopkins, 118 U.S. 356 (1886) (finding unlawful discrimination when an ordinance prohibiting washing of clothes in public laundries after 10 P.M. was enforced only against Chinese owners).

91. For a thoughtful examination of the subject, see Scott Burris, *Rationality Review and the Politics of Public Health,* 34 VILL. L. REV. 933 (1989).

92. Berman v. Parker, 348 U.S. 26 (1954).

93. Railway Express Agency, Inc. v. New York, 336 U.S. 106 (1949) (upholding regulation of vehicle advertising as a traffic safety measure).

94. Williamson v. Lee Optical, 348 U.S. 483 (1955) (upholding a state law favoring ophthalmologists over optometrists to ensure proper diagnosis of eye disease).

95. Jacobson v. Massachusetts, 197 U.S. 11 (1905).

96. Heller v. Doe, 509 U.S. 312, 321 (1993) (courts accept "a legislature's generalizations even when there is an imperfect fit between means and ends").

97. Berger v. City of Mayfield Heights, 154 F.3d 621 (6th Cir. 1998) (finding an ordinance requiring certain lots to be clear-cut of all vegetation over eight inches arbitrary).

98. Euclid v. Ambler Realty Co., 272 U.S. 365, 395 (1926) (persons adversely affected by public health regulation carry the burden of proving that the law is "arbitrary and unreasonable, having no substantial relation to the public health, safety, morals, or general welfare"); Lehnhausen v. Lake Shore Auto Parts Co., 410 U.S. 356, 364 (1973) ("The burden is on the one attacking the legislative arrangement to negate every conceivable basis which might support it.").

99. FCC v. Beach Communications, 508 U.S. 307, 313 (1993).

100. Nordlinger v. Hahn, 505 U.S. 1, 11 (1992).

101. *Beach Communications,* 508 U.S. at 313.

102. Heller v. Doe, 509 U.S. 312, 320 (1993) (upholding statutes requiring "clear and convincing" evidence to civilly commit the mentally retarded, but "beyond a reasonable doubt" to commit the mentally ill).

103. *Beach Communications,* 508 U.S. at 307.

104. Metropolis Theatre Co. v. Chicago, 228 U.S. 61, 69 (1913).

105. Local 1812, American Fed'n of Gov't Employees v. United States Dep't of State, 662 F. Supp. 50 (D.D.C. 1987) (upholding government's mandatory HIV testing program for foreign service personnel).

106. Reynolds v. McNichols, 488 F.2d 1378 (10th Cir. 1973) (finding no equal protection violation when female sex workers were detained and treated, but not johns).

107. Pro-Eco v. Board of Comm'rs of Jay County, Indiana, 57 F.3d 505 (7th Cir. 1995) (holding that depositing garbage in landfills is not a fundamental right and concern for public health is a sufficient reason to regulate landfills).

108. New York State Trawlers Ass'n v. Jorling, 16 F.3d 1303 (2d Cir. 1994) (upholding a conservation law that prohibited trawlers from possessing lobsters in Long Island Sound).

109. United States v. Carolene Prods. Co., 304 U.S. 144, 152, n.4 (1938): "It is unnecessary to consider now whether legislation which restricts those political processes which can ordinarily be expected to bring about repeal of undesirable legislation, is to be subjected to more exacting scrutiny. . . . Nor need we enquire . . . whether prejudice against discrete and insular minorities may be a special condition, which tends seriously to curtail the operation of those political processes ordinarily to be relied upon to protect minorities, and which may call for a correspondingly more searching judicial inquiry."

110. City of Cleburne v. Cleburne Living Ctr., 473 U.S. 432 (1985). *But see* Heller v. Doe, 509 U.S. 312 (1993) (finding that the higher standard of proof for involuntary commitment of the mentally ill, as opposed to the mentally retarded, had a rational basis).

111. Romer v. Evans, 517 U.S. 620 (1996).

112. *Id.* at 632.

113. *Id.*

114. United States Dep't of Agriculture v. Moreno, 413 U.S. 528, 534 (1973) (finding denial of food stamps if a household includes unrelated persons unconstitutional under rationality review).

115. Burris, *supra* note 91.

116. United States v. Virginia, 518 U.S. 515 (1996) (using intermediate scrutiny to invalidate the maintenance of an all-male military college).

117. New Jersey Welfare Rights Org. v. Cahill, 411 U.S. 619 (1973) (using intermediate scrutiny to strike down a law that limited benefits to families with two individuals of the opposite sex "ceremoniously married").

118. Mississippi Univ. for Women v. Hogan, 458 U.S. 718 (1982) (using intermediate scrutiny to invalidate the policy of excluding men from state nursing school).

119. Craig v. Boren, 429 U.S. 190, 197 (1976) (holding that gender-based classifications on legal drinking age must serve state interests and be substantially related to achievement of state objectives).

120. *Virginia*, 518 U.S. at 526.

121. Reynolds v. McNichols, 488 F.2d 1380, 1383 (10th Cir. 1973) (upholding the enforcement of the city's "hold and treat" ordinance requiring testing and treatment of persons reasonably suspected of having an STD against a female sex worker, but not the john: "[T]he ordinance is aimed at the primary source of venereal disease and the . . . prostitute was the potential source, not her would-be customer."); Illinois v. Adams, 597 N.E.2d 574 (Ill. 1992) (finding that mandatory HIV testing of prostitutes does not violate equal protection

because it draws no distinction between male and female offenders, and the legislature had no intent to disadvantage females).

122. See case study, chapter 7.

123. *See, e.g.,* Loving v. Virginia, 388 U.S. 1 (1967) (invalidating Virginia's miscegenation law that made it a crime for a white person to marry outside the Caucasian race).

124. *See, e.g.,* Korematsu v. United States, 323 U.S. 214 (1944) (applying strict scrutiny to uphold the military curfew for persons of Japanese descent during World War II).

125. Classifications based on alienage involve discrimination against persons who are not United States citizens. *See, e.g.,* Bernal v. Fainter, 467 U.S. 216 (1984) (invalidating a law requiring that a notary public be a U.S. citizen).

126. So-called "positive" discrimination benefiting racial minorities also triggers strict scrutiny. *See, e.g.,* Regents of Univ. of Cal. v. Bakke, 438 U.S. 265 (1978) (invalidating the University of California's affirmative action program for medical school admission).

127. Skinner v. Oklahoma, 316 U.S. 535 (1942) (striking down a statute authorizing the sterilization of habitual criminals).

128. *Loving,* 388 U.S. at 1.

129. Shapiro v. Thompson, 394 U.S. 618 (1969) (invalidating the residency requirements for welfare programs).

130. Cruzan v. Director, Mo. Dep't of Health, 497 U.S. 261, 278 (1990) ("[T]he principle that a competent person has a constitutionally protected liberty interest in refusing unwanted medical treatment may be inferred from our prior decisions."); Washington v. Harper, 494 U.S. 210, 221–22 (1990) (finding that a mentally ill prisoner has a "significant liberty interest in avoiding the unwanted administration of antipsychotic drugs").

131. Planned Parenthood v. Casey, 505 U.S. 833, 851 (1992).

132. In *New York City Transit Authority v. Beazer,* 440 U.S. 568, 575 (1979), the Court upheld an ordinance that excluded persons in methadone maintenance from employment with the transit authority despite the substantial overinclusiveness. Presumably, if this regulation had interfered with liberty instead of employment, it would have failed a strict scrutiny analysis.

133. *See, e.g.,* San Antonio Independent Sch. Dist. v. Rodriguez, 411 U.S. 1, 109–110 (1973) (Marshall, J., dissenting) (finding that a principled constitutional analysis would apply a spectrum of standards depending on the nature of the right and the discriminatory effects).

134. Fullilove v. Klutznick, 448 U.S. 448 (1980) (Marshall, J., concurring).

135. Bowers v. Hardwick, 478 U.S. 186 (1986) (applying rational basis test to uphold a state statute prohibiting sodomy).

136. Heller v. Doe, 509 U.S. 312 (1993) (applying rational basis test to uphold civil commitment for mentally ill and mentally retarded persons under different standards); City of Cleburne v. Cleburne Living Ctr., 473 U.S. 432 (1985) (using rational basis test to invalidate a zoning ordinance that prevented the construction of a group home for persons with mental retardation).

137. *Rodriguez,* 411 U.S. at 1.

138. Whalen v. Roe, 429 U.S. 589 (1977) (upholding a state statute requiring that the state be provided with every prescription for certain types of drugs).

139. Washington v. Glucksberg, 521 U.S. 702, 711 (1997) (upholding a state statute prohibiting the causation or assistance of suicide).

4. PUBLIC HEALTH REGULATION:
A SYSTEMATIC EVALUATION

SOURCES FOR CHAPTER EPIGRAPHS: Page 85: JOHN STUART MILL, ON LIBERTY 13 (1856). Page 94: NATIONAL RESEARCH COUNCIL, UNDERSTANDING RISK: INFORMING DECISIONS IN A DEMOCRATIC SOCIETY 215–216 (Paul C. Stern & Harvey V. Fineberg eds., 1996). Page 97: Amartya Sen, *Freedoms and Needs: An Argument for the Primacy of Political Rights,* NEW REPUBLIC, Jan. 10, 1994, at 31, 32–33.

1. Norman Daniels, *Health-Care Needs and Distributive Justice,* 10 PHIL. & PUB. AFF. 146 (1981); NORMAN DANIELS, JUST HEALTH CARE (1985); Lawrence O. Gostin, *Securing Health or Just Health Care? The Effect of the Health Care System on the Health of America,* 39 ST. LOUIS U. L.J. 7–43 (1994).

2. Joel Feinberg, in a series of influential books on *The Moral Limits of the Criminal Law,* examines the sorts of conduct that the state may appropriately proscribe. Among the "liberty-limiting" principles he discusses are harm to others (the "harm principle") and offense to others (the "offense principle"). The "liberal position" holds that the harm and offense principles between them exhaust the class of good reasons for legal prohibitions. Liberals exclude harm to the person himself (paternalism) as a sufficient justification for legal prohibitions. *See* 3 JOEL FEINBERG, THE MORAL LIMITS OF THE CRIMINAL LAW: HARM TO SELF 27 (1986).

3. Derived from the Greek *autos* ("self") and *nomos* ("law," "rule," or "governance"), meaning "the having or making of one's own laws." *See id.*

4. TOM L. BEAUCHAMP & JAMES F. CHILDRESS, PRINCIPLES OF BIOMEDICAL ETHICS (1977).

5. BERNARD GERT ET AL., BIOETHICS: A RETURN TO FUNDAMENTALS 77–79 (1997).

6. EMMANUEL KANT, CRITIQUE OF PRACTICAL REASON AND OTHER WRITINGS IN MORAL PHILOSOPHY (1949).

7. JOHN STUART MILL, ON LIBERTY 13 (1856).

8. *See, e.g.,* Simon v. Sargent, 409 U.S. 1020, *aff'g* 346 F. Supp. 277 (D. Mass. 1972) (finding that the state can constitutionally require unwilling motorcyclists to wear protective headgear); Benning v. Vermont, 641 A.2d 757 (Vt. 1994) (finding that the motorcycle helmet regulation did not violate the state constitutional right of "enjoying and defending liberty"); Everhardt v. City of New Orleans, 217 So. 2d 400, 402 (La. 1968) (holding that driving upon public highways is a privilege and not a right and, in the field of public safety, the city council could regulate motorcycle helmets).

9. *See, e.g.,* Illinois v. Kohrig, 498 N.E.2d 1158 (Ill. 1986) (holding that the legislature could rationally determine that a seatbelt use law would serve public safety and welfare); Ohio v. Batsch, 541 N.E.2d 475 (Ohio Ct. App. 1988) (finding that

seat belts promote the state's interest in protecting the health, safety, and welfare of its citizens); Wells v. New York, 495 N.Y.S.2d 591 (Sup. Ct. Steuben Cty. 1985) (holding that seat belts save lives and therefore come within state police power).

10. *See, e.g.,* Lewis v. United States, 348 U.S. 419 (1955) (upholding a tax affecting gamblers as a valid exercise of taxing power); Martin v. Trout, 199 U.S. 212 (1905) (subjecting the property owner where gaming was carried on to payment of judgments for money lost there at play).

11. *See, e.g.,* Minnesota State Bd. of Health v. Brainerd, 241 N.W.2d 624, 629–30 (Minn. 1976) (holding that it is not the court's function to second-guess the scientific accuracy of legislation based on the fact that fluoridation prevents dental caries); Froncek v. City of Milwaukee, 69 N.W.2d 242, 247 (Wis. 1955) (upholding fluoridation of the city's water supply in the interest of promoting public health and welfare); Readey v. St. Louis Water Co., 352 S.W.2d 622 (Mo. 1961) (finding that fluoridation of water did not deny residents freedom of choice in matters relating to bodily care and health).

12. DANIEL I. WIKLER, ETHICAL ISSUES IN GOVERNMENTAL EFFORTS TO PROMOTE HEALTH (1978). Paternalism is also used as a justification for protecting a class of persons other than the class subject to the regulation. For example, health professional licensing requirements and FDA approval of pharmaceuticals are intended to protect consumers. Consumers cannot purchase unapproved drugs or the services of unlicensed practitioners even if they are informed of, and willingly assume, the risks.

13. Gerald Dworkin, *Paternalism, in* PHILOSOPHY OF LAW 271 (Joel Feinberg & Jules Coleman eds., 6th ed. 2000).

14. Ian Kennedy's definition exposes the problematic assumptions of paternalism: "Decisions concerning a particular person's fate are better made *for* him than *by* him, because others wiser than he are more keenly aware of his best interests than he can be." Ian Kennedy, *The Legal Effect of Requests by the Terminally Ill and Aged Not to Receive Further Treatment,* 1976 CRIM. L. REV. 217, 219.

15. For the philosophical perspective, *see* Dworkin, *supra* note 13, at 278 ("[W]e are all aware of our irrational propensities, deficiencies in cognitive and emotional capacities, and avoidable and unavoidable ignorance, lack of willpower, and psychological and sociological pressures."). For the law and economics perspective, see Christine Jolls et al., *A Behavioral Approach to Law and Economics,* 50 STAN. L. REV. 1471–1550 (1998) (individual capacity to pursue utility is constrained by "bounded rationality," "bounded willpower," and "bounded self-interest").

16. There are at least two possible social meanings in condom use. First, imagine a world where condom use is the exception, such that asking another to use it, or proposing its use, signals the belief that there is a special reason to use a condom and interrupt sex. Second, imagine a world where people ordinarily use condoms and where an ordinary part of sex is the use of a condom. Lawrence Lessig, *The Regulation of Social Meaning,* 62 U. CHI. L. REV. 943, 1022–23 (1995).

17. Barbara A. Israel et al., *Health Education and Community Empowerment: Conceptualizing and Measuring Perceptions of Individual,*

Organizational, and Community Control, 21 HEALTH EDUC. Q. 149 (1994); Daniel Stokols, *Establishing and Maintaining Healthy Environments: Toward a Social Ecology of Health Promotion,* 47 AM. PSYCHOLOGIST 6 (1992); Daniel Stokols, *Translating Social Ecological Theory into Guidelines for Community Health Promotion,* 10 AM. J. HEALTH PROMOTION 282 (1996).

18. Everhardt v. City of New Orleans, 217 So. 2d 400, 403 (La. 1968) ("loose stones on the highway kicked up by passing vehicles . . . could so affect the operator of a motorcycle [without a helmet] as to cause him momentarily to lose control and thus become a menace to other vehicles on the highways"); Benning v. Vermont, 641 A.2d 757, 758 (Vt. 1994) ("[A]n unprotected motorcycle operator could be affected by roadway hazards, temporarily lose control and become a menace to other motorists.").

19. Lawrence O. Gostin, *The Legal Regulation of Smoking (and Smokers): Public Health or Secular Morality?, in* MORALITY AND HEALTH, 331 (Allan M. Brandt & Paul Rozin eds., 1997); Michael Brauer & Andrea 't Mannetje, *Restaurant Smoking Restrictions and Environmental Tobacco Smoke Exposure,* 88 AM. J. PUB. HEALTH 1834 (1998); Ronald M. Davis, *Exposure to Environmental Tobacco Smoke: Identifying and Protecting Those at Risk,* 280 JAMA 1947 (1998).

20. *Benning,* 641 A.2d at 762 ("Whether in taxes or insurance rates, our costs are linked to the actions of others and are driven up when others fail to take preventive steps that would minimize health care consumption."); *Everhardt,* 217 So. 2d at 403 ("[T]he legislature is [not] powerless to prohibit individuals from pursuing a course of conduct which could conceivably result in their becoming public charges.").

21. Simon v. Sargent, 346 F. Supp. 277, 279 (D. Mass. 1972).

22. Richard J. Bonnie, *The Efficacy of Law as a Paternalistic Instrument, in* NEBRASKA SYMPOSIUM ON MOTIVATION 131 (1985).

23. NATIONAL RESEARCH COUNCIL, UNDERSTANDING RISK: INFORMING DECISIONS IN A DEMOCRATIC SOCIETY 215 (Paul C. Stern & Harvey V. Fineberg eds., 1996).

24. Scott Burris, *Law and the Social Risk of Health Care: Lessons from HIV Testing,* 61 ALB. L. REV. 831 (1998).

25. Risk analysis is the application of scientific and other methods to evaluate risk. Its aim is to increase understanding of the substantive qualities, seriousness, likelihood, and conditions of a hazard and the options for managing it. *See, e.g.,* JOHN J. COHRSSEN & VINCENT T. COVELLO, RISK ANALYSIS: A GUIDE TO PRINCIPLES AND METHODS FOR ANALYZING HEALTH AND ENVIRONMENTAL RISKS (1989); NATIONAL RESEARCH COUNCIL, ISSUES IN RISK ASSESSMENT (1993); KENNETH J. ARROW ET AL., BENEFIT-COST ANALYSIS IN ENVIRONMENTAL, HEALTH, AND SAFETY REGULATION: A STATEMENT OF PRINCIPLES (1996).

26. Risk perception is the study of the diverse ways that different communities perceive risk, and the use of these perceptions to select (and prioritize) a regulatory agenda to reduce risk. Many scholarly examinations of risk perception are concerned with differences between expert and lay perspectives of risk. *See, e.g.,* J.A. Bradbury, *The Policy Implications of Differing Concepts of Risk,* 14 SCI., TECH. & HUM. VALUES 380 (1989); G.A. Cole & S.B. Whithey,

Perspective on Risk Perception, 1 RISK ANALYSIS 143 (1981); William R. Freudenburg, *Perceived Risk, Real Risk: Social Science and the Art of Probabilistic Risk Assessment,* 241 SCI. 44 (1988).

27. Risk characterization typically has been seen as a summary of scientific information as an aid to policy formulation. NATIONAL RESEARCH COUNCIL, RISK ASSESSMENT IN THE FEDERAL GOVERNMENT: MANAGING THE PROCESS 20 (1983). The National Research Council later emphasized the importance of consultation in a democratic society: "Risk characterization is a synthesis and summary of information about a potentially hazardous situation that addresses the needs and interests of decision makers and of interested and affected parties. Risk characterization is a prelude to decision making and depends on an iterative, analytic-deliberative process." *See* NATIONAL RESEARCH COUNCIL, *supra* note 23, at 27.

28. Risk communication is the process by which policymakers explain the nature and seriousness of risks to the public. Risk communication is concerned with the effectiveness with which messages are presented to the public: Are they understandable? Do they over- or undersimplify? Do they accurately explain the scientific evidence or the scientific uncertainties? *See, e.g.,* RISK COMMUNICATION AND PUBLIC HEALTH (Peter Bennett & Kenneth Calman eds., 1999); NATIONAL RESEARCH COUNCIL, IMPROVING RISK COMMUNICATION (1989); Caron Chess et al., *Improving Risk Communication in Government: Research Priorities,* 15 RISK ANALYSIS 127 (1995); Dorothy Nelkin, *Communicating Technological Risk: The Social Construction of Risk Perception,* 10 ANN. REV. OF PUB. HEALTH 95 (1989).

29. Risk management is a study of the various policies that could be adopted in response to risk. What policy options exist and how likely are they to prevent harm, reduce the probabilities that harm will occur, or ameliorate harms once they have occurred? Risk management may have to grapple with competing risks—for example, the risks of acting or not acting, and the risk from one source or another source. *See, e.g.,* SHEILA JASANOFF, RISK MANAGEMENT AND POLITICAL CULTURE (1986).

30. This risk analysis borrows from disability discrimination law and Justice Brennan's decision in *School Board of Nassau County v. Arline,* 480 U.S. 273, 285 (1987). Titles I and III of the ADA permit discrimination in employment and public accommodations if a person with a disability poses "a direct threat to the health or safety of others," providing reasonable accommodations or modifications will not eliminate that threat. 42 U.S.C. §§ 12113(b), 12182(b)(3)(1994).

31. *See* Industrial Union Dep't, AFL-CIO v. American Petroleum Inst., 448 U.S. 607, 644 (1980) (lowering benzene exposure levels required proof of "a significant risk of harm and therefore a probability of significant benefits"). For an argument about the efficiency advantages of better information and evidence, see W. KIP VISCUSI, RISKS BY CHOICE: REGULATING HEALTH AND SAFETY IN THE WORK PLACE (1983).

32. For excellent historical works that chronicle the invidious discrimination and prejudiced attitudes toward illness and disease, see, e.g., SUSAN SONTAG, ILLNESS AS A METAPHOR (1986); ALLAN M. BRANDT, NO MAGIC BULLET:

A SOCIAL HISTORY OF VENEREAL DISEASE IN THE UNITED STATES SINCE 1880 (1985).

33. STEPHEN BREYER, BREAKING THE VICIOUS CIRCLE: TOWARD EFFECTIVE RISK REGULATION 9–10 (1993).

34. Transgenic plants and animals have created concerns in Europe and North America despite the absence of scientific evidence about risks to human health. See NATIONAL RESEARCH COUNCIL, GENETICALLY-MODIFIED PEST-PROTECTED PLANTS: SCIENCE AND REGULATION (2000); ROYAL SOCIETY OF MEDICINE, GENETICALLY MODIFIED PLANTS FOR FOOD USE (1998); Othmar Kappeli & Lillian Auberson, How Safe Is Safe Enough in Plant Genetic Engineering? 3 TRENDS IN PLANT SCI. 276–281 (1998); Allison A. Snow & Pedro Moran Palma, Commercialization of Transgenic Plants: Potential Ecological Risks, 47 BIO/SCI. 86–96 (1997); Michael Pollan, Fried, Mashed or Zapped with DNA, N.Y. TIMES MAG., Feb. 25, 1998, at 44.

35. Lawrence O. Gostin, The Resurgent Tuberculosis Epidemic in the Era of AIDS: Reflections on Public Health, Law, and Society, 54 MD. L. REV. 1, 102–108 (1995).

36. For a perversion of the significant risk standard, see Onishea v. Hopper, 171 F.3d 1289 (11th Cir. 1999) (en banc), cert. denied sub nom. Davis v. Hopper, 120 S. Ct. 931 (2000) (holding that because HIV infection carries grave consequences, even a theoretical risk of transmission is sufficient to justify segregation of HIV-infected prisoners).

37. Harold P. Green, The Law-Science Interface in Public Policy Decisionmaking, 51 OHIO ST. L.J. 375 (1990).

38. Frank B. Cross, The Public Role in Risk Control, 24 ENVTL. L. 887, 888 (1994).

39. See, e.g., HOWARD MARGOLIS, DEALING WITH RISK 1 (1996); BREYER, supra note 33, at 35–39; Cass R. Sunstein, Selective Fatalism, 27 J. LEGAL STUD. 799 (1998); R. Krutzer & C. Arnesen, The Scientific Assessment and Public Perception of Risk, 1 CURRENT ISSUES PUB. HEALTH 102 (1995).

40. Rachel Novak, Flesh-Eating Bacteria: Not New, but Still Worrisome, 264 SCI. 1665 (1994).

41. Eliot Marshall, A Is For Apple, Alar, and . . . Alarmist? Two Years Ago Environmentalists Branded Alar the Most Dangerous Chemical Residue in Children's Food; Since Then, the Official Risk Estimates Have Fallen, 254 SCI. 5028 (1991).

42. See, e.g., BREYER, supra note 33, at 9–10.

43. These kinds of lay distinctions are far from simple. Cass R. Sunstein, A Note on "Voluntary" Versus "Involuntary" Risks, 8 DUKE ENVTL. L. & POL'Y J. 173 (1997). Why, for example, is air travel thought to be involuntary, but automobile travel voluntary? Why do people feel that they can avert accidents through skillful and careful driving, even though the data show otherwise? See Neil D. Weinstein, Optimistic Biases About Personal Risks, 246 SCI. 1232 (1989).

44. Lawrence O. Gostin et al., Water Quality Laws and Waterborne Diseases: Cryptosporidium and Other Emerging Pathogens, 90 AM. J. PUB. HEALTH 847 (2000).

45. Cass R. Sunstein, *Health-Health Tradeoffs*, 63 U. CHI. L. REV. 1533 (1996).

46. The following cases illustrate court decisions that refrain from a means-tested analysis in reaching a conclusion. Vernonia School Dist. v. Acton, 515 U.S. 646 (1995) (finding that the public school district's student athlete drug testing policy did not violate the students' constitutional rights); People v. Adams, 149 Ill. 2d. 331 (Ill. 1992) (upholding mandatory HIV testing of persons convicted of prostitution as constitutional).

47. Allan M. Brandt et al., *Routine Hospital Testing for HIV: Health Policy Considerations, in* AIDS AND THE HEALTH CARE SYSTEM 125 (Lawrence O. Gostin ed., 1990).

48. INSTITUTE OF MEDICINE, IMPROVING HEALTH IN THE COMMUNITY: A ROLE FOR PERFORMANCE MONITORING 5 (Jane S. Durch et al. eds., National Academy Press 1997). See INSTITUTE OF MEDICINE, HEALTH PERFORMANCE MEASUREMENT IN THE PUBLIC SECTOR (1999); INSTITUTE OF MEDICINE, USING PERFORMANCE MONITORING TO IMPROVE COMMUNITY HEALTH (2 vols. 1996); Centers for Disease Control & Prevention, *Framework for Program Evaluation in Public Health*, 48 MORBID. & MORTAL. WKLY. REP. 1 (1999).

49. Quality-adjusted life-years (QUALYs) are a measure of health needs that encompass not only length of life, but also the quality of that life (e.g., in symptoms and ability to function). In the context of vaccines, *see* INSTITUTE OF MEDICINE, VACCINES FOR THE 21ST CENTURY: A TOOL FOR DECISION-MAKING (1999) (reviewing cost-effectiveness and ethical concerns regarding QUALYs).

50. *See, e.g.,* W. KIP VISCUSI, FATAL TRADEOFFS: PUBLIC AND PRIVATE RESPONSIBILITIES FOR RISK (1992); Cass R. Sunstein, *Paradoxes of the Regulatory State*, 57 U. CHI. L. REV. 407 (1990); Kenneth J. Arrow et al., *Is There a Role for Benefit-Cost Analysis in Environmental, Health, and Safety Regulation*, 272 SCI. 221 (1996); W. Kip Viscusi, *Regulating the Regulators*, 63 U. CHI. L. REV. 1423 (1996).

51. COST-EFFECTIVENESS IN HEALTH AND MEDICINE (Marthe R. Gold ed., 1996); Louise B. Russell et al., *The Role of Cost-Effectiveness Analysis in Health and Medicine*, 276 JAMA 1172 (1996); Joanna E. Siegel et al. *Recommendations for Reporting Cost-Effectiveness Analysis*, 276 JAMA 1339 (1996); Milton C. Weinstein et al., *Recommendations*, 276 JAMA 1253 (1996).

52. Perhaps the most famous critique of the regulatory state was offered by Stephen Breyer before he was appointed to the Supreme Court. BREYER, *supra* note 33, at 10–29.

53. Craig Gannett, *Congress and the Reform of Risk Regulation*, 107 HARV. L. REV. 2095 (1994) (reviewing STEPHEN BREYER, *supra* note 33.).

54. United States v. Ottati & Goss, 900 F.2d 429 (1st Cir. 1990).

55. Here are some of the costs per lives saved (thousands) in John F. Morrall's famous table comparing various risk-reducing regulations: unvented space heaters ($100), passive restraints/belts ($300), alcohol and drug control ($500), asbestos ($104,200), benzene/ethylbenzenol styrene ($483,000), formaldehyde ($72,000,000). John F. Morrall III, *A Review of the Record,* REGULATION 30 (Nov./Dec. 1986). For a powerful critique of Morrall's methods, see Lisa Heinzerling, *Regulatory Costs of Mythic Proportions*, 107 YALE

L.J. 1981, 2042 (1998) [hereinafter *Regulatory Costs*]; Lisa Heinzerling, *The Rights of Statistical People*, 24 HARV. ENVTL. L. REV. 189 (2000).

56. Heinzerling, *Regulatory Costs*, supra note 55, at 2042.

57. Ellen K. Silbergeld, *The Risks of Comparing Risks*, 3 N.Y.U. ENVTL. L.J. 405 (1995).

58. Heinzerling, *Regulatory Costs*, supra note 55, at 1981 (arguing that the assumptions made in cost-benefit analyses are far from value-neutral).

59. Another way of thinking about fairness, advocated by many scholars in the fields of law and economics, is that costs and burdens might justifiably be placed not only on those who cause risk, but also on those who can best afford to incur regulatory costs or burdens (see chapter 10).

60. LAWRENCE O. GOSTIN & ZITA LAZZARINI, HUMAN RIGHTS AND PUBLIC HEALTH IN THE AIDS PANDEMIC (1997).

61. Jonathan M. Mann et al., *Health and Human Rights*, 1 J. HEALTH & HUM. RTS. 6, 19 (1994).

62. While not disputing the disincentives engendered by fear of discrimination, Professor Burris observes that law reform, in and of itself, is insufficient to reassure persons to come forward for testing and treatment. Burris, *supra* note 24, at 831.

63. For a case study on named HIV reporting, see chapter 5.

64. Jonathan M. Mann, *Medicine and Public Health, Ethics and Human Rights*, 27 HASTINGS CENTER RPT. 6, 9–11 (1997).

65. REBECCA J. COOK, WOMEN'S HEALTH AND HUMAN RIGHTS: THE PROMOTION AND PROTECTION OF WOMEN'S HEALTH THROUGH INTERNATIONAL HUMAN RIGHTS LAW (1994).

5. PUBLIC HEALTH INFORMATION: PERSONAL PRIVACY

SOURCES FOR CHAPTER EPIGRAPHS: Page 113: WILLIAM FARR, VITAL STATISTICS: A MEMORIAL VOLUME OF SELECTIONS FROM THE REPORTS AND WRITINGS WITH A BIOGRAPHICAL SKETCH (Scarecrow Press, 1975) (1885); *see* Mervyn Susser & Abraham Adelstein, *An Introduction to the Work of William Farr: An Abridged Version of the Introduction to the Reprinting of Reference 1 by the New York Academy of Medicine*, 101 AM. J. EPIDEMIOL. 469 (1975); Alexander D. Langmuir, *William Farr: Founder of Modern Concepts of Surveillance*, 5 INT'L. J. EPIDEMIOL. 13, 15 (1976); *see also* MAJOR GREENWOOD, MEDICAL STATISTICS FROM GRAUNT TO FARR (1948). Page 117: MILTON J. ROSENAU, PREVENTIVE MEDICINE AND HYGIENE 1002 (1917). Page 121: Thomas Parran, *The Eradication of Syphilis as a Practical Public Health Objective*, 92 JAMA 73 (1931). Page 136: Marion C. Potter, *Venereal Prophylaxis*, 7 AM. J. NURSING, 340, 349–50 (1907).

1. Denis J. Protti, *The Application of Information Science, Information Technology, and Information Management to Public Health, in* OXFORD TEXTBOOK OF PUBLIC HEALTH 419 (Roger Detels et al. eds., 3d ed. 1997) [hereinafter OXFORD TEXTBOOK OF PUBLIC HEALTH].

2. INSTITUTE OF MEDICINE, THE FUTURE OF PUBLIC HEALTH 44 (1988) (the core public health function of "assessment" includes surveillance).

3. WAYNE W. DANIEL, BIOSTATISTICS: A FOUNDATION FOR ANALYSIS IN THE HEALTH SCIENCES 1 (5th ed. 1991).

4. JUDITH S. MAUSNER ET AL., MAUSNER & BAHN EPIDEMIOLOGY—AN INTRODUCTORY TEXT 1 (2d ed. 1985); Roger Detels, *Epidemiology: The Foundation of Public Health, in* OXFORD TEXTBOOK OF PUBLIC HEALTH at 501; THE DICTIONARY OF EPIDEMIOLOGY 55–56 (Int'l Epidemiological Ass'n ed., 3d ed. 1995); Nancy D. Pearce, *Traditional Epidemiology, Modern Epidemiology, and Public Health,* 86 AM. J. PUB. HEALTH 68 (1996). See chapter 1 for a further discussion of epidemiology.

5. Lawrence O. Gostin et al., *The Public Health Information Infrastructure: A National Review of the Law on Health Information Privacy,* 275 JAMA 1921, 1922 (1996).

6. *See, e.g.,* INSTITUTE OF MEDICINE, HEALTH DATA IN THE INFORMATION AGE: USE, DISCLOSURE, AND PRIVACY (1994); NATIONAL RESEARCH COUNCIL, FOR THE RECORD: PROTECTING ELECTRONIC HEALTH INFORMATION (1997).

7. Lawrence O. Gostin, *Health Information Privacy,* 80 CORNELL L. REV. 451, 482–84 (1995).

8. JANLORI GOLDMAN & DENNIS MULLIGAN, PRIVACY AND HEALTH INFORMATION SYSTEMS: A GUIDE TO PROTECTING PATIENT CONFIDENTIALITY (1997).

9. THE OXFORD ENGLISH DICTIONARY 309, vol. XVII (2d ed. 1989) (General Becker was the officer who was charged with the surveillance of Bonaparte); *see* W.J. EYLENBOSCH & N.D. NOAH, SURVEILLANCE IN HEALTH AND DISEASE 9 (1988); Ruth L. Berkelman et al., *Public Health Surveillance, in* OXFORD TEXTBOOK OF PUBLIC HEALTH, *supra* note 1, at 735.

10. Stephen B. Thacker & Ruth L. Berkelman, *Public Health Surveillance in the United States,* 10 EPIDEMIOL. REV. 164 (1988); Alexander D. Langmuir, *The Surveillance of Communicable Diseases of National Importance,* 268 NEW ENG. J. MED. 182 (1963); Stephen B. Thacker et al., *The Science of Public Health Surveillance,* 10 J. PUB. HEALTH POL'Y 187 (Summer 1989).

11. Stephen B. Thacker, *Historical Development, in* PRINCIPLES AND PRACTICE OF PUBLIC HEALTH SURVEILLANCE 4 (Steven M. Teutsch & R. Elliott Churchill eds., 1994).

12. Henry Ingersoll Bowditch et al., *Letter from Massachusetts State Board of Health to Physicians,* 30 (Suppl. 12) PUB. HEALTH REP. 31 (1915).

13. VITAL STATISTICS OF THE UNITED STATES, 1958 (1959).

14. CENTERS FOR DISEASE CONTROL, MANUAL OF PROCEDURES FOR NATIONAL MORBIDITY REPORTING AND PUBLIC HEALTH SURVEILLANCE ACTIVITIES (1985).

15. JAMES A. TOBEY, PUBLIC HEALTH LAW 109 (1926).

16. Langmuir, *supra* note 10.

17. Donald A. Henderson, *Surveillance of Smallpox,* 5 INT. J. EPIDEMIOL. 19 (1976).

18. Centers for Disease Control, *Kaposi's Sarcoma and Pneumocystis Pneumonia Among Homosexual Men—New York City and California,* 30 MORB. MORT. WKLY. REP. 305 (1981).

19. Brian Hjelle et al., *Emergence of Hanta-Viral Disease in the Southwestern United States,* 161 WEST. J. MED. 467 (1994).

20. CENTERS FOR DISEASE CONTROL & PREVENTION, ADDRESSING EMERGING INFECTIOUS DISEASE THREATS: A PREVENTION STRATEGY FOR THE UNITED STATES (1994); Centers for Disease Control & Prevention, *Preventing Emerging Infectious Diseases: A Strategy for the 21st Century,* 47 MORB. MORT. WKLY. REP. 1 (1998); David P. Fidler, *Return of the Fourth Horseman: Emerging Infectious Diseases and International Law,* 81 MINN. L. REV. 771 (1997).

21. Anthony G. Macintyre et al., *Weapons of Mass Destruction: Events with Contaminated Casualties,* 238 JAMA 242 (2000); Donald A. Henderson, *The Looming Threat of Bioterrorism,* 283 SCI. 1279 (1999); Centers for Disease Control & Prevention, *Bioterrorism Alleging Use of Anthrax and Interim Guidelines for Management,* 281 JAMA 787 (1999).

22. *See, e.g.,* Centers for Disease Control & Prevention, *Youth Risk Behavior Surveillance—United States, 1997,* 47 MORB. MORT. WKLY. REP. 1 (Supp. 1998).

23. CENTERS FOR DISEASE CONTROL & PREVENTION, TRANSLATING ADVANCES IN HUMAN GENETICS INTO PUBLIC HEALTH ACTION—A STRATEGIC PLAN, (1997); Muin J. Khoury, *From Genes to Public Health: The Applications of Genetic Technology in Disease Prevention,* 86 AM. J. PUB. HEALTH 1717 (1996); Scott Burris & Lawrence O. Gostin, *Genetic Screening from a Public Health Perspective: Some Lessons from the HIV Experience, in* GENETIC SECRETS: PROTECTING PRIVACY AND CONFIDENTIALITY IN THE GENETIC ERA 137 (Mark A. Rothstein ed., 1997).

24. Nancy D. Pearce, *Information Resources in the United States, in* OXFORD TEXTBOOK OF PUBLIC HEALTH, *supra* note 1, at 435.

25. Ruth L. Berkelman et al., *Infectious Disease Surveillance: A Crumbling Foundation,* 264 SCI. 368 (1994); Michael T. Osterholm et al., *Impediments to Public Health Surveillance in the 1990s: The Lack of Resources and the Need for Priorities,* 2 PUB. HEALTH MGMT. PRAC. 11 (1996).

26. Whalen v. Roe, 429 U.S. 589 (1977) (upholding the New York reporting requirement for prescriptions for certain dangerous drugs).

27. Lawrence O. Gostin et al., *The Law and the Public's Health: A Study of Infectious Disease Law in the United States,* 99 COLUM. L. REV. 59 (1999).

28. New York State Soc'y of Surgeons v. Axelrod, 572 N.E.2d 605 (N.Y. 1991).

29. Terence L. Chorba et al., *Mandatory Reporting of Infectious Diseases by Clinicians,* 262 JAMA 3018 (1989).

30. Centers for Disease Control, *Mandatory Reporting of Infectious Disease by Clinicians,* 39 MORB. MORT. WKLY. REP. 1 (1990).

31. Sandra Roush et al., *Mandatory Reporting of Diseases and Conditions by Health Care Providers and Laboratories,* 282 JAMA 164 (1999).

32. COUNCIL FOR STATE AND TERRITORIAL EPIDEMIOLOGISTS, REPORTING REQUIREMENTS OF DISEASE AND CONDITIONS UNDER NATIONAL SURVEILLANCE (visited May 15, 2000), <http://www.cste.org>. CSTE regularly updates the current list of reportable diseases at its web site.

33. Centers for Disease Control & Prevention, *Case Definitions for Infectious Conditions Under Public Health Surveillance,* 46 MORB. MORT. WKLY. REP. 1 (1997).

34. Daniel M. Fox, *Social Policy and City Politics: Tuberculosis Reporting in New York, 1889–1900*, BULL. HIST. OF MED. (1975); Daniel M. Fox, *The Politics of Public Health in New York City: Contrasting Styles Since 1920*, in HIVES OF SICKNESS: PUBLIC HEALTH AND EPIDEMICS IN NEW YORK CITY 197 (David Rosner ed., 1995).

35. Daniel M. Fox, *From TB to AIDS: Value Conflicts in Reporting Disease*, HASTINGS CENTER REP. 11 (Dec. 1986).

36. RONALD BAYER, PRIVATE ACTS, SOCIAL CONSEQUENCES: AIDS AND THE POLITICS OF PUBLIC HEALTH 117–23 (1991).

37. Lawrence O. Gostin et al., *National HIV Case Reporting for the United States: A Defining Moment in the History of the Epidemic*, 337 NEW ENG. J. MED. 1162 (1997); Lawrence O. Gostin & James G. Hodge Jr., *The "Names Debate:" The Case for National HIV Reporting in the United States*, 61 ALB. L. REV. 679 (1998).

38. AMERICAN CIVIL LIBERTIES UNION, HIV SURVEILLANCE AND NAME REPORTING (1998).

39. Sue Landry, *AIDS List Is Out: State Investigating Breach*, ST. PETERSBURG TIMES, Sept. 20, 1996, at A1.

40. 410 ILCS 305/12 (West 1999); *see also id.* at 325/8.

41. AIDS ACTION FOUNDATION, SHOULD HIV TEST RESULTS BE REPORTABLE? A DISCUSSION OF THE KEY POLICY QUESTIONS (1993).

42. Studies indicate that persons at risk of HIV are not deterred from seeking testing in states that provide alternative sites offering anonymous testing. Andrew B. Bindman et al., *Multistate Evaluation of Anonymous HIV Testing and Access to Care,* 280 JAMA 1416 (1998). Surveys also demonstrate that most people are not even aware of state reporting requirements and, therefore, are unlikely to be influenced by them. Centers for Disease Control & Prevention, *HIV Testing Among Populations at Risk for HIV Infection—9 States, November 1995–December 1996*, 47 MORB. MORT. WKLY. REP. 1086 (1998); Frederick M. Hecht et al., *Named Reporting of HIV: Attitudes and Knowledge of Those at Risk*, 12 J. GEN. INTERNAL MED. 108 (1997).

43. Lynda Richardson, *AIDS Group Urges New York to Start Reporting of HIV*, N.Y. TIMES, Jan. 13, 1998, at A1.

44. Centers for Disease Control & Prevention, *Evaluation of HIV Case Surveillance through the Use of Non-Name Unique Identifiers—Maryland and Texas, 1994–1996*, 46 MORB. MORT. WKLY. REP. 1254 (1998); David Osmond et al., *Name-Based Surveillance and Public Health Interventions for Persons with HIV Infection*, 131 ANNALS INTERNAL MED. 775 (1999).

45. Centers for Disease Control & Prevention, *Guidelines for National HIV Case Surveillance*, 48 MORB. MORT. WKLY. REP. 1 (1999).

46. Ronald Bayer & Kathleen E. Toomey, *HIV Prevention and the Two Faces of Partner Notification*, 82 AM. J. PUB. HEALTH 1158 (1992); Lawrence O. Gostin & James G. Hodge, Jr., *Piercing the Veil of Secrecy in HIV/AIDS and Other Sexually Transmitted Diseases: Theories of Privacy and Disclosure in Partner Notification*, 5 DUKE J. GENDER L. & POL'Y 9, 14–51 (1998).

47. VERLA L. BULLOUGH, THE HISTORY OF PROSTITUTION 166–72 (1964); GEORGE ROSEN, A HISTORY OF PUBLIC HEALTH 73 (1993).

48. The Contagious Disease Acts of 1864 and 1866 adopted partner notification as a method of controlling STDs in the military. The statutes also ordered confinement for up to six months for prostitutes. *See* Michael J. Adler, *The Terrible Peril: A Historical Perspective on the Venereal Diseases*, 281 BRIT. MED. J. 206 (1980).

49. ALLAN M. BRANDT, NO MAGIC BULLET: A SOCIAL HISTORY OF VENEREAL DISEASE IN THE UNITED STATES SINCE 1880 (1987).

50. Army Appropriations Act, 40 Stat. 855, 856 (1918), *amended by* the National Venereal Disease Act, 52 Stat. 439, 439–40 (1938). *See* Public Health Service Act, ch. 373, 58 Stat. 667, 693–94 (1944) (granting funds to the states for prevention, treatment, and control of venereal diseases).

51. *See* Gostin et al., *supra* note 27.

52. Jon K. Andrus et al., *Partner Notification: Can it Control Syphilis?*, 112 ANNALS INTERNAL MED. 539 (1990).

53. The CDC requires federally funded contact tracing programs to provide a comprehensive set of supplemental services, including testing, medical treatment, and counseling, in addition to notification assistance. CENTERS FOR DISEASE CONTROL & PREVENTION, HIV PARTNER NOTIFICATION SUPPORT SERVICES OPERATIONAL GUIDANCE OUTLINE 1–8 (1997).

54. For a detailed table of state laws authorizing contact tracing, see Gostin & Hodge, *supra* note 46, at 28–32.

55. Early federal law on the control of STDs did not mention contact tracing, but created a Division of Venereal Diseases within the Bureau of the Public Health Service. Army Appropriations Act, 40 Stat. 855, 856 (1918), *amended by* the National Venereal Disease Act, 52 Stat. 439, 439–40 (1938). *See* Public Health Service Act, ch. 373, 58 Stat. 667, 693–94 (1944) (funding states for prevention, treatment, and control of venereal diseases).

56. Although Surgeon General Parran incorporated contact tracing into mainstream public health in the 1930s, the term was not enumerated in federal law until 1972 when Congress passed the Communicable Disease Control Amendments Acts, Pub. L. No. 92-449, sec. 203 § 318(d)(1)(B), 86 Stat. 751, 870–72 (1972) (authorizing the Secretary to fund case finding including contact tracing). The Acts were amended by the Public Health Service Act of 1976, Pub. L. 94-317, sec. 203 § d(1)(B), 90 Stat. 695, 703–04 (codified as amended 42 U.S.C. § 247c (1997)) (authorizing the Secretary to make project grants for routine testing). The Acts were further amended by the Preventative Health Amendments of 1984, Pub. L. No. 98-555, sec. 3 § (d)(6)(A–B), 98 Stat. 2854, 2855 (1984) (adding STDs in addition to syphilis and gonorrhea, and replacing the antiquated term "venereal disease" with "sexually transmitted disease").

57. AIDS Emergency Act of 1990, Pub. L. No. 101-381, title III, § 301(a), 104 Stat. 597, 602 (codified as 42 U.S.C. § 300(f)(f)-46 (1994)).

58. Pub. L. No. 104-146 S41, 110 Stat. 1346 (codified at 42 U.S.C. § 201 (Supp. 1996)).

59. CENTERS FOR DISEASE CONTROL & PREVENTION, 1993 SEXUALLY TRANSMITTED DISEASES TREATMENT GUIDELINES: PARTNER NOTIFICATION AND MANAGEMENT OF SEX PARTNERS (1993); Frances M. Cowan et al., *The Role and*

Effectiveness of Partner Notification in STD Control: A Review, 72 GENITOURINARY MED. 247 (1996).

60. Brandt, *supra* note 49.

61. *See* Bayer, *supra* note 36 (the gay community characterized partner notification as "Orwellian"); Chandler Burr, *The AIDS Exception: Privacy vs. Public Health,* ATLANTIC MONTHLY, June 1997, at 57–67.

62. Karen H. Rothenberg & Stephen J. Paskey, *The Risk of Domestic Violence and Women with HIV Infection: Implications for Partner Notification, Public Policy, and the Law,* 85 AM. J. PUB. HEALTH 1569 (1990).

63. The evidence is accumulated in Gostin & Hodge, *supra* note 46, at 72–82.

64. John M. Last, *Epidemiology and Ethics,* 19 LAW MED. & HEALTH CARE 166 (1991).

65. JAMES H. JONES, BAD BLOOD: THE TUSKEGEE SYPHILIS EXPERIMENT (expanded ed. 1993). In 1997, President Clinton publicly apologized to the subjects of the Tuskegee experiments. Allison Mitchell, *Clinton Regrets "Clearly Racist" U.S. Study,* N.Y. TIMES, May 17, 1997, at A10.

66. ADVISORY COMMITTEE ON HUMAN RADIATION EXPERIMENTS, FINAL REPORT (1996).

67. Marlene Simmons, *CDC Says It Erred in Measles Study: Agency Failed to Tell Parents That One of Two Vaccines Used on Infants in L.A. During Epidemic Was Experimental,* L.A. TIMES, June 17, 1996, at A11.

68. Marcia Angell, *The Ethics of Clinical Research in the Third World,* 337 NEW ENG. J. MED. 847 (1997); Peter Lurie & Sidney M. Wolfe, *Unethical Trials of Interventions to Reduce Perinatal Transmission of the Human Immunodeficiency Virus in Developing Countries,* 337 N. ENG. J. MED. 853 (1997). For a more recent ethical discussion of a clinical trial in rural Uganda, see Marcia Angell, *Investigators' Responsibilities for Human Subjects in Developing Countries,* 342 NEW ENG. J. MED. 967 (2000).

69. Harold Varmus & David Satcher, *Ethical Complexities of Conducting Research in Developing Countries,* 337 NEW ENG. J. MED. 1003 (1997).

70. NATIONAL BIOETHICS ADVISORY COMMISSION, RESEARCH INVOLVING PERSONS WITH MENTAL DISORDERS THAT MAY AFFECT DECISIONMAKING CAPACITY (1998).

71. NATIONAL COMMISSION FOR THE PROTECTION OF HUMAN SUBJECTS OF BIOMEDICAL AND BEHAVIORAL RESEARCH, ETHICAL PRINCIPLES AND GUIDELINES FOR THE PROTECTION OF HUMAN SUBJECTS OF RESEARCH (April 18, 1979).

72. Nuremberg Code 1947, *reprinted in* TRIALS OF WAR CRIMINALS BEFORE THE NUREMBERG MILITARY TRIBUNALS UNDER CONTROL COUNCIL LAW NO. 10, vol. II 181–82 (1949) ("The voluntary consent of the human subject is absolutely essential.").

73. WORLD MEDICAL ASSOCIATION DECLARATION OF HELSINKI: RECOMMENDATIONS GUIDING MEDICAL DOCTORS IN BIOMEDICAL RESEARCH INVOLVING HUMAN SUBJECTS, *adopted by* the 18th World Medical Assembly (WMA), Helsinki, Finland, 1964; *revised by* the 29th WMA, Tokyo, Japan, 1975; 35th WMA in Venice, Italy, 1983; and the 41st WMA in Hong Kong, 1989. ("In research on man, the interest of science and society should never take precedence over considerations related to the wellbeing [sic] of the subject."). *See* Medical

Ethics Committee, *Proposed Revision of the World Medical Association Declaration of Helsinki* (WMA Document 17.C/Rev. 1/98, 1999); Robert J. Levine, *The Need to Revise the Declaration of Helsinki*, 341 NEW ENG. J. MED. 531 (1999).

74. COUNCIL OF INT'L ORG. OF MED. SCI., PROPOSED INTERNATIONAL GUIDELINES FOR BIOMEDICAL RESEARCH INVOLVING HUMAN SUBJECTS (1982).

75. COUNCIL OF INT'L ORG. OF MED. SCI., INTERNATIONAL GUIDELINES FOR ETHICAL REVIEW OF EPIDEMIOLOGIC STUDIES (1991), *reprinted in* Bernard M. Dickens et al. (eds.), *Research on Human Populations: National and International Ethical Guidelines*, 19 LAW MED. & HEALTH CARE 247 (1991).

76. Larry Gostin, *Ethical Principles for the Conduct of Human Subject Research: Population-Based Research and Ethics*, 19 LAW, MED. & HEALTH CARE 191 (1991).

77. *See, e.g.,* ETHICS IN EPIDEMIOLOGY AND PUBLIC HEALTH PRACTICE: COLLECTED WORKS (Steven S. Coughlin ed., 1997); STEVEN S. COUGHLIN & TOM L. BEAUCHAMP, ETHICS AND EPIDEMIOLOGY (1996); Alexander M. Capron, *Protection of Research Subjects: Do Special Rules Apply in Epidemiology?*, 44 J. CLIN. EPIDEMIOL. 81–89 (1991).

78. Protection of Human Subjects, 45 C.F.R. §§ 46.101–.404 (1993) [also known as the "Common Rule"]. The Federal Food and Drug Administration (FDA) operates its own rules for protection of human subjects that are similar, but not identical, to the Common Rule.

79. DEPARTMENT OF HEALTH & HUM. SERVS. OFFICE OF INSPECTOR GEN., INSTITUTIONAL REVIEW BOARDS: THEIR ROLE IN REVIEWING APPROVED RESEARCH (1998); DEPARTMENT OF HEALTH & HUM. SERVS. OFFICE OF INSPECTOR GEN., INSTITUTIONAL REVIEW BOARDS: THE EMERGENCE OF INDEPENDENT BOARDS (1998); DEPARTMENT OF HEALTH & HUM. SERVS. OFFICE OF INSPECTOR GEN., INSTITUTIONAL REVIEW BOARDS: A TIME FOR REFORM (1998).

80. 45 C.F.R. § 46.111(a)(7) (1993).

81. *Id.* at § 46.116(a)(5).

82. 42 U.S.C. § 241(d) (1994).

83. Protection is available upon application for a named project and is conferred in the form of a "certificate of confidentiality" issued directly by the Assistant Secretary for Health. The certificate provides legal authority to resist compulsory demands for identifiable research subject information. An investigator with a certificate has a legal defense against subpoena or court order similar to the physician-patient privilege. The defense applies only to information about individual subjects, not aggregate data. ASSISTANT SECRETARY FOR HEALTH, INTERIM POLICY STATEMENT (June 8, 1989).

84. However, if the researcher seeks a certificate to avoid reporting a communicable disease, the Assistant Secretary requires a special demonstration of how the research would be impaired by the reporting. *Id.*

85. *Id.*

86. ROBERT J. LEVINE, ETHICS AND REGULATION OF CLINICAL RESEARCH 3–7 (2d ed. 1986).

87. 45 C.F.R. § 46.102(d) (1993). Classifying an activity as research does not automatically require IRB review. Once an activity is classified as research,

two additional determinations must be made: Does the research involve "human subjects" and, if so, is the research "exempt" from IRB review? As to the meaning of "human subject," see *id.* at § 46.102(f)(1),(2). As to the categories of research that are exempt from IRB review, see *id.* at § 46.101(b).

88. For a thoughtful review, see MAJORIE SPEARS, GUIDELINES FOR DEFINING PUBLIC HEALTH RESEARCH AND PUBLIC HEALTH NON-RESEARCH (Centers for Disease Control & Prevention, unpublished background paper, March 1999).

89. Wendy K. Mariner, *Public Confidence in Public Health Research Ethics,* 112 PUB. HEALTH REPS. 33 (1997).

90. Dixie E. Snider & Donna F. Stroup, *Defining Research When It Comes to Public Health,* 112 PUB. HEALTH REPS. 29 (1997).

91. Lawrence O. Gostin, *Personal Privacy in the Health Care System: Employer-Sponsored Insurance, Managed Care, and Integrated Delivery Systems,* 7 KENNEDY INST. OF ETHICS J. 361, 363–64 (1997).

92. *See, e.g.,* ANITA L. ALLEN, UNEASY ACCESS: PRIVACY FOR WOMEN IN A FREE SOCIETY 11, 31–34 (1987); Ruth Gavison, *Privacy and the Limits of Law, in* PHILOSOPHICAL DIMENSIONS OF PRIVACY: AN ANTHOLOGY 346 (Ferdinand D. Schoeman ed., 1984).

93. Samuel D. Warren & Louis D. Brandeis, *The Right to Privacy,* 4 HARV. L. REV. 193 (1890).

94. U.S. INFO. INFRASTRUCTURE TASK FORCE, PRIVACY AND THE NATIONAL INFORMATION INFRASTRUCTURE: PRINCIPLES FOR PROVIDING AND USING PERSONAL INFORMATION (1995).

95. NATIONAL RESEARCH COUNCIL, *supra* note 6; Gostin, *supra* note 91.

96. There is no settled view as to how difficult it must be to determine the person's identity in order to classify the record as "identifiable." Human subject regulations, for example, exempt research involving data recorded in such a manner that "subjects cannot be identified, directly or through identifiers linked to the subjects." Protection of Human Subjects, 45 C.F.R. §§ 46.101(b)(4) (1993). A record is "individually identifiable" if "the identity of the subject is or may readily be ascertained by the investigator or associated with the information." *Id.* at 46.102(f). *See* SECRETARY OF HEALTH & HUM. SERVS., CONFIDENTIALITY OF INDIVIDUALLY IDENTIFIABLE HEALTH INFORMATION: RECOMMENDATIONS OF THE SECRETARY OF HEALTH AND HUMAN SERVICES, PURSUANT TO SECTION 264 OF THE HEALTH INSURANCE PORTABILITY AND ACCOUNTABILITY ACT OF 1996 (September 11, 1997) ("covered" information "identifies the individual, or with respect to which there is a reasonable basis to believe that the information can be used to identify the patient").

97. NATIONAL BIOETHICS ADVISORY COMM'N, RESEARCH INVOLVING HUMAN BIOLOGICAL MATERIALS: ETHICAL ISSUES AND POLICY (1999).

98. Madison Powers, *Justice and Genetics: Privacy Protection and the Moral Basis of Public Policy, in* GENETIC SECRETS: PROTECTING PRIVACY AND CONFIDENTIALITY IN THE GENETIC ERA 355 (Mark A. Rothstein ed., 1997).

99. Lawrence O. Gostin & Jack Hadley, *Editorial: Health Services Research—Public Benefits, Personal Privacy, and Proprietary Interests,* 129 ANNALS OF INTERNAL MED. 833–35 (1998).

100. Howard Minkof & Anne Willoughby, *Pediatric HIV Disease, Zidovudine in Pregnancy, and Unblinding Heelstick Surveys: Reframing the Debate on Prenatal HIV Testing*, 274 JAMA 1165 (1995).

101. ALLEN, *supra* note 92; TOM L. BEAUCHAMP & JAMES F. CHILDRESS, PRINCIPLES OF BIOMEDICAL ETHICS 406–29 (4th ed. 1994); ALAN F. WESTIN, PRIVACY AND FREEDOM (1967).

102. *See e.g.*, BEAUCHAMP & CHILDRESS, *supra* note 101, at 422–24.

103. *See e.g.*, AMITAI ETZIONI, THE LIMITS OF PRIVACY (1999).

104. *See, e.g.*, Seth F. Kreimer, *Sunlight, Secrets, and Scarlet Letters: The Tension Between Privacy and Disclosure in Constitutional Law*, 140 U. PA. L. REV. 1 (1991); Francis S. Chlapowski, *The Constitutional Protection of Informational Privacy*, 71 B.U. L. REV. 133 (1991).

105. 429 U.S. 589 (1977). In *Nixon v. Administrator of General Services*, 433 U.S. 425 (1977), decided four months after *Whalen*, the Court also hesitantly acknowledged a narrow right to privacy. *See also* Planned Parenthood v. Danforth, 428 U.S. 52, 80 (1976) (recognizing the right to privacy, but upholding reporting and record-keeping requirements that were reasonably directed to the preservation of maternal health and properly respected a patient's privacy).

106. *Whalen*, 429 U.S. at 605.

107. *Id.*

108. Rasmussen v. South Fla. Blood Serv., Inc., 500 So. 2d 533 (Fla. 1987) (finding that a person with AIDS is not entitled to a subpoena to assist him in proving that he was infected during a blood transfusion).

109. 638 F.2d 570, 578 (3d Cir. 1980).

110. Individuals asserting a constitutional right to informational privacy are unlikely to obtain a remedy except in cases where the state fails to assert any significant interest or is particularly careless in disclosing highly sensitive information. *See* Doe v. Borough of Barrington, 729 F. Supp. 376 (D.N.J. 1990) (holding that a police officer violated the constitutional right to privacy by disclosing that a person was infected with HIV); Woods v. White, 689 F. Supp. 874 (W.D. Wis. 1988) (extending the constitutional right to privacy to disclosure of prisoner's HIV status by prison medical service personnel), *aff'd*, 899 F.2d 17 (7th Cir. 1990).

111. 18 U.S.C. § 24 (West 1994).

112. DEPT. OF HEALTH & HUM. SERVS. PROPOSED STANDARDS FOR PRIVACY OF INDIVIDUALLY IDENTIFIABLE HEALTH INFORMATION (1999); *see* SECRETARY OF HEALTH & HUM. SERVS *supra* note 96.

113. 5 U.S.C. § 552(b)(1)–(3), (6) (1994).

114. *Id.* at § 552a(a)(7). Health agencies have used this concept to justify many further uses of personally identifiable information. For example, the Health Care Financing Administration (HCFA) releases to researchers data collected from patient records by Medicare Peer Review Organizations, with patient names and provider identifiers intact. Notice of New System of Records, 56 Fed. Reg. 67,078 (1991).

115. 5 U.S.C. § 552 (1994).

116. *See, e.g.*, 13 U.S.C. § 9 (1994) (raw census data); 42 U.S.C. § 290dd-2 (1994) (drug abuse records); 38 U.S.C. § 5701 (1994) (claimants' medical

and insurance records); 42 U.S.C. § 242m(d) (Supp. V 1993) (identifiable health statistics); 42 U.S.C. § 247c(e)(5) (1994) (venereal disease records).

117. *But see* Washington Post v. United States Dep't of Health & Hum. Servs., 690 F.2d 252, 258 (D.C. Cir. 1982) (finding that data exempt from disclosure under FOIA may still be subject to discovery). Courts balance privacy interests against the parties' interests in the administration of justice, and sometimes fashion creative protective orders that permit discovery while limiting privacy infringements. Lampshire v. Procter & Gamble Co., 94 F.R.D. 58, 60 (N.D. Ga. 1982); Farnsworth v. Procter & Gamble Co., 101 F.R.D. 355, 357 (N.D. Ga. 1984), *aff'd*, 758 F.2d 1545 (11th Cir. 1985); Rasmussen v. South Fla. Blood Serv., Inc., 500 So. 2d 533, 535 (Fla. 1987).

118. United States Dep't of State v. Washington Post, 456 U.S. 595, 599 (1982) (exempting medical files from the FOIA because disclosure would invade privacy).

119. Gostin et al., *supra* note 5, at 1921.

120. For a review of these statutes, see Gostin, *supra* note 7, at 451, 499–508.

121. WORKGROUP FOR ELEC. DATA INTERCHANGE, DEPARTMENT OF HEALTH & HUM. SERVS. OBSTACLES TO EDI IN THE CURRENT HEALTH CARE INFRASTRUCTURE , app. 4 at iii (1992).

122. 42 U.S.C. § 290dd-2 (1994) (upholding strict confidentiality for oral and written communications of "[r]ecords of the identity, diagnosis, prognosis, or treatment").

123. Harold Edgar & Hazel Sandomire, *Medical Privacy Issues in the Age of AIDS: Legislative Options*, 16 AM. J.L. & MED. 155 (1990).

124. Thomas H. Murray, *Genetic Exceptionalism and "Future Diaries": Is Genetic Information Different from Other Medical Information?*, in GENETIC SECRETS *supra* note 18, at 137; Lawrence O. Gostin & James G. Hodge, Jr., *Genetics Privacy and the Law: An End to Genetics Exceptionalism*, 40 JURIMETRICS 21 (1999).

125. Restatement (Second) of Torts § 4 (1965). See chapter 10.

126. *See, e.g.*, Alberts v. Devine, 479 N.E.2d 113, 118 (Mass. 1985) (holding that privacy was violated when a physician disclosed health information to a patient's employer).

127. Alan B. Vickery, *Breach of Confidence: An Emerging Tort*, 82 COLUM. L. REV. 1426 (1982).

128. Hague v. Williams, 181 A.2d 345, 349 (N.J. 1962) (finding that public and private interest militates against an obligation of privacy with respect to disclosure of a child's condition to an insurer).

129. Bratt v. International Bus. Mach. Corp., 785 F.2d 352 (1st Cir. 1986) (holding that an employer has violated an employee's right to privacy when the intrusion on employee's privacy outweighs employer's legitimate business interest in the information). *See* Ellen E. Schultz, *Medical Data Gathered by Firms Can Prove Less than Confidential*, WALL ST. J., May 18, 1994, at A1 (documenting numerous instances of disclosures by EAP professionals to employers and insurers).

130. Humphers v. First Interstate Bank of Or., 696 P.2d 527, 530 (Or. 1985) ("[O]nly one who holds the information in confidence can be charged with a breach of confidence.").

131. The duty to warn applies to physicians and psychotherapists, but not necessarily to all health care professionals. *See* Bradley v. Ray, 904 S.W.2d 302 (Mo. Ct. App. 1995) (extending *Tarasoff* to cover other health care professionals); *In re* Sealed Case, 67 F.3d 965 (D.C. Cir. 1995) (refusing to extend the duty to warn third parties to a lab technician).

132. *See, e.g.,* Alberts v. Devine, 479 N.E.2d 113, 115 (Mass. 1985) (recognizing an exception to the duty of confidentiality where there is serious danger to the patient or others).

133. For a summary of state laws, see Gostin & Hodge, *supra* note 46, at 47.

134. For a review of court cases, see John C. Williams, Annotation, *Liability of One Treating Mentally Afflicted Patient for Failure to Warn or Protect Third Persons Threatened by Patient,* 83 A.L.R.3d 1201 (1995); Alan A. Stone, *The Tarasoff Decisions: Suing Psychotherapists to Safeguard Society,* 90 HARV. L. REV. 358 (1976).

135. 551 P.2d 334 (Cal. 1976). Interestingly, the precedent for *Tarasoff* was from old infectious disease cases. *See, e.g.,* Davis v. Rodman, 227 S.W. 612 (Ark. 1921) (upholding a physician's duty to advise family members likely to be exposed to a patient's typhoid fever); Skillings v. Allen, 173 N.W. 663 (Minn. 1919) (finding a physician negligent to advise the plaintiff's wife that it was safe to visit a child known to have scarlet fever). These cases, however, are different from *Tarasoff* because they involve *misdiagnosis* of an infectious condition so that family members were placed at risk, or *misinformation* so that physicians incorrectly informed the family that the disease was not infectious.

136. The case involved the murder of Tatiana Tarasoff, who was the former acquaintance of Prosenjit Poddar, a mentally deranged patient of psychotherapist, Dr. Lawrence Moore. In therapy sessions Poddar conveyed to Dr. Moore his intent to kill a girl whom he did not specifically name, although it was evident to the doctor that the intended victim was Tarasoff. Dr. Moore did not warn Tarasoff or her parents, but instead asked the campus police to pick up Poddar. Although the police detained Poddar initially, he was later released on his recognizance after being advised to stay away from Tarasoff. Two months later, Poddar murdered Tarasoff.

137. Lipari v. Sears, Roebuck & Co., 497 F. Supp. 185 (D. Neb. 1980) (establishing liability by the existence of foreseeable danger to any member of a targeted class of people).

138. Lemon v. Stewart, 682 A.2d 1177 (Md. Ct. Spec. App. 1996) (denying recovery to a family who unknowingly cared for an HIV-infected man because there was no possibility of transmission).

139. *See, e.g.,* Cairl v. State, 323 N.W.2d 20, 26 (Minn. 1982) (finding that the duty requires warning only insofar as latent dangers posed to identifiable, specific persons).

140. *See, e.g.,* Garcia v. Santa Rosa Health Care Corp., 925 S.W.2d 372, 377 (Tex. App. 1996) (health care workers "who discover some disease . . . owe a duty to reasonably warn the third party").

141. Gammill v. United States, 727 F.2d 950 (10th Cir. 1984) (denying that a person has a duty to protect another except when a special relationship exists,

or when the first person placed the other in peril); see Derrick v. Ontario Comm. Hosp., 47 Cal. App. 3d 145 (Cal. Ct. App. 4d 1975) (finding that a hospital has no duty to warn the general public that a patient with a contagious disease is being released).

142. Hofmann v. Blackmon, 241 So. 2d 752, 753 (Fla. Dist. Ct. App. 1970) (finding a doctor liable to persons infected by his patient for negligent failure to diagnose a contagious disease). Contra Britton v. Soltes, 563 N.E.2d 910 (Ill. App. 1990) (finding that negligent failure to diagnose tuberculosis does not give rise to action by a third party who became infected through contact with the patient).

143. Wojcik v. Aluminum Co. of Am., 183 N.Y.S.2d 351, 357–58 (Sup. Ct. 1959) (placing a doctor under duty to warn members of the patient's family after diagnosing a contagious disease).

144. Reisner v. Regents of the Univ. of Calif., 37 Cal. Rptr. 2d 518, 523 (Ct. App. 1995) ("[W]e believe that a doctor who knows he is dealing with the 20th Century version of Typhoid Mary ought to have a very strong incentive to tell his patient what she ought to do and not do and how she ought to comport herself in order to prevent the spread of her disease."); see also Lawrence O. Gostin, Hospitals, Health Care Professionals, and AIDS: The "Right to Know" the Health Status of Professionals and Patients, 48 MD. L. REV. 12, 48–50 (1989).

145. See, e.g., Mussivand v. David, 544 N.E.2d 265 (Ohio 1989) (finding that people with an STD have a duty to use reasonable care to avoid infecting others with whom they have had sex); Meany v. Meany, 639 So. 2d 229 (La. 1994); see also Douglas W. Baruch, AIDS in the Courts—Tort Liability for the Sexual Transmission of Acquired Immunodeficiency Syndrome, 22 TORT & INS. L.J. 165 (1987); Eric L. Schulman, Sleeping with the Enemy: Combatting [sic] the Sexual Spread of HIV-AIDS through a Heightened Legal Duty, 29 JOHN MARSHALL L. REV. 957 (1996).

146. No. C 574153 (Cal. Super. Ct. Feb. 17, 1989).

147. Aetna Casualty & Sur. Co. v. Sheft, 989 F.2d 1105 (9th Cir. 1993) (holding that a man's misrepresentation that he did not have AIDS to induce his lover to engage in sex was inherently harmful conduct).

148. Doe v. Johnson, 817 F. Supp. 1382 (W.D. Mich. 1993) (sustaining the claim for negligent transmission of HIV if the defendant knew he was infected or that a prior sex partner was infected).

149. LAWRENCE O. GOSTIN & JAMES G. HODGE, JR., MODEL STATE PUBLIC HEALTH PRIVACY ACT (visited May 15, 2000), <http://www.critpath.org/msphpa/privacy.htm>.

6. HEALTH, COMMUNICATION, AND BEHAVIOR: FREEDOM OF EXPRESSION

SOURCES FOR CHAPTER EPIGRAPHS: Page 146: Abrams v. United States, 250 U.S. 616, 630 (1919) (Holmes, J., dissenting). Page 148: American Booksellers Ass'n. v. Hudnut, 771 F.2d 323, 327–28 (7th cir. 1985), quoting

West Virginia State Bd. of Educ. v. Barnette, 319 U.S. 624, 642 (1943). Page 154: WASH. POST, March 7, 1999, at B1. Page 000: DAN E. BEAUCHAMP, THE HEALTH OF THE REPUBLIC: EPIDEMICS, MEDICINE, AND MORALISM AS CHALLENGES TO DEMOCRACY 147 (1988). Page 154: Virginia State Bd. of Pharmacy v. Virginia Citizens Consumer Council, 425 U.S. 748, 763 (1976). Page 165: Riley v. National Fed'n of the Blind of N.C., 487 U.S. 781, 796–97 (1988).

1. Barbara A. Israel et al., *Health Education and Community Empowerment: Conceptualizing and Measuring Perceptions of Individual, Organizational, and Community Control*, 21 HEALTH EDUC. QUART. 149 (1994).

2. *See generally* NANCY SIGNORIELLI, MASS MEDIA IMAGES AND IMPACT ON HEALTH (1993) (the success of health education campaigns depends on the broader cultural context and is shaped predominantly by mass media).

3. Steve Younger, *Alcoholic Beverage Advertising on the Airwaves: Alternatives to a Ban or Counter-Advertising*, 34 UCLA L. REV. 1139 (1987).

4. ERWIN CHEMERINSKY, CONSTITUTIONAL LAW: PRINCIPLES AND POLICIES 751–56 (1997).

5. C. Edwin Baker, *Scope of the First Amendment Freedom of Speech*, 25 UCLA L. REV. 964, 994 (1978).

6. ALEXANDER MEIKLEJOHN, FREE SPEECH AND ITS RELATION TO SELF-GOVERNMENT (1948); ALEXANDER MEIKLEJOHN, POLITICAL FREEDOM (1960); Alexander Meiklejohn, *The First Amendment is an Absolute*, 1961 SUP. CT. REV. 245 (1961).

7. For an argument that political speech should be the foremost, if not the only, expression deserving of First Amendment protection, see Robert Bork, *Neutral Principles and Some First Amendment Problems*, 47 IND. L.J. 1 (1971); CASS R. SUNSTEIN, DEMOCRACY AND THE PROBLEM OF FREE SPEECH (1993).

8. JOHN MILTON, AREOPAGITICA—A SPEECH FOR THE LIBERTY OF UNLICENSED PRINTING, TO THE PARLIAMENT OF ENGLAND (1644) ("And though all the winds of doctrine were let loose to play upon the earth, so Truth be in the field, we do injuriously, by licensing and prohibiting, to misdoubt her strength. Let her and Falsehood grapple; who ever knew Truth put to the worst, in a free and open encounter?") 32 GREAT BOOKS OF THE WESTERN WORLD 409 (Robert Maynard Hutchins ed., 1952).

9. JOHN STUART MILL, ON LIBERTY 76 (1859) (The "peculiar evil of silencing the expression of an opinion is that it is robbing the human race, posterity as well as the existing generation—those who dissent from the opinion, still more than those who hold it.").

10. GERALD GUNTHER & KATHLEEN M. SULLIVAN, CONSTITUTIONAL LAW 1025 (1997) (summarizing the Millian theory of free expression).

11. Abrams v. United States, 250 U.S. 616, 630 (1919) (Holmes, J., dissenting).

12. Ronald Bayer et al., *Trades, AIDS, and the Public's Health: The Limits of Economic Analysis*, 83 GEO. L.J. 79, 82 (1995) ("Public health is therefore interventionist, taking the prevailing pattern of morbidity-related choices and their outcomes as both the beginning of the analysis and as the prod for public policy.").

13. C. Edwin Baker, *Scope of the First Amendment Freedom of Speech*, 25 UCLA L. REV. 964, 978 (1978) ("[T]he marketplace of ideas appears improperly biased in favor of presently dominant groups."); Jerome A. Barron, *Access to the Press—A New First Amendment Right*, 80 HARV. L. REV. 1641, 1648 (1967) ("[A] right of expression is somewhat thin if it can be exercised only at the sufferance of the managers of mass communications."); Stanley Ingber, *The Marketplace of Ideas: A Legitimizing Myth*, 1984 DUKE L.J. 1, 5 (regulation is needed to correct "communicative market failures").

14. LAURENCE H. TRIBE, AMERICAN CONSTITUTIONAL LAW 786 (2d ed. 1988).

15. Space limitations prevent me from examining two additional areas of public health regulation that affect First Amendment values. First, government regulation of public places implicates the right to freedom of expression and association. For example, courts have upheld the closure of bathhouses and adult cinemas or bookstores to control anonymous sex, which risks HIV or STD transmission. *See, e.g.*, New York v. New St. Mark's Baths, 130 Misc. 2d 911 (N.Y. Sup. Ct. 1986), *aff'd*, 122 A.D.2d 747 (N.Y. 1986) (finding that closure of a bathhouse did not violate the patrons' freedom of association); Ben Rich Trading v. City of Vineland, 126 F.3d 155 (3d Cir. 1997) (finding that an ordinance requiring viewing booths in bookstores to be open and visible did not violate the patrons' freedom of expression). Second, government controls access to public property ("public forums") for the presentation of health-related messages. For example, courts have required transportation authorities to provide nondiscriminatory access to condom advertisements to prevent HIV transmission. *See, e.g.*, AIDS Action Comm. of Massachusetts v. Massachusetts Bay Transp. Auth., 42 F.3d 1 (1st Cir. Mass. 1994). Similarly, the Supreme Court has heard a number of cases involving restricted access to the vicinity around abortion clinics (traditional public forums). *See, e.g.*, Madsen v. Women's Health Ctr., 512 U.S. 753, 764–65 (1994) (denying that an injunction establishing a 36-foot buffer zone around abortion clinic entrances violates the First Amendment).

16. For a definition of health communication campaigns, see William Paisley, *Public Communication Campaigns: The American Experience, in* PUBLIC COMMUNICATION CAMPAIGNS 7 (Ronald E. Rice & Charles K. Atkin eds., 2d ed. 1989) "purposive attempts to inform, persuade, or motivate behavior changes in a relatively well-defined and large audience, generally for noncommercial benefits to the individuals and/or society at large, typically within a given time period, by means of organized communication activities involving mass media and often complemented by interpersonal support."

17. Pub. L. No. 100–102, § 514(a), 101 Stat. 1329–289 (1988) (the Helms Amendment).

18. Mark V. Tushnet, *Talking to Each Other: Reflections on Yudof's* When Government Speaks, 1984 WIS. L. REV. 129, 132.

19. For intriguing examinations of government and individual constructions of social norms, see Lawrence Lessig, *The Regulation of Social Meaning*, 62 U. CHI. L.REV. 943–1045 (1995); Cass R. Sunstein, *Social Norms and Social Roles*, 96 COLUM. L. REV. 903 (1996). *See also* DAVID BUCHANAN, AN ETHIC FOR HEALTH PROMOTION: RETHINKING THE SOURCES OF HUMAN WELL-BEING (2000);

PROMOTING HEALTH BEHAVIOR: HOW MUCH FREEDOM? WHOSE RESPONSIBILTY? (Daniel Callahan ed., 2000).

20. Another way to think about health education campaigns is that they are designed to instill fear in people about the harmful effects of their behavior. R.F. Soames Job, *Effective and Ineffective Use of Fear in Health Promotion Campaigns*, 78 AM. J. PUB. HEALTH 163 (1988).

21. Health communication campaigns can pose social risks in more subtle ways. For example, campaigns that associate smoking with impotence portray impotent men in mocking or derogatory ways. Campaigns can also imply that people who fail to comply with the health message are stupid or antisocial (e.g., "Listen to a Dummy—Buckle Up").

22. Government health messages may be hurtful to discrete groups or populations. In 1995, the CDC revised guidelines that had recommended that women infected with HIV "should consider not having children" after community groups of women and African-Americans protested that the recommendation was stigmatizing and insensitive.

23. For an insightful examination, see Ruth R. Faden, *Ethical Issues in Government Sponsored Public Health Campaigns*, 14 HEALTH EDUC. QUART. 27, 33–34 (1987).

24. David S. Alberts et al., *Lack of Effect of a High-Fiber Cereal Supplement on the Recurrence of Colorectal Adenomas*, 342 New ENG. J. MED. 1156 (2000).

25. Linda Villeross, *New Fatness Guidelines Spur Debate on Fitness*, N.Y. TIMES, June 23, 1998, at F7.

26. *Compare* Stephen A. Feig, *Increased Benefit From Shorter Screening Mammography Intervals for Women Ages 40–49 Years*, 80 CANCER 2091 (1997) (supporting screening of women aged 40–49) *with* National Institutes of Health, *Breast Cancer Screening for Women Ages 40–49*, 15 NIH CONSENSUS STATEMENT ONLINE 1 (1997) (finding that evidence of effectiveness for screening women aged 40–49 is inconclusive).

27. Daniel Wikler & Dan E. Beauchamp, *Health Promotion and Health Education*, *in* 2 ENCYCLOPEDIA OF BIOETHICS 1126, 1128 (Warren Thomas Reich ed., 1995).

28. Campaigns are difficult to evaluate because of the diffuse nature of the target audience, the low salience of the campaign's subject matter, and the complexity of the causal relationship between the campaign and behavior change. Brian R. Flay & Thomas D. Cook, *Three Models for Summative Evaluation of Prevention Campaigns with a Mass Media Component*, *in* PUBLIC COMMUNICATION CAMPAIGNS, *supra* note 16, at 175. Moreover, researchers suggest that many of the campaigns that are evaluated appear to have limited effectiveness. *See generally* Charles K. Atkin, *Formative Evaluation Research in Campaign Design, id.* at 131.

29. *See, e.g.,* THOMAS I. EMERSON, THE SYSTEM OF FREEDOM OF EXPRESSION 697–716 (1970); MARK G. YUDOF, WHEN GOVERNMENT SPEAKS: POLITICS, LAW, AND GOVERNMENT EXPRESSION IN AMERICA (1983); Frederick Schauer, *Is Government Speech a Problem?*, 35 STAN. L.REV. 373 (1983).

30. TRIBE, *supra* note 14, at 807.

31. The Supreme Court is quite prepared to defend government speech, even when government registers "official" disapproval of privately held ideas.

For example, in *Meese v. Keene,* 481 U.S. 465 (1987), the Court upheld a Department of Justice classification of three foreign films as "political propaganda"—one concerning the environmental hazards of nuclear war and the other two concerning acid rain.

32. Kathleen Sullivan, *Unconstitutional Conditions,* 102 HARV. L. REV. 1415 (1989).

33. Speiser v. Randall, 357 U.S. 513, 517 (1958) ("To deny a [tax] exemption to claimants who engage in certain forms of speech is in effect to penalize them for such speech.").

34. Professors Sullivan and Gunther offer the following distinction between an unconstitutional condition and a constitutionally permissible subsidy. Under this distinction, government may not use "a subsidy to induce recipients to refrain from speech they would otherwise engage in with their own resources, but it may refrain from paying for speech with which it disagrees." KATHLEEN M. SULLIVAN & GERALD GUNTHER, FIRST AMENDMENT LAW 310 (1999).

35. Rust v. Sullivan, 500 U.S. 173, 193-94 (1991).

36. Jon S. Vernick et al., *Regulating Firearm Advertisements That Promise Home Protection,* 277 JAMA 1391 (1997) (LADIES HOME JOURNAL advertisement: "Self-protection is more than your right . . . it's your responsibility."). *See also* GAREN J. WINTEMUTE, ADVERTISING FIREARMS AS PROTECTION (1995).

37. Stuart Elliot, *Liquor Industry Ends Its Ad Ban in Broadcasting,* N.Y. TIMES, Nov. 8, 1996, at A1.

38. Nutritional Health Alliance v. Shalala, 144 F.3d 220 (2d Cir.), *cert. denied,* 525 U.S. 1040 (1998) (upholding the FDA requirement for prior approval of health claims on dietary supplement labels because of health and safety risks); National Council for Improved Health v. Shalala, 122 F.3d 878 (10th Cir. 1997) (same); Pearson v. Shalala, 164 F.3d 650 (D.C. Cir.), *denying petition for rehearing en banc,* 172 F.3d 72 (D.C. Cir. 1999) (invalidating the same regulation because the FDA was required to consider whether inclusion of appropriate disclaimers would negate potentially misleading health claims). *See* David C. Vladeck, *Devaluing Truth—Unverified Health Claims in the Aftermath of* Pearson v. Shalala, 54 FOOD & DRUG L.J. 535 (1999).

39. In a settlement between twelve attorneys general and SmithKline Beecham, the company agreed to cease using its misleading "The Power to Quit" slogan for antismoking products Nicorette and NicoDermCQ after evidence emerged that consumers start smoking again one year after they quit. CHEMICAL BUSINESS NEWSBASE, Dec. 22, 1998, *available in* WL 21881828. *See also* Washington Legal Foundation v. Friedman, 13 F. Supp. 2d 51 (D.D.C. 1998) (invalidating FDA restriction on use of journal reprints and educational seminars to promote off-label prescription drug uses).

40. Central Hudson Gas & Elec. Corp. v. Public Serv. Comm'n, 447 U.S. 557, 561 (1980).

41. Virginia State Bd. of Pharmacy v. Virginia Citizens Consumer Council, Inc., 425 U.S. 748, 762 (1976).

42. In *Bad Frog Brewery, Inc. v. New York State Liquor Auth.,* 134 F.3d 87 (2d Cir. 1998), the Second Circuit found that a beer label displaying a frog giving an insulting gesture was commercial speech, but not the more fully pro-

tected social commentary or political speech. Bad Frog labels meet the three criteria for commercial speech and the purported noncommercial message was not "inextricably intertwined" enough to merit full First Amendment protection. *Id.* at 97.

43. Bolger v. Youngs Drug Prods. Corp., 463 U.S. 60, 67 (1983).

44. In *New York Times Co. v. Sullivan*, 376 U.S. 254 (1964), the Court expressly rejected the argument that the First Amendment did not apply to "paid" commercial advertisements. Corporate speech can amount to fully protected political speech, such as when a company advocates its business interests in a political referendum campaign. *See also* First Nat'l Bank of Boston v. Bellotti, 435 U.S. 765 (1978) (invalidating a state statute prohibiting corporations from advertising designed to influence votes submitted to the electorate other than one materially affecting the corporation's business).

45. N.Y. TIMES, Sept. 26, 1995, at A17 (paid for by R.J. Reynolds and Philip Morris).

46. In 1985, R.J. Reynolds paid for editorial-style advertisements that appeared in twenty-five publications including the *New York Times*. In the so-called advertorial "Of Cigarettes and Science," the company asserted that the Multiple Risk Factor Intervention Trial ("Mr. Fit") failed to find a relationship between smoking and heart disease. The FTC agreed to settle charges of false advertising, while the company pledged not to misrepresent scientific studies in the future. Barry Meier, *Selling or Advising? Dispute Settled on Tobacco Ads*, N.Y. TIMES, Oct. 21, 1989, at A50.

47. For a discussion of the issue, see Peter S. Arno et al., *Tobacco Industry Strategies to Oppose Federal Regulation*, 275 JAMA 1258 (1996).

48. Valentine v. Chrestensen, 316 U.S. 52, 54 (1942).

49. Bigelow v. Virginia, 421 U.S. 809, 826 (1975) (invalidating a state statute making it a crime to sell or circulate any publication that encourages or prompts the procuring of an abortion).

50. *Id.*

51. Carey v. Population Servs. Int'l, 431 U.S. 678 (1977) (invalidating a New York ban on advertising nonprescription contraceptives).

52. Virginia State Bd. of Pharmacy v. Virginia Citizens Consumer Council, Inc., 425 U.S. 748 (1976).

53. Indeed, the Court has said that commercial speech enjoys no special procedural protections, such as the strict scrutiny of prior restraints or overly broad regulation. *Id.*, at 771–72; Bates v. State Bar of Arizona, 433 U.S. 350, 380–81 (1977). *But see* New York Magazine v. MTA, 136 F.3d 123, 131 (2d Cir. 1998) ("Although the Supreme Court has indicated that commercial speech may qualify as one of the exceptions to the bar on prior restraints, we see no reason why the requirement of procedural safeguards [in prior restraint cases] should be relaxed whether speech is commercial or not."); Nutritional Health Alliance v. Shalala, 144 F.3d 220 (2d Cir. 1998) (holding that the FDA requirement for prior approval of health claims on dietary supplement labels is not an unconstitutional prior restraint of commercial speech).

54. Ohralik v. Ohio State Bar Assn., 436 U.S. 447, 455–56 (1978).

55. Central Hudson Gas v. Public Serv. Comm'n, 447 U.S. 557, 563 (1980).

56. *Id.* at 566.

57. Greater New Orleans Broadcasting Ass'n v. United States, 527 U.S. 173, 188 (1999).

58. Florida Bar v. Went For It, Inc., 515 U.S. 618, 623 (1995).

59. Edenfield v. Fane, 507 U.S. 761, 770–71 (1993).

60. Pittsburgh Press Co. v. Pittsburgh Comm'n on Hum. Relations, 413 U.S. 376 (1973) (denying First Amendment protection to illegal gender-based classification in help wanted ads).

61. For example, the Supreme Court allows tort litigation by smokers based on claims that cigarette manufacturers engaged in fraudulent misrepresentation or conspiracy to misrepresent or conceal material facts. Cipollone v. Liggett Group, Inc., 505 U.S. 504 (1992).

62. Sylvia Law, *Addiction, Autonomy and Advertising,* 77 IOWA L. REV. 909 (1992).

63. Peter Michael Fischer et al., *Recall and Eye Tracking Study of Adolescents Viewing Tobacco Advertisements,* 261 JAMA 84 (1989). *See also* Kathleen J. Lester, *Cowboys, Camels, and Commercial Speech: Is the Tobacco Industry's Commodification of Childhood Protected by the First Amendment?,* 24 N. KY. L. REV. 615 (1997).

64. In the mid-1950s, L & M Filters were advertised as the new "miracle product": the "alpha cellulose" filter is "just what the doctor ordered." R.J. Reynolds similarly advertised: "More doctors smoke Camels than any other cigarette." THOMAS WHITESIDE, SELLING DEATH: CIGARETTE ADVERTISING AND PUBLIC HEALTH (1971).

65. Ohralik v. Ohio State Bar Ass'n, 436 U.S. 447, 462 (1978).

66. Friedman v. Rogers, 440 U.S. 1, 13 (1979) ("[T]here is a significant possibility that trade names will be used to mislead the public.").

67. *See Ohralik,* 436 U.S. at 465 (holding that face-to-face attorney solicitation inherently risks that clients will be deceived and pressured). However, in a contradictory ruling the Court found that personal solicitations by accountants is constitutionally protected. Edenfield v. Fane, 507 U.S. 761 (1993). And attorneys may constitutionally engage in truthful, nondeceptive advertising of their services provided it does not involve face-to-face solicitation. Bates v. State Bar of Ariz., 433 U.S. 350 (1977); Shapero v. Kentucky Bar Ass'n, 486 U.S. 466 (1988). *But see* Florida Bar v. Went for It, Inc., 515 U.S. 618 (1995) (upholding the prohibition of attorney mail solicitation for thirty days after an accident).

68. Vincent Blasi & Henry Paul Monaghan, *The First Amendment and Cigarette Advertising,* 256 JAMA 502 (1986).

69. Metromedia, Inc. v. City of San Diego, 453 U.S. 490 (1981) (upholding an ordinance prohibiting outdoor displays [relating to commercial, but not political, speech] because they pose a traffic hazard). *But see* City of Cincinnati v. Discovery Network, Inc., 507 U.S. 410 (1993) (invalidating an ordinance prohibiting commercial newspapers from being distributed on news racks while allowing other kinds of newspapers to be sold).

70. Rubin v. Coors Brewing Co., 514 U.S. 476, 485 (1995) (finding that the state has a significant interest in "preventing brewers from competing on the

basis of alcohol strength, which could lead to greater alcoholism and its attendant social costs." The regulation, however, was found unconstitutional because it was more intrusive than necessary to achieve its goals.).

71. Posadas de P.R. Assocs. v. Tourism Co. of P.R., 478 U.S. 328, 341 (1986) (in upholding a ban on advertising casino gambling directed to residents, the Court had "no difficulty" finding state interest in health constitutes a "substantial interest"); United States v. Edge Broadcasting Co., 509 U.S. 418 (1993) (upholding a federal law prohibiting lottery advertising by radio stations located in states that did not operate lotteries). However, the Court subsequently struck down this federal statute as applied to states where gambling was lawful. Greater New Orleans Broadcasting Ass'n v. United States, 527 U.S. 173 (1999).

72. Oklahoma Telecasters Ass'n v. Crisp, 699 F.2d 490, 501 (10th Cir. 1983), rev'd on other grounds sub nom. Capital Cities Cable v. Crisp, 467 U.S. 691 (1984) (e.g., it is not "constitutionally unreasonable for the State . . . to believe that advertising will increase sales . . . of alcoholic beverages").

73. 478 U.S. at 341–42. Chief Justice Rehnquist in Posadas made a now discredited argument that the greater power to completely ban a product necessarily includes the lesser power to regulate advertising of that product: "It would surely . . . be a strange constitutional doctrine which would concede to the legislature the authority to totally ban a product or activity, but deny to the legislature the authority to forbid the stimulation of demand for the product or activity." Id. at 346. This "greater includes the lesser" theory would give public health authorities virtually plenary authority to suppress advertising of tobacco, alcoholic beverages, and gambling. However, Rehnquist's argument assumes wrongly that speech restrictions are the lesser included power. Arguably, product prohibitions on health or safety grounds would be less offensive to the Constitution than speech prohibitions. See 44 Liquormart, Inc. v. Rhode Island, 517 U.S. 484, 513–514 (1996) (rejecting the argument that the power to restrict speech about certain socially harmful activities was as broad as the power to prohibit such conduct); Greater New Orleans Broadcasting, 527 U.S. at 193 ("[T]he power to prohibit or to regulate particular conduct does not necessarily include the power to prohibit or regulate speech about that conduct.").

74. Coors Brewing, 514 U.S. at 488–89.

75. 44 Liquormart, 517 U.S. at 505–07.

76. 527 U.S. at 173 (finding that exemptions in the government's gambling policy prevent it from directly and materially advancing the asserted interests in reducing the social costs of casino gambling and assisting states that prohibit it within their own borders).

77. Id. at 174.

78. Id. at 173.

79. After 44 Liquormart, the level of proof required to demonstrate that a commercial speech regulation directly advances the state's interest is unclear. No single standard has the support of the majority of the Court. Justice Steven's plurality opinion in 44 Liquormart requires an evidentiary showing that the advertising regulation would significantly reduce demand for a hazardous product. However, Justice O'Connor, writing for four members of the Court, pointedly

declined to adopt Justice Steven's approach on the third prong of *Central Hudson*, 517 U.S. at 530. In *Greater New Orleans Broadcasting*, 527 U.S at 190, the Court said it was not necessary on the facts of the case to resolve the evidentiary dispute within the Court because the flaw in the government's case is more fundamental.

80. Edenfield v. Fane, 507 U.S. 761, 770 (1993).

81. *See, e.g.*, Dunagin v. City of Oxford, Miss., 718 F.2d 738, 751 (5th Cir. 1983) (en banc), *cert. denied*, 467 U.S. 1259 (1984); Queensgate Invest. Co. v. Liquor Control Comm'n, 433 N.E.2d 138 (Ohio), *cert. denied*, 459 U.S. 807 (1982).

82. 492 U.S. 469, 477 (1989) (upholding a university regulation restricting the operation of commercial enterprises on campus).

83. *Id.* at 480 (citations omitted).

84. In *Coors Brewing*, the Court noted a number of alternative ways of preventing strength wars so the government's interest could be achieved "in a manner less intrusive to . . . First Amendment rights." 514 U.S. at 491. In *44 Liquormart*, the plurality opinion concluded that "it is perfectly obvious that alternative forms of regulation that would not involve any restriction on speech would be more likely to achieve the State's goal of promoting temperance." 517 U.S. at 507. And in *Greater New Orleans Broadcasting*, the Court said, "There surely are practical and non–speech related forms of regulation . . . that could more directly and effectively alleviate some of the social costs of casino gambling." 527 U.S. at 192.

85. *44 Liquormart*, 517 U.S. at 501 (not "*all* commercial speech regulations are subject to a similar form of constitutional review")(emphasis in original).

86. Zauderer v. Office of Disciplinary Counsel, 471 U.S. 626, 647 (1985). *See also* Bad Frog Brewery, Inc. v. New York State Liquor Auth., 134 F.3d 87, 96–97 (2d Cir. 1998) (holding that the label displaying a frog giving a well-known insulting gesture was reasonably understood as conveying the source of the product so that it contains some useful consumer information).

87. *Compare* David A. Strauss, *Persuasion, Autonomy and Freedom of Expression*, 91 COLUM. L. REV. 334 (1991) *with* Law, *supra* note 62, at 909.

88. *44 Liquormart*, 517 U.S. at 501 (citations omitted):

> [W]hen a State entirely prohibits the dissemination of truthful, nonmisleading commercial messages for reasons unrelated to the preservation of a fair bargaining process, there is far less reason to depart from the rigorous review that the First Amendment generally demands. [Complete] speech bans, unlike content-neutral restrictions on the time, place, or manner of expression, are particularly dangerous because they all but foreclose alternative means of disseminating certain information.

89. Greater New Orleans Broadcasting Ass'n v. United States, 527 U.S. 173 191 (1999)("[T]he government is committed to prohibiting accurate product information, not commercial enticements of all kinds, and then only conveyed over certain forms of media and for certain types of gambling.").

90. Anheuser-Busch, Inc. v. Schmoke, 101 F.3d 325, 329 (4th Cir. 1996) (upholding an ordinance prohibiting the placement of a stationary outdoor alcohol beverage advertisements in certain areas where children walk to school or play because it merely restricts "time, place, and manner" and "does not

foreclose the plethora of newspaper, magazine, radio, television, direct mail, Internet, and other media"). *See* Penn Advertising, Inc. v. Mayor of Baltimore, 101 F.3d 332 (4th Cir. 1996) (upholding an ordinance banning billboard advertisements for cigarettes in areas children frequent).

91. The *Schmoke* case, for example, distinguished between alcoholic beverage advertisements targeted to adults (as in 44 *Liquormart*) and those targeted to children.

92. Where advertising reaches both a lawful and unlawful audience, the Court grants the commercial speech constitutional protection, but arguably at a lower level. United States v. Edge Broadcasting Co., 509 U.S. 418, 428 (1993). The government's interest in protecting children does not justify an unnecessarily broad suppression of speech addressed to adults. Reno v. American Civil Liberties Union, 521 U.S. 844, 875 (1997) (invalidating a statute prohibiting transmission of obscene or indecent communications through the Internet to persons under age 18).

93. *See, e.g.,* Ginsberg v. New York, 390 U.S. 629, 636 (1968) (rejecting the assertion that "the scope of the constitutional freedom of expression . . . cannot be made to depend on whether the citizen is an adult or a minor"); FCC v. Pacifica Found., 438 U.S. 726, 749 (1978) (upholding the FCC finding that indecent speech "in an afternoon broadcast when children are in the audience was patently offensive"); Denver Area Educ. Telecomm. Consortium, Inc. v. FCC, 518 U.S. 727, 744–45 (1996) (upholding cable television restrictions as a means of protecting children from indecent programming).

94. *Schmoke,* 101 F.3d at 329.

95. Rubin v. Coors Brewing, 514 U.S. 476, 482 (1995).

96. Cincinnati v. Discovery Network, Inc., 507 U.S. 410, 424–30 (1993).

97. William M. Sage, *Regulating through Information: Disclosure Laws and American Health Care,* 100 COLUM. L. REV. 1701 (1999).

98. California Proposition 65, for example, requires businesses to provide a "clear and reasonable" warning before knowingly exposing anyone to a listed chemical carcinogen. Safe Drinking Water and Toxic Enforcement Act of 1986, CAL. HEALTH & SAFETY CODE §§ 25249.5–.13 (West 1992 & Supp. 1999). *See* Clifford Rechtschaffen, *The Warning Game: Evaluating Warnings under California's Proposition 65,* 23 ECOLOGY L.Q. 303 (1996).

99. *Groups Petition FCC for Alcohol Counter-Ads,* ALCOHOLISM & DRUG WKLY., May 26, 1997 (discussing counter-advertising proposals made by the National Council on Alcoholism and Drug Dependence, Mothers Against Drunk Driving, and twenty-two other organizations); Kathryn Murphy, *Can the Budweiser Frogs Be Forced to Sing a New Tune?: Compelled Commercial Counter-Speech and the First Amendment,* 84 VA. L. REV. 1195 (1998).

100. Vango Media, Inc. v. City of N.Y., 829 F. Supp. 572 (S.D.N.Y. 1993) (finding that a New York City administrative law requiring the display of one public health message for every four tobacco advertisements on city property was preempted under the Federal Cigarette Labeling and Advertising Act of 1965, 15 U.S.C. §§ 1331–1340 (2000)).

101. In August 1995 the FDA proposed to compel tobacco companies to establish a national education program, using television as its predominant medium,

to discourage youth smoking (60 FR 41314). Later, the FDA reexamined its statutory authority, but still proposed to require industry to inform the public of the
health risks. See Lisa Goitein et al., *Developments in Policy: The FDA's Tobacco
Regulations,* 15 YALE L. & POL'Y REV. 399 (1996). In 2000, the Supreme Court
held that the FDA lacked jurisdiction to regulate cigarettes. FDA v. Brown &
Williamson Tobacco Corp., 120 S. Ct. 1291 (2000).

102. The "fairness doctrine" (47 U.S.C. § 315 (1994)) required broadcasters to air public issues and give each side fair coverage. In 1972, Congress expanded the doctrine from political campaigns to "controversial matters of public importance." See Red Lion Broadcasting Co. v. FCC, 395 U.S. 367 (1969)
(validating the fairness doctrine under the First Amendment because government licenses broadcasters to use scarce resources).

103. See In re Television Station WCBS, N.Y.: Applicability of the Fairness
Doctrine to Cigarette Advertising, 9 F.C.C.2d 921 (1967) (applying the fairness
doctrine to cigarette advertising, recognizing that tobacco is a controversial
issue and emphasizing public health); Banzhaf v. F.C.C., 405 F.2d 1082 (D.C.
Cir. 1968), *cert. denied, sub nom.* Tobacco Inst., Inc. v FCC, 396 U.S. 842
(1969) (applying the fairness doctrine to tobacco advertising is constitutional);
Larus & Brother Co. v. FCC, 447 F.2d 876 (4th Cir. 1971) (holding that tobacco is no longer a "controversial issue" for the purposes of the fairness doctrine). The FCC abandoned the fairness doctrine in 1987. *In re* Complaint of
Syracuse Peace Council against Television Station WTUH, 2 F.C.C.R 5043
(1987).

104. Wooley v. Maynard, 430 U.S. 705, 714 (1977) ("[T]he right of freedom of thought protected by the First Amendment against state action includes
both the right to speak freely and the right to refrain from speaking at all.").
As a corollary principle, government may not compel individuals to subsidize
speech by private organizations such as trade unions and bar associations. See,
e.g., Abood v. Detroit Bd. of Educ., 431 U.S. 209 (1977) (compelled contributions to union's agency shops); Keller v. State Bar of Cal., 496 U.S. 1 (1990)
(state-compelled dues to an integrated bar association to advance political
causes).

105. West Virginia State Bd. of Educ. v. Barnette, 319 U.S. 624 (1943).

106. 430 U.S. at 705.

107. Talley v. California, 362 U.S. 60 (1960).

108. McIntyre v. Ohio Elections Comm., 514 U.S. 334 (1995).

109. Similarly, the Court has overturned state laws requiring groups to disclose their membership lists because they may discourage individuals from associating with an unpopular group. Gibson v. Florida Legislative Investigation
Comm., 372 U.S. 539 (1963); NAACP v. Alabama, 357 U.S. 449 (1958). And
the Court has invalidated state laws requiring parade organizers to include gay
marchers because it may discourage the organizers from holding the parade at
all. Hurley v. Irish-American Gay, Lesbian and Bisexual Group of Boston, Inc.,
515 U.S. 557 (1995).

110. In *Glickman v. Wileman Bros. & Elliot, Inc.,* 521 U.S. 437 (1997), the
Court upheld federal marketing orders requiring California fruit producers to
fund a generic advertising program. The Court characterized the orders as eco-

nomic regulation that did not impinge on First Amendment rights. *See* Nicole B. Casarez, *Don't Tell Me What to Say: Compelled Commercial Speech and the First Amendment*, 63 Mo. L. Rev. 929 (1998). In *Riley v. National Fed'n of the Blind of N.C.*, 487 U.S. 781, 796 (1988), the Court declined to utilize a commercial speech test in striking down a statute mandating professional fundraisers to disclose the percentage of charitable contributions actually turned over to the charity. "[E]ven assuming . . . that [the mandated] speech in the abstract is merely 'commercial,' we do not believe that the speech retains its commercial character when it is inextricably intertwined with the otherwise fully protected speech [involved in charitable solicitations]."

111. *See, e.g.*, 44 Liquormart v. Rhode Island, 517 U.S. 484, 501 (1996).

112. *See, e.g.*, United States v. Sullivan, 332 U.S. 689, 693 (1948) (upholding a federal law requiring warning labels on "harmful foods, drugs and cosmetics").

113. Virginia State Bd. of Pharmacy v. Virginia Citizens Consumer Council, Inc., 425 U.S. 748, 772 (1976).

114. *Id.*, at 771 n. 24 ("It is appropriate to require that a commercial message appear in such a form, or include such additional information, warnings and disclaimers as are necessary to prevent its being deceptive.").

115. Bates v. State Bar of Ariz., 433 U.S. 350, 384 (1977). *See In re* R.M.J., 455 U.S. 191, 201 (1982) ("[A] warning or disclaimer might be appropriately required . . . in order to dissipate the possibility of consumer confusion or deception.").

116. Zauderer v. Office of Disciplinary Counsel, 471 U.S. 626 (1985).

117. *Id.* at 651. *But see* Ibanez v. Florida Dep't of Bus. & Prof. Regulation, 512 U.S. 136, 146–47 (1994) (finding the exhaustive disclaimer required in certain accountant advertisements overbroad).

118. 92 F.3d 67 (2d Cir. 1996). *See* Cal-Almond, Inc., v. United States Dep't of Agriculture, 14 F.3d 429 (9th Cir. 1993) (finding a marketing program requiring almond handlers to pay assessments toward advertising unconstitutional); United States v. Frame, 885 F.2d 119 (3d Cir. 1989), *cert. denied*, 493 U.S. 1094 (1990) (upholding a federal law requiring businesses to participate administratively and financially in the promotion of beef—"desirable, healthy, nutritious"—as constitutional).

119. International Dairy Foods Ass'n v. Amestoy, 92 F.3d 67, 73 (2d Cir. 1996).

120 *Id.* at 74 ("Were consumer interest alone sufficient, there is no end to the information that states could require manufacturers to disclose about their production methods."). But see the passionate dissent of Circuit Judge Leval arguing that Vermont had legitimate concerns about human and animal health, novel biotechnology, and the survival of small dairy farms. *Id.* at 76. *See also* Caren Schmulen Sweetland, *The Demise of a Workable Commercial Speech Doctrine: Dangers of Extending First Amendment Protection to Commercial Disclosure Requirements*, 76 Tex. L. Rev. 471, 477 (1997).

121. *Zauderer*, 471 U.S. at 651.

122. Riley v. National Fed'n of the Blind, 487 U.S. 781, 797–98 (1988).

123. *See* Glickman v. Wileman Bros. & Elliott, Inc., 521 U.S. 457, 471 (1997).

124. DEPARTMENT OF HEALTH, EDUC. & WELFARE, SURGEON GENERAL'S REPORT ON SMOKING AND HEALTH (1964).

125. Lawrence O. Gostin et al., *FDA Regulation of Tobacco Advertising and Youth Smoking: Historical, Social, and Constitutional Perspectives*, 277 JAMA 410 (1997); Lawrence O. Gostin & Allan M. Brandt, *Criteria for Evaluating a Ban on the Advertisement of Cigarettes: Balancing Public Health Benefits with Constitutional Burdens*, 269 JAMA 904 (1993).

126. Pub. L. No. 89–92, §4, 79 Stat. 283 (1965). The original warning label read, "Caution: Cigarette Smoking May Be Hazardous to Your Health." The labeling act was substantially amended in 1970 to read, "The Surgeon General Has Determined that Cigarette Smoking Is Dangerous to Your Health." Pub. L. No. 21–222, §2, 84 Stat 88 (1970). It was amended again in 1984 by the Comprehensive Smoking Education Act to include four warnings on a rotational basis. 15 U.S.C. §1333 (1994).

127. Capitol Broadcasting Co. v. Acting Attorney Gen., 405 U.S. 1000 (1972) (mem) aff'ing sub nom. Capitol Broadcasting Co. v. Mitchell, 333 F. Supp. 582 (D.D.C. 1971).

128. *In re* Lorillard, 80 FTC 455 (1972). Congress imposed a similar requirement in 1984. 15 U.S.C. §1334 (1994).

129. FTC REPORT TO CONGRESS FOR 1996 (1998) ("The tobacco industry spent $5.1 billion for domestic advertising and promotional activities in 1996.").

130. FDA, REGULATIONS RESTRICTING THE SALE AND DISTRIBUTION OF CIGARETTES AND SMOKELESS TOBACCO TO PROTECT CHILDREN AND ADOLESCENTS, FINAL RULE, 21 CFR 897.2. *See* David A. Kessler et al., *The Food and Drug Administration's Rule on Tobacco: Blending Science and Law*, 99 PEDIATRICS 884 (1997); Leonard Glantz, *Controlling Tobacco Advertising: The FDA Regulations and the First Amendment*, 87 AM. J. PUB. HEALTH 446 (1997); *Developments in Policy, The FDA's Tobacco Regulations*, 15 YALE L. & POL'Y REV. 399 (1996).

131. FDA v. Brown & Williamson Tobacco Corp., 120 S. Ct. 1291 (2000).

132. Barry Meier, *Lost Horizons: The Billboard Prepares to Give Up Smoking*, N.Y. TIMES, April 19, 1999, at A1, A20. (For a discussion of tobacco litigation, see chapter 9.)

133. For an excellent review, see KENNETH E. WARNER, SELLING SMOKE: CIGARETTE ADVERTISING AND PUBLIC HEALTH 85–96 (1986).

134. Martin H. Redish, *Tobacco Advertising and the First Amendment*, 81 IOWA L. REV. 589 (1996); Howard Jeruchimowitz, *Tobacco Advertisements and Commercial Speech Balancing: A Cancer to Truthful, Nonmisleading Advertisements of Lawful Products*, 82 CORNELL L. REV. 432 (1997); David C. Vladeck & John Cary Sims, *Why the Supreme Court Will Uphold Strict Controls on Tobacco Advertising*, 22 SO. ILL. L.J. 651 (1998).

135. MATTHEW L. MEYERS ET AL., FEDERAL TRADE COMMISSION STAFF REPORT ON THE CIGARETTE ADVERTISING INVESTIGATION (1981); FTC, REPORT TO CONGRESS PURSUANT TO THE PUBLIC HEALTH CIGARETTE SMOKING ACT (1979).

136. John Schwartz, *1973 Cigarette Company Memo Proposed New Brand for Teens*, WASH. POST, Oct. 4, 1995, at A2.

137. Kwechansky Marketing Research. Project Plus/Minus-3 or Cry 11 (Montreal, Que., Canada: Imperial Tobacco. May 7, 1982).

138. John P. Pierce et al., *Does Tobacco Advertising Target Young People to Start Smoking?*, 266 JAMA 3154–58 (1991); Joseph R. DiFranza & B.F. Aisquith, *Does the Joe Camel Campaign Preferentially Reach 18–24 Year Old Adults?*, 4 TOBACCO CONTROL 367–71 (1995).

139. David G. Altman et al., *Tobacco Promotion and Susceptibility to Tobacco Use among Adolescents Aged 12 through 17 Years in a Nationally Representative Sample*, 86 AM. J. PUB. HEALTH 1590 (1996); Fischer et al., *supra* note 63 at 84.

140. GEORGE H. GALLUP INTERNATIONAL INSTITUTE, TEENAGE ATTITUDES AND BEHAVIOR CONCERNING TOBACCO: REPORT OF THE FINDINGS (1992); William H. Redmond, *Effects of Sales Promotion on Smoking among U.S. Ninth Graders*, 28 PREV. MED. 243 (1999).

141. John P. Pierce et al., *Tobacco Industry Promotion of Cigarettes and Adolescent Smoking*, 279 JAMA 511 (1998) (a longitudinal study showing that tobacco promotional activities are causally related to the onset of smoking); John P. Pierce, *Sharing the Blame: Smoking Experimentation and Future Smoking—Attributable Mortality Due to Joe Camel and Marlboro Advertising and Promotions*, 8 TOBACCO CONTROL 37–41 (1999).

142. Centers for Disease Control & Prevention, *Tobacco Use and Usual Source of Cigarettes among High School Students—United States, 1995*, 45 MORB. MORT. WKLY. REP. 413 (1996); Centers for Disease Control & Prevention, *Cigarette Smoking Among High School Students—11 States, 1991–1997*, 48 MORB. MORTAL. WKLY. REP. 686 (1999).

143. Joseph R. DiFranza & Joe B. Tye, *Who Profits from Tobacco Sales to Children?*, 263 JAMA 2784–87 (1990); Centers for Disease Control & Prevention, *Incidence of Initiation of Cigarette Smoking—United States, 1965–1996*, 47 MORB. MORTAL. WKLY. REP. 837 (1998) (1,226,000 persons aged less than 18 years became regular daily smokers in 1996).

144. DEPARTMENT OF HEALTH & HUM. SERVS., PREVENTING TOBACCO USE AMONG YOUNG PEOPLE: A REPORT OF THE SURGEON GENERAL (1994).

145. Emanuela Taioli & Ernst L. Wynder, *Effect of the Age at which Smoking Begins on Frequency of Smoking in Adulthood*, 325 NEW ENG. J. MED. 968–69 (1991). Scott L. Tomar & Gary A. Giovino, *Incidence and Predictors of Smokeless Tobacco Use Among U.S. Youth*, 88 AM. J. PUB. HEALTH 20 (1998).

146. DEPARTMENT OF HEALTH & HUM. SERVS., REDUCING THE HEALTH CONSEQUENCES OF SMOKING: 25 YEARS OF PROGRESS: A REPORT OF THE SURGEON GENERAL (1989).

147. DEPARTMENT OF HEALTH & HUM. SERVS., THE HEALTH CONSEQUENCES OF SMOKING, NICOTINE ADDICTION: A REPORT OF THE SURGEON GENERAL (1988).

148. Diane R. Gold et al., *Effects of Cigarette Smoking on Lung Function in Adolescent Boys and Girls*, 335 NEW ENG. J. MED. 931–37 (1996).

149. Centers for Disease Control & Prevention, *Cigarette Smoking among Adults—United States, 1990*, 42 MORB. MORTAL. WKLY. REP. 645–49 (1993); Centers for Disease Control & Prevention, *Projected Smoking Related Deaths Among Youth—United States*, 45 MORB. MORTAL. WKLY. REP. 971 (1996).

150. GROWING UP TOBACCO FREE: PREVENTING NICOTINE ADDICTION IN CHILDREN AND YOUTHS (Barbara S. Lynch & Richard J. Bonnie eds., 1994).

151. Centers for Disease Control & Prevention, *Achievements in Public Health 1900–1999: Tobacco Use—United States, 1900–1999*, 48 MORB. MORTAL. WKLY. REP. 986 (1999).

152. *Id.*

7. IMMUNIZATION, TESTING AND SCREENING:
    BODILY INTEGRITY

SOURCES FOR CHAPTER EPIGRAPHS: Page 175: PAUL DE KRUIF, MICROBE HUNTERS 115 (1996) (describing Robert Koch's scientific observation of the bacterial cause of anthrax). Page 180: EDWARD JENNER, THE ORIGIN OF THE VACCINE INOCULATION (1801). Page 181: GEORGE ROSEN, A HISTORY OF PUBLIC HEALTH 162–65 (Johns Hopkins expanded ed., 1993). Page 185: Walter R. Dowdle, *The 1976 Experience*, 176 (Supp. 1) J. INFECTIOUS DISEASE S69 (1997). Page 188: REDUCING THE ODDS: PREVENTING PERINATAL TRANSMISSION OF HIV IN THE UNITED STATES 37 (Michael A. Stoto et al. eds., 1999). Page 197: School Bd. of Nassau County v. Arline, 480 U.S. 273, 284 (1987).

1. *See, e.g.,* Joseph H. Bates & William W. Stead, *The History of Tuberculosis as a Global Epidemic*, 77 MED. CLINICS OF N.A. 1205 (1993) (TB was initially a disease of lower mammals, and the etiologic agent probably preceded the development of man on earth).

2. *See generally,* GEORGE ROSEN, A HISTORY OF PUBLIC HEALTH (1993).

3. Jenner's original work was self-published in 1798 under the title, *An Inquiry into the causes and effects of the variolae vaccinae, a disease discovered in some of the western counties of England, particularly Gloucestershire, and known by the name of the Cow pox.* Jenner's work was not a radical departure from a long-standing practice known as variolation—traced to China in the early twelfth century and introduced in Europe and North America in the early eighteenth century. Variolation consisted of an inoculation into the skin of a small amount of material taken from a pustule or scab of a smallpox patient, inducing a milder form of smallpox that afforded immunity against more serious infection acquired by the respiratory route. Jenner's innovation was the use of pustular material from a cowpox lesion. Donald A. Henderson, *Edward Jenner's Vaccine*, 112 PUB. HEALTH REP. 116 (1997). Indeed, perhaps the earliest European law on inoculation predated Jenner. Switzerland (Berne), Decree No. 119 of 21 March 1777 on Inoculation Against Smallpox: ("To prevent any further, uninterrupted spread of the epidemic of smallpox, it is hereby prescribed that inoculation against smallpox or 'children-pox' should be made available to everyone, subject to the following restriction being observed namely that inoculation will not be carried out in towns but only in the countryside, and only during the spring and autumn.").

4. ROSEN, *supra* note 2, at 304–07.

5. *See generally,* RENE DUBOS, PASTEUR AND MODERN SCIENCE (Thomas Brock ed., 1998). The germ theory, of course, predated the pioneering microbiologists of the late nineteenth century. Gerolamo Fracastoro, influenced by the syphilis epidemic, published his work *De Contagiounibus* in 1546. In 1675, Antoni van Leeuwenhoek was the first person to observe "animalcules" (proto-

zoa) with a microscope. ABRAHAM SCHIERBEEK, MEASURING THE INVISIBLE WORLD: THE LIFE AND WORKS OF ANTONI VAN LEEUWENHOEK 60 (1959). Fracastoro and Leeuwenhoek both believed in the connection between microbes and disease, but the doctrine of living contagion soon lost hold on the public and medicine so that by the early ninteenth century the idea was discredited. JOHN M. EAGER, FIGHTING TRIM: THE IMPORTANCE OF RIGHT LIVING 23 (1917).

6. Robert Koch, *A Further Communication on a Cure for Tuberculosis*, in FROM CONSUMPTION TO TUBERCULOSIS: A DOCUMENTARY HISTORY 300 (Barbara Guttmann Rosenkrantz ed., 1994).

7. Alexander Fleming, *On the Antibacterial Action of Cultures of a Penicillium with Special Reference to Their Use in the Isolation of H. Influenzae*, 10 BRIT. J. EXPER. PATHOLOGY 226 (1929).

8. Robert T. Rolfs et al., *Treatment of Syphillus*[sic], *1989*, 12 REV. INFECTIOUS DISEASES 590–609 (Supp. 1990).

9. Alexander Fleming, *Chemotherapy: Yesterday, To-day, To-morrow*, THE LINACRE LECTURES 32 (1946).

10. Jon N. Hays, THE BURDENS OF DISEASE: EPIDEMICS AND HUMAN RESPONSE IN WESTERN HISTORY 212–39 (1998).

11. Michael H. Vodkin et al., *Mosquito Productivity and Surveillance for St. Louis Encephalitis Virus in Chicago During 1993*, 11 J. AM. MOSQUITO CONTROL ASS'N 302 (1995).

12. Mark D. Sobsey, *Inactivation of Health-Related Microorganisms in Water by Disinfection Processes*, 21 WATER SCI. TECH. 179 (1989).

13. American Pub. Health Ass'n, *Policy Statement 9303: Evaluating Federal Meat, Poultry, and Seafood Inspection*, 84 AM. J. PUB. HEALTH 513 (1994).

14. *See, e.g.*, Centers for Disease Control & Prevention, *Youth Risk Behavior Surveillance—United States, 1997*, 48 MORB. MORT. WKLY. REP. 1 (Supp. 1998).

15. Scott Burris, *The Invisibility of Public Health: Population-Level Measures in a Politics of Market Individualism*, 87 AM. J. PUB. HEALTH 1607, 1609 (1997).

16. Mervyn Susser & Ezra Susser, *Choosing a Future for Epidemiology: II. From Black Box to Chinese Boxes and Eco-epidemiology*, 86 AM. J. PUB. HEALTH 674 (1996).

17. Bruce G. Link & Jo Phelan, *Social Conditions as Fundamental Causes of Disease*, 1995 J. HEALTH & SOC. BEHAVIOR 87 ("The fundamental social causes of disease . . . include money, knowledge, power, prestige, and the kinds of interpersonal resources embodied in the concepts of social support and social network."); ANNE PLATT, INFECTING OURSELVES: HOW ENVIRONMENTAL AND SOCIAL DISRUPTIONS TRIGGER DISEASE 26–30 (1996) (poverty limits individual education, lifestyle choices, and mobility, thereby creating "breeding grounds" for infectious diseases).

18. CENTERS FOR DISEASE CONTROL & PREVENTION, ADDRESSING EMERGING INFECTIOUS DISEASE THREATS: A PREVENTION STRATEGY FOR THE UNITED STATES (1994); Joshua Lederberg, *Infectious Diseases as an Evolutionary Paradigm*, 3 EMERGING INFECTIOUS DISEASES 417 (1997).

19. Lawrence O. Gostin, *The Law and Communicable Diseases: The Role of Law in an Era of Microbial Threats*, 49 INT'L DIG. HEALTH LEGIS. 221 (1998).

20. MEREDETH TURSHEN, POLITICS OF PUBLIC HEALTH 57–64 (1989).

21. JOHN DUFFY, THE SANITARIANS: A HISTORY OF AMERICAN PUBLIC HEALTH 93–108 (1990).

22. On the use of vaccination as a treatment, see Donald S. Burke, *Vaccine Therapy for HIV: A Historical Review of the Treatment of Infectious Diseases by Active Specific Immunization with Microbe-Derived Antigens*, 11 VACCINE 883 (1993).

23. DORLAND'S ILLUSTRATED MEDICAL DICTIONARY 1787 (1980). The terms "vaccination" and "immunization" are often used interchangeably. Immunization is the more inclusive term, denoting the process of inducing or providing immunity artificially by administering an immunobiologic. Immunization can be passive or active. Passive immunization involves the administration of antibodies produced by an immune animal or human, conferring short-term protection against infection. In active immunization (vaccination), the vaccine induces the host's own immune system to provide protection against the pathogen. W. Michael McDonnell & Frederick K. Askari, *Immunization*, 278 JAMA 2000 (1997).

24. Centers for Disease Control & Prevention, *Ten Great Public Health Achievements, 1900–1999: Impact of Vaccines Universally Recommended for Children*, 48 MORB. MORT. WKLY. REP. 241, 243–48 (1999).

25. Thomas Jefferson was an active supporter of Dr. Benjamin Waterhouse, an American disciple of Jenner, who actively practiced vaccination. ROSEN, *supra* note 2, at 165.

26. These claims were evident as the Supreme Court struggled with the issue of vaccination in *Jacobson v. Massachusetts*, 197 U.S. 11 (1905): "[S]ome physicians of great skill and repute do not believe that vaccination is a preventive" (quoting *Viemeister v. White*) (*Jacobson*, 197 U.S. at 34); "vaccination quite often caused serious and permanent injury to the health of the person vaccinated" (quoting Henning Jacobson) (*id.* at 36); compulsory vaccination is "hostile to the inherent right of every freeman to care for his own body and health" (quoting Henning Jacobson) (*id.* at 15–16, 26).

27. WILLIAM PACKER PRENTICE, POLICE POWERS ARISING UNDER THE LAW OF OVERRULING NECESSITY 132 (1993) ("Compulsory vaccination has been instituted . . . by the laws of several States, in respect to minors. City ordinances regulate it, but the indirect methods of excluding children not vaccinated from schools and factories, or, in case of immigrants, insisting upon quarantine, and the offer of free vaccination . . . are more effective."); Charles L. Jackson, *State Laws on Compulsory Immunization in the United States*, 84 PUB. HEALTH REP. 787, 792–94 (1969) (Massachusetts enacted the first mandatory vaccination law in 1809).

28. 197 U.S. 11 (1905); Viemeister v. White, 179 N.Y. 235 (1904) (upholding a N.Y. statute excluding from public schools all children who had not been vaccinated): "Nearly every state in the Union has statutes to encourage, or directly or indirectly to require, vaccination; and this is true of most nations of Europe." *Id.* at 239–40; William Fowler, *Principal Provisions of Smallpox*

Vaccination Laws and Regulations in the United States, 56 PUB. HEALTH REP. 325 (1942) (only six states did not have a smallpox vaccination statute). It was not until the late 1930s that compulsory immunization laws pertaining to other diseases were enacted. William Fowler, *State Diphtheria Immunization Requirements,* 57 PUB. HEALTH REP. 325 (1942).

29. Centers for Disease Control & Prevention, *Measles and School Immunization Requirements—United States, 1978,* 27 MORB. MORT. WKLY. REP. 303 (1978) (states which strictly enforced vaccination laws had measles incidence rates more than 50 percent lower than in other states); *see* Kenneth B. Robbins et al., *Low Measles Incidence: Association with Enforcement of School Immunization Laws,* 71 AM. J. PUB. HEALTH 270 (1981) (states with low incidence rates were significantly more likely to have, and enforce, laws requiring immunization of the entire school population).

30. John P. Middaugh & Lawrence D. Zyla, *Enforcement of School Immunization Law in Alaska,* 239 JAMA 2128 (1978).

31. Walter A. Orenstein & Alan R. Hinman, *The Immunization System in the United States—The Role of School Immunization Laws,* presented to the 4TH EUROPEAN CONFERENCE ON VACCINOLOGY, MARCH 17–19, 1999, Brighton, U.K.

32. Advisory Comm. on Immunization Practices (ACIP), *Combination Vaccines for Childhood Immunization,* 48 MORB. MORT. WKLY. REP. 1 (1999). Current CDC recommendations are available at <http://www. cdc.gov>.

33. Lawrence O. Gostin & Zita Lazzarini, *Childhood Immunization Registries: A National Review of Public Health Information Systems and the Protection of Privacy,* 274 JAMA 1793, 1795–96 (1995).

34. The language of religious exemptions varies from a strict standard ("recognized church or denomination" whose teaching forbids vaccination ARK. CODE ANN. § 6-18-702 (Michie 1997)) to a more vague standard ("belief in relation to a Supreme being" DEL. CODE ANN. tit. 14 § 131 (1997)). As of the 1999/2000 school year, only two states, West Virginia and Mississippi, did not have a religious exemption. W. VA. CODE § 16-3-4 (1999) (two religious exemption bills failed in the state House and Senate. *See* S. B. 442 (W. Va. 1999); H. B. 2302 (W. Va. 1999); MISS. CODE. ANN. § 41-23-37 (Supp. 1994) (the state Supreme Court held the religious exemption was unconstitutional in Brown v. Stone, 378 So. 2d 218 (Miss. 1979), *cert. denied,* 449 U.S. 887 (1980)).

35. As of the 1999/2000 school year, fifteen states had exemptions for nonreligious objections, such as moral, philosophical, or personal beliefs. ARIZ. REV. STAT. ANN. § 15-872 (West 1998), CAL. HEALTH & SAFETY CODE § 120365 (Deering 1999), IDAHO CODE § 39-4802 (1998), IND. CODE ANN. § 20-8.10-7-2 (1998), LA. REV. STAT. ANN. § 17:170(E) (West 1999), ME. REV. STAT. ANN. tit. 20-A, § 6355 (West 1999), MICH. COMP. LAWS ANN. § 333.9215 (West 1998), MINN. STAT. § 121A.15 (1998), NEB. REV. STAT. § 79-221 (1999), N.D. CENT. CODE § 23-07-17.1 (1999), OHIO REV. CODE. ANN. § 3313.671 (Anderson 1998), OKLA. STAT. tit. 70, § 1210.192 (1998), VT. STAT. ANN. tit. 18, § 1122 (1999), WASH. REV. CODE § 28A.210.090 (1998), and WIS. STAT. § 252.04 (1998).

36. NATIONAL VACCINE ADVISORY COMM., REPORT OF THE NVAC WORKING GROUP ON PHILOSOPHICAL EXEMPTIONS (1998) (total exemptions in 1994–95 school year were less than 1 percent of school entrants).

37. Thomas Novotny et al., *Measles Outbreaks in Religious Groups Exempt from Immunization Laws*, 103 PUB. HEALTH REP. 49 (1988).

38. The first case upholding vaccination was *Hazen v. Strong*, 2 Vt. 427 (1830) (finding that the power of selectmen extends to incurring the expense of vaccinating inhabitants when exposed, even though there were no cases in town). *See* JAMES A. TOBEY, PUBLIC HEALTH LAW: A MANUAL OF LAW FOR SANITARIANS 89–98 (1947) (assembling sixty-seven court cases, almost always upholding state power to vaccinate); James A. Tobey, *Vaccination and the Courts*, 83 JAMA 462 (1924).

39. Jacobson v. Massachusetts, 197 U.S. 11 (1905).

40. *See, e.g.*, Cude v. State, 377 S.W.2d 816 (Ark. 1964) (citing numerous precedents); Maricopa County Health Dep't v. Harmon, 750 P.2d 1364 (Ariz. Ct. App. 1987); Brown v. Stone, 378 So. 2d 218 (Miss. 1979), *cert. denied*, 449 U.S. 887 (1980).

41. 260 U.S. 174 (1922). State supreme courts also routinely upheld school vaccination. *See, e.g.*, People *ex rel.* Hill v. Board of Educ. of the City of Lansing, 195 N.W. 95 (Mich. 1923).

42. *Jacobson*, 197 U.S. at 38–39.

43. *See, e.g.*, *Brown*, 378 So. 2d at 223 ("The protection of the great body of school children . . . against the horrors of crippling and death resulting from [vaccine-preventable disease] demand that children who have not been immunized should be excluded from school. . . . To the extent that it may conflict with the religious beliefs of a parent, however sincerely entertained, the interests of the school children must prevail."); Cude, 377 S.W.2d at 819 ("[A]ccording to the great weight of authority, it is within the police power of the State to require that school children be vaccinated . . . and that . . . it does not violate the constitutional rights of anyone, on religious grounds or otherwise.").

44. Employment Div. v. Smith, 494 U.S. 872 (1990).

45. 321 U.S. 158, 166–67 (1944).

46. Wright v. De Witt Sch. Dist., 385 S.W.2d 644, 648 (Ark. 1965).

47. *Brown*, 378 So. 2d at 223 (holding that a religious exemption violates equal protection of the law because it "discriminates against the great majority of children whose parents have no such religious convictions. To give it effect would . . . expose [the great body of school children] . . . to the hazard of associating in school with children exempted . . . who had not been immunized.").

48. *See, e.g.*, Mason v. General Brown Cent. Sch. Dist., 851 F.2d 47 (2d Cir. 1988); Berg v. Glen Cove City Sch. Dist., 853 F. Supp. 651 (E.D.N.Y. 1994).

49. *In re* Elwell, 284 N.Y.S.2d 924, 932 (N.Y. Fam. Ct. 1967) (finding that, although the parents were members of a recognized religion, their objections to the polio vaccine were not based on the tenets of their religion); McCartney v. Austin, 293 N.Y.S.2d 188 (Sup. Ct. 1968) (finding that the vaccination statute did not interfere with the freedom of worship of Roman Catholic faith, which

does not have a proscription against vaccination); Brown v. City Sch. Dist., 429 N.Y.S.2d 355 (Sup. Ct. 1980) (entitling a parent to a religious exemption given the genuineness and sincerity of the parent's religious beliefs and the absence of risk to the public); *but see Berg,* 853 F. Supp. at 655 (finding that although nothing in the Jewish religion prohibited vaccination, the parents still had a sincere religious belief).

50. Hanzel v. Arter, 625 F. Supp. 1259 (S.D. Ohio 1985) (denying exemption to parents with objections to vaccination based on "chiropractic ethics"); *Mason,* 851 F.2d at 47 (finding the parents' sincerely held belief that immunization was contrary to the "genetic blueprint" was a secular, not a religious, belief).

51. As to the establishment clause argument, *compare* Sherr v. Northport-East Northport Union Free Sch. Dist., 672 F. Supp. 81, 91, 97 (E.D.N.Y. 1987) (upholding exemption for children of parents with "sincere religious beliefs," but finding that the provision requiring them to be "bona fide members of a recognized religious organization" violates the establishment clause) *with* Kleid v. Board of Educ., 406 F. Supp. 902, 904 (W.D. Ky. 1976) (finding that the exemption for a "nationally recognized and established church or religious denomination" does not violate the establishment clause). As to the equal protection argument, see Dalli v. Board of Educ., 267 N.E.2d 219 (Mass. 1971) (holding that the exemption for objectors who subscribe to "tenets and practice of a recognized church or religious denomination" violates equal protection by extending preferred treatment to these groups while denying it to others with sincere religious objections).

52. Centers for Disease Control & Prevention, *Update: Childhood Vaccine-Preventable Diseases—United States, 1994,* 43 MORB. MORT. WKLY. REP. 718 (1994).

53. Kristine M. Severyn, Jacobson v. Massachusetts: *Impact on Informed Consent and Vaccine Policy,* 5 J. PHARM. & LAW 249, 260–61 (1996); Charles L. Jackson, *State Laws on Compulsory Immunization in the United States,* 84 PUB. HEALTH REP. 787, 792–94 (1969).

54. INSTITUTE OF MEDICINE, RISK COMMUNICATION AND VACCINATION: WORKSHOP SUMMARY 11 (1997).

55. INSTITUTE OF MEDICINE, VACCINES FOR THE 21ST CENTURY: A TOOL FOR DECISIONMAKING (1999).

56. *Poliomyelitis Prevention: Recommendations for Use of Inactivated Polio Virus Vaccine and Live Oral Poliovirus Vaccine,* 99 AM. ACAD. PEDIATRICS COMM. INFECTIOUS DISEASES, PEDIATRICS 300, 303 (1997) (since 1979 nearly all U.S. cases of paralytic poliomyelitis have been vaccine associated). The government, in 1999, announced that it will cease the use of live attenuated polio vaccine. *Change in Polio Vaccines is Recommended,* N.Y. TIMES, June 9, 1999, at A12. *See* Centers for Disease Control & Prevention, *Poliomyelitis Prevention in the United States* 49 MORB. MORT. WKLY. REP. 1 (2000).

57. Under the principle of herd immunity, a population becomes resistant to attack by a disease if a large proportion of its members are immune. This concept explains why some members of a group can remain unvaccinated and the group can still remain protected against disease. LEON GORDIS, EPIDEMIOLOGY 18 (1996).

58. Garrett Hardin, *The Tragedy of the Commons*, 162 SCIENCE 1243 (1968).

59. 42 U.S.C. § 300aa-1 (1994); *see* Derry Ridgway, *No-Fault Vaccine Insurance: Lessons from the National Vaccine Injury Compensation Program*, 24 J. HEALTH POL., POL'Y & L. 59 (1999).

60. The NCVIA, particularly the compensation program, has been controversial. Although it has sharply reduced litigation, the "no-fault" adjudication system has been time-consuming, costly, and adversarial; a high percentage of the cases have been dismissed. *See* Wendy Mariner, *The National Vaccine Injury Compensation Program*, 11 HEALTH AFF. 262 (1992).

61. INSTITUTE OF MEDICINE, VACCINE SAFETY FORUM (1997).

62. Centers for Disease Control & Prevention, *Measles—United States, 1992*, 42 MORB. MORT. WKLY. REP. 378 (1993); National Vaccine Advisory Committee, *The Measles Epidemic: The Problems, Barriers, and Recommendations*, 266 JAMA 1547 (1991).

63. Centers for Disease Control & Prevention, *Reported Vaccine-Preventable Diseases—United States, 1993, and the Childhood Immunization Initiative*, 43 MORB. MORT. WKLY. REP. 57 (1994); GENERAL ACCOUNTING OFFICE, VACCINES FOR CHILDREN: CRITICAL ISSUES IN DESIGN AND IMPLEMENTATION (1994).

64. GENERAL ACCOUNTING OFFICE, PREVENTIVE HEALTH CARE FOR CHILDREN: EXPERIENCE FROM SELECTED FOREIGN COUNTRIES (1993).

65. Centers for Disease Control & Prevention, *Vaccination Coverage of 2-Year-Old Children—United States, 1991–92*, 271 JAMA 260 (1994).

66. Centers for Disease Control & Prevention, *Impact of Missed Opportunities to Vaccinate Preschool-Aged Children on Vaccination Coverage Levels—Selected U.S. Sites, 1991–1992*, 38 MORB. MORT. WKLY. REP. 709 (1994).

67. NATIONAL VACCINE ADVISORY COMMITTEE, DEVELOPING A NATIONAL CHILDHOOD IMMUNIZATION SYSTEM: REGISTRIES, REMINDERS, AND RECALL (1994); Gostin & Lazzarini, *supra* note 33, at 1795–96.

68. Immunization coverage in the United States in the year ending June 30, 1998 for 19–35-month-old children was over 90 percent for most individual vaccines; only varicella had coverage below 80 percent. Centers for Disease Control & Prevention, unpublished data (1999).

69. *See* RICHARD E. NEUSTADT & HARVEY FINEBERG, THE EPIDEMIC THAT NEVER WAS: POLICY-MAKING AND THE SWINE FLU AFFAIR (1983); Walter R. Dowdle, *The 1976 Experience*, 176 (Supp. 1) J. INFECTIOUS DISEASE S69 (1997).

70. Louis Weinstein, *Influenza—1918, A Revisit?* 294 NEW ENG. J. MED. 1058 (1976).

71. Cyril Wecht, *The Swine Flu Immunization Program: Scientific Venture or Political Folly*, 3 AM. J. L. & MED. 425 (1977); *but see* Nicholas Wade, *1976 Swine Flu Campaign Faulted, Yet Principals Would Do It Again*, 202 SCIENCE 849 (1978).

72. NEUSTADT & FINEBERG, *supra* note 69.

73. Jonathan E. Fielding, *Managing Public Health Risks: The Swine Flu Immunization Program Revisited*, 4 AM. J. L. & MED. 35 (1978).

74. Donald A. Henderson et al., *Smallpox as a Biological Weapon: Medical and Public Health Management*, 281 JAMA 2127 (1999); Thomas V. Inglesby, et al., *Anthrax as a Biological Weapon: Medical and Public Health Management*, 281 JAMA 1735 (1999).

75. Ronald Bayer et al., *HIV Antibody Screening: An Ethical Framework for Evaluating Proposed Programs*, 256 JAMA 1768 (1986).

76. William C. Black & Gilbert Welch, *Screening for Disease*, 168(1) AM. J. ROENTGENOLOGY 3 (1997).

77. REDUCING THE ODDS: PREVENTING PERINATAL TRANSMISSION OF HIV IN THE UNITED STATES 22 (Michael A. Stoto et al. eds., 1999) [hereinafter REDUCING THE ODDS].

78. *See, e.g.,* Holcomb v. Armstrong, 239 P2d 545 (Wash. 1952) (TB screening of university students); Conlon v. Marshall, 59 N.Y.S. 2d 52 (Sup. Ct. 1945) (TB screening of public school teachers).

79. Katherine L. Acuff & Ruth R. Faden, *A History of Prenatal and Newborn Screening Programs: Lessons for the Future, in* AIDS, WOMEN, AND THE NEXT GENERATION: TOWARDS A MORALLY ACCEPTABLE PUBLIC POLICY FOR HIV TESTING OF PREGNANT WOMEN AND NEWBORNS 59 (Ruth R. Faden et al. eds., 1991) [hereinafter AIDS, WOMEN, AND THE NEXT GENERATION].

80. THEODORE M. HAMMETT ET AL., 1992 UPDATE: HIV/AIDS IN CORRECTIONAL FACILITIES—ISSUES AND OPTIONS (1994).

81. Martha A. Field, *Testing for AIDS: Uses and Abuses*, 16 AM. J. L. & MED. 34, 35 (1990).

82. For criteria to evaluate screening see UNITED STATES PREVENTIVE SERVICES TASK FORCE, GUIDE TO CLINICAL PREVENTIVE SERVICES (1989). In the context of HIV screening, *see* Allan M. Brandt et al., *Routine Hospital Testing for HIV: Health Policy Considerations, in* AIDS AND THE HEALTH CARE SYSTEM 125 (Lawrence O. Gostin ed., 1990); Lawrence O. Gostin & William J. Curran, *The Case against Compulsory Case Finding in Controlling AIDS: Testing, Screening and Reporting*, 12 AM. J. LAW & MED. 1 (1987).

83. JUDITH S. MAUSNER & SHIRA KRAMER, EPIDEMIOLOGY—AN INTRODUCTORY TEXT 217 (2d ed. 1985).

84. The positive PV is the proportion of those with the disease among those with a positive test and the negative PV is the proportion of those who are healthy among those with a negative test.

85. *See, e.g.,* Inger Torhild Gram et al., *Quality of Life Following a False Positive Mammogram*, 62 BRIT. J. CANCER 1018 (1990); Centers for Disease Control & Prevention, *Update—HIV Counseling and Testing Using Rapid Tests*, 47 MORB. MORT. WKLY. REP. 211–15 (1998).

86. Bernard J. Turnock & Chester J. Kelly, *Mandatory Premarital Testing for Human Immunodeficiency Virus: The Illinois Experience*, 261 JAMA 3415, 3418 (1989) (the Illinois program was later repealed); *see* Paul D. Cleary et al., *Compulsory Premarital Screening for the Human Immunodeficiency Virus: Technical and Public Health Considerations*, 258 JAMA 1757 (1987).

87. JOHN MAXWELL, GLOVER WILSON & GUNNAR JUNGNER, PRINCIPLES AND PRACTICE OF SCREENING FOR DISEASE (1968).

88. RONALD BAYER, PRIVATE ACTS, SOCIAL CONSEQUENCES: AIDS AND THE POLITICS OF PUBLIC HEALTH (1989).

89. Ruth R. Faden et al., *Warrants for Screening Programs: Public Health, Legal and Ethical Frameworks, in* AIDS, WOMEN, AND THE NEXT GENERATION, *supra* note 79, at 3.

90. *See* NATIONAL CONFERENCE OF STATE LEGISLATURES, SEXUALLY TRANSMITTED DISEASES: A POLICYMAKER'S GUIDE AND SUMMARY OF STATE LAWS (1998); NATIONAL CONFERENCE OF STATE LEGISLATURES, HIV/AIDS: FACTS TO CONSIDER (1999) [hereinafter NCSL: HIV/AIDS].

91. *See, e.g.,* VT. STAT. ANN. tit. 18, § 1092 (1982) (authorizing testing of any person reasonably suspected of being infected with a venereal disease).

92. *See, e.g.,* N.C. GEN. STAT. § 15A-615 (1997) (authorizing STD testing of sex offenders who have had alleged sexual contact with a minor).

93. *See, e.g.,* N.J. STAT. ANN. § 26:4-49.6 (West 1996) (requiring migrant laborers to submit to syphilis and gonorrhea testing).

94. As of 1999, at least eleven states mandated HIV testing of persons convicted of prostitution. NCSL: HIV/AIDS, *supra* note 90, at 78.

95. *See, e.g.,* OHIO REV. CODE ANN. § 3701.49 (Anderson 1997) (requiring syphilis and gonorrhea testing of specimens taken from pregnant women).

96. *See, e.g.,* N.Y. PUB. HEALTH LAW § 2500-f (McKinney 1999) (mandating HIV testing of newborns and notification of parent of the results).

97. *See, e.g.,* VA. CODE § 32.1-59 (Michie 1997) (requiring venereal disease testing for any person admitted to a state correctional institution or state hospital).

98. As of 1999, twenty-one states permitted mandatory testing of patients who expose health care workers, emergency personnel, or law enforcement officers to HIV. NCSL: HIV/AIDS, *supra* note 90, at 62.

99. *See, e.g.,* N.Y. PUB. HEALTH LAW § 2301 (McKinney 1993) (authorizing a health officer to apply to a court for an order to test for an STD).

100. *See, e.g.,* GA. CODE ANN. § 19-3-40 (Michie 1991) (requiring a syphilis test prior to issuing a marriage license).

101. Lawrence O. Gostin, *Controlling the Resurgent Tuberculosis Epidemic: A Fifty State Survey of Tuberculosis Statutes and Proposals for Reform,* 269 JAMA 255 (1993).

102. Lawrence O. Gostin et al., *Screening and Exclusion of International Travelers and Immigrants for Public Health Purposes: An Evaluation of United States Policy,* 322 NEW ENG. J. MED. 1743 (1990).

103. RUTH R. FADEN & TOM L. BEACHAMP, A HISTORY AND THEORY OF INFORMED CONSENT 25 (1986).

104. Canterbury v. Spence, 464 F.2d 772 (D.C. Cir. 1972).

105. See chapters 2 and 3.

106. Government-authorized testing must also conform to the Fourteenth Amendment protection of due process and equal protection of the law. *See* Hill v. Evans, 62 U.S. L.W. 2355 (M.D. Ala. 1993) (finding mandatory HIV testing of "high-risk" persons unconstitutional because it is not rationally related to the state's interest in public health).

107. Schmerber v. California, 384 U.S. 757, 767–68 (1966).

108. Skinner v. Railway Labor Executives' Ass'n, 489 U.S. 602, 613–14 (1989) (upholding drug tests following major train accidents for employees who violate safety rules, even without reasonable suspicion of impairment); National Treasury Employees Union v. Von Raab, 489 U.S. 656 (1989) (upholding suspicionless drug testing by U.S. Customs Service due to government's "compelling" interest in safeguarding borders and public safety); see also Diana Chapman Walsh et al., Worksite Drug Testing, 13 Ann. Rev. Publ. Health 197 (1992).

109. Skinner, 489 U.S. at 625.

110. See, e.g., Veronia Sch. Dist. 47J v. Acton, 515 U.S. 646 (1995) (upholding random urinalysis for participation in interscholastic athletics).

111. Anonymous Fireman v. City of Willoughby, 779 F. Supp. 402 (N.D. Ohio 1991) (upholding mandatory HIV testing for firefighters and paramedics because they are "high-risk" employees).

112. Plowman v. United States Dep't of Army, 698 F. Supp. 627 (E.D. Va. 1988) (upholding HIV testing of federal civilian employees).

113. Local 1812, Am. Fed'n of Gov't Employees v. United States Dep't of State, 662 F. Supp. 50 (D.D.C. 1987) (upholding HIV testing of foreign service employees).

114. Haitian Ctrs. Council v. Sale, 823 F. Supp. 1028 (E.D.N.Y. 1993).

115. In re Juveniles A, B, C, D, E, 847 P.2d 455 (Wash. 1993) (upholding mandatory HIV testing for juveniles convicted of sexual offenses).

116. Donna I. Dennis, HIV Screening and Discrimination: The Federal Example, in AIDS Law Today 187 (Scott Burris et al. eds., 1993).

117. But see Glover v. Eastern Neb. Community Office of Retardation, 686 F. Supp. 243 (D. Neb. 1988), aff'd, 867 F.2d 461 (9th Cir. 1989) (invalidating on Fourth Amendment grounds chronic infectious disease policy mandating HIV and HBV screening of employees); see also Steven Eisenstat, An Analysis of the Rationality of Mandatory Testing for the HIV Antibody: Balancing Public Health Interest with the Individual's Privacy Interest, 52 U. Pitt. L. Rev. 327 (1991).

118. Americans with Disabilities Act of 1990, 42 U.S.C. §§ 12101–12201 (1992).

119. Id. at § 12102(2).

120. See, e.g., New York State Ass'n for Retarded Children v. Carey, 612 F.2d 644 (2d Cir. 1979) (finding that mentally retarded carriers of serum hepatitis B could not be excluded from public school); Kohl v. Woodhaven Learning Ctr., 865 F.2d 930 (8th Cir. 1989) (finding inoculation of school staff for hepatitis not a "reasonable accommodation").

121. United States Equal Employment Opportunity Commission v. AIC Sec. Investigations, Ltd., 823 F. Supp. 571 (N.D. Ill. 1993) (finding unlawful the termination of a person after diagnosis of brain cancer that did not affect his job performance).

122. Bragdon v. Abbott, 524 U.S. 624 (1998); see Lawrence O. Gostin et al., Disability Discrimination in America: HIV/AIDS and Other Health Conditions, 281 JAMA 745 (1999); George J. Annas, Protecting Patients from Discrimination—the Americans with Disabilities Act and HIV Infection, 339 New Eng. J. Med. 1255 (1998).

123. 42 U.S.C. §§ 12102(2)(B), (2)(C) (1994).

124. Lawrence O. Gostin, *The Americans with Disabilities Act and the U.S. Health Care System*, 11 HEALTH AFFAIRS 248 (1992).

125. Albertsons, Inc. v. Kirkingburg, 527 U.S. 555 (1999) (holding that persons with monocular vision must prove a limitation on a major life activity, not merely that they see "differently" than persons with normal eyesight).

126. Sutton v. United Air Lines, Inc., 526 U.S. 1036 (1999) (finding myopic twin sisters who function normally with corrective measures not disabled under ADA); Murphy v. United Parcel Serv., Inc., 527 U.S. 516 (1999) (finding a driver whose blood pressure is normal when corrected by medication not disabled under ADA).

127. ROBERT L. BURGDORF, JR., MEMORANDUM TO FRIENDS OF THE DISABILITY RIGHTS COMMUNITY: THE SUPREME COURT'S ASSAULT ON THE ADA AND WHERE TO FROM HERE (July 16, 1999); *see* Robert L. Burgdoff, Jr., *"Substantially Limited" Protection from Disability Discrimination: The Special Treatment Model and Misconstruction of the Definition of Disability*, 42 VILL. L. REV. 409 (1997). The Court's fourth ADA decision in its 1999 term was more nuanced. Olmstead v. L.C., 525 U.S. 1062 (1999) (finding that the state must place a mentally disabled person in a community setting when it is medically appropriate, if the person does not oppose the transfer from institutional care and the placement can be reasonably accommodated taking into account the state's resources and needs of others with mental disabilities).

128. 42 U.S.C. § 12113(b) (1994).

129. *Id.* at § 12112(b)(5)(A).

130. Kohl v. Woodhaven Learning Ctr., 865 F.2d 930 (8th Cir. 1989) (finding that a school for persons with mental retardation was not obliged to vaccinate employees to accommodate a student with HBV).

131. 42 U.S.C. § 12112(d) (1994).

132. The reasons that Title II governs public health powers exercised by health authorities are explained in Lawrence O. Gostin, *The Resurgent Tuberculosis Epidemic in the Era of AIDS: Reflections on Public Health, Law, and Society*, 54 MD. L. REV. 1, 92–94 (1995). *See* City of Newark v. J.S., 652 A.2d 265, 273 (N.J. Super. Ct. Law Div. 1993) (applying the ADA not only to employment but also to the exercise of public health powers such as compulsory confinement).

133. 42 U.S.C. § 12181(7)(F) (1994) (defining public accommodation to include a pharmacy, the professional office of a health care provider, a hospital, or another service establishment).

134. Catherine Peckham & Diana Gibb, *Mother-to-Child Transmission of the Human Immunodeficiency Virus*, 298 NEW ENG. J. MED. 333 (1995).

135. *Recommendations of the U.S. Public Health Service Task Force on the Use of Zidovudine to Reduce Perinatal Transmission of Human Immunodeficiency Virus*, 43 MORB. MORT. WKLY. REP. 1 (1994); *Public Health Service Task Force's Recommendations for the Use of Antiviral Drugs in Pregnant Women Infected with HIV-1 for Maternal Health and for Reducing Perinatal HIV-1 Transmission in the United States*, 47 MORB. MORT. WKLY. REP. 1 (1998) (updating the 1994 guidelines); CENTERS FOR DISEASE CONTROL & PREVENTION, GUIDELINES FOR THE USE OF ANTIRETROVIRAL AGENTS IN PEDIATRIC HIV INFECTION (1999).

136. *U.S. Public Health Service Recommendations for Human Immuno-deficiency Virus Counseling and Voluntary Testing for Pregnant Women,* 44 MORB. MORT. WKLY. REP. 1 (1995).

137. Ryan White Comprehensive AIDS Resources Emergency (Care) Act Amendments, P.L. 104–46. 42 U.S.C. § 300ff (1994).

138. N.Y. PUB. HEALTH LAW § 2500-f (McKinney 1994); *see also* David Abramson, *Passing the Test: New York's Newborn HIV Testing Policy, 1987–1997, in* REDUCING THE ODDS, *supra* note 77, at 313 (providing a political and social account of the passage of the New York newborn screening law).

139. Miriam Davis, *Workshop I Summary, in* REDUCING THE ODDS, *supra* note 77, at 190, 197 (quoting Assemblywoman Mayersohn).

140. Ronald Bayer, *Rethinking the Testing of Babies and Pregnant Women for HIV Infection,* 7 J. CLINICAL ETHICS 85 (1996).

8.   RESTRICTIONS OF THE PERSON: AUTONOMY, LIBERTY, AND BODILY INTEGRITY

SOURCES FOR CHAPTER EPIGRAPHS: Page 203: ALBERT CAMUS, THE PLAGUE 34 (Stuart Gilbert trans., 1948). Page 208: *Quoted in* Ronald Bayer & Amy Fairchild-Carrino, *AIDS and the Limits of Control: Public Health Orders, Quarantine, and Recalcitrant Behavior,* 83 AM. J. PUB. HEALTH 1471, 1476 (1993). Page 216: Union Pac. Ry. Co. v. Botsford, 141 U.S. 250, 251 (1891). Page 224: IV COMMENTARIES ON THE LAWS OF ENGLAND, PUBLIC WRONGS (1869).

1. Prevailing theories of disease ranged from foul air or soil to hereditary causes; scientists sometimes flatly rejected theories of contagion. Erwin H. Ackerknecht, *Anti-Contagionism between 1821 and 1867,* 22 BULL. HIST. MED. 562 (1948); Charles Rosenberg, *The Bitter Fruit: Heredity, Disease, and Social Thought in 19th Century America, in* FROM CONSUMPTION TO TUBERCULOSIS: A DOCUMENTARY HISTORY 154 (Barbara Guttmann Rosenkrantz ed., 1994); JOHN MACAULEY EAGER, THE EARLY HISTORY OF QUARANTINE: ORIGIN OF SANITARY MEASURES DIRECTED AGAINST YELLOW FEVER 5–15 (1903).

2. A pest is any deadly epidemic disease or a pestilence, notably bubonic plague, derived from the French *peste,* the Old French *pestilence,* or the Latin *pestis.* 11 OXFORD ENGLISH DICTIONARY 622 (2d ed. 1989).

3. 8 OXFORD ENGLISH DICTIONARY 738; *see also lazar-house,* meaning a house for lazars or diseased persons, and *lazar,* meaning a poor and diseased person, usually one afflicted with a loathsome disease. *Id.* (quoting Byron (1820), "Thou must be cleansed of the black blood which makes thee a lazar-house of tyranny"; and G. Meredith (1880), "Their house would be a lazar-house, they would be condemned to seclusion").

4. EAGER, *supra* note 1, at 4–5.

5. OLEG P. SCHEPIN & WALDEMAR V. YERMAKOV, INTERNATIONAL QUARANTINE 11 (Boris Meerovich & Vladimir Bobrov trans., 1991); GEORGE ROSEN, A HISTORY OF PUBLIC HEALTH 40 (expanded ed. 1993).

6. ROSEN, *supra* note 5, at 41–43; EAGER, *supra* note 1, at 5–6; SCHEPIN & YERMAKOV, *supra* note 5, at 10.

7. EAGER, *supra* note 1, at 16–18; ROSEN, *supra* note 5, at 43–44.

8. Frank Gerard Clemow, *Origin of Quarantine*, BRIT. MED. J. 122 (1929).

9. EAGER, *supra* note 1, at 18, 20–21.

10. Elizabeth C. Tandy, *Local Quarantine and Inoculation for Smallpox in the American Colonies (1620–1775)*, 13 AM. J. PUB. HEALTH 203 (1923).

11. DONALD HOPKINS, PRINCES AND PEASANTS: SMALLPOX IN HISTORY 238–39 (1983); James A. Tobey, *Public Health and the Police Power*, 4 N.Y.U. L. REV. 126 (1927); SCHEPIN & YERMAKOV, *supra* note 5, at 17–18.

12. 1 ACTS AND RESOLVES OF THE PROVINCE OF MASS. BAY 467–70, ch. 9 (1701–02).

13. 3 COLONIAL LAWS OF N.Y. 1071–73, ch. 9973 (1755).

14. Wendy E. Parmet, *AIDS and Quarantine: The Revival of an Archaic Doctrine*, 14 HOFSTRA L. REV. 53, 55–58 (1985).

15. Sandeep Jauhar, *Leper Home to Fade but Not Memories of Prejudice*, HOUS. CHRON., June 29, 1998, at D5 (a federal statute transferred control of the Gillis W. Long Hansen's Disease Center, called the "Louisiana Leper Home" or "Carville," from the United States to the state; the state plans to close the hospital).

16. Act of May 27, 1796, ch. 31, 1 Stat. 474 (repealed 1799); Edwin Maxey, *Federal Quarantine Law*, 43 AM. L. REV. 382, 383 (1909).

17. Act of Feb. 25, 1799, ch. 12, 1 Stat. 619.

18. ERNEST FREUND, THE POLICE POWER: PUBLIC POLICY AND CONSTITUTIONAL RIGHTS 124–30 (1904); Blewett H. Lee, *Limitations Imposed by the Federal Constitution on the Right of the States to Enact Quarantine Laws*, 2 HARV. L. REV. 267, 270–82 (1889). A conflict regarding quarantine, of course, can also ensue among different states. *See* Louisiana v. Texas, 176 U.S. 1 (1900) (Louisiana complaining about a Texas quarantine on goods coming from New Orleans, where yellow fever had been reported).

19. Hennington v. Georgia, 163 U.S. 299, 309 (1896) (upholding state police power regulation affecting commerce until superseded by Congress); *see also* Cowles, *State Quarantine Laws and the Federal Constitution*, 25 AM. L. REV. 45 (1891).

20. Gibbons v. Ogden, 22 U.S. 1, 205–06 (1824) ("[C]ongress may control the state [quarantine] laws . . . for the regulation of commerce"); Compagnie Française de Navigation á Vapeur v. Louisiana State Bd. of Health, 186 U.S. 380, 388 (1902) ("[W]henever Congress shall undertake to provide . . . a general system of quarantine . . . all state laws on the subject will be abrogated").

21. 42 U.S.C. § 243(a). As to federal quarantine powers and duties, *see id.* at §§ 266–72 (1994).

22. SCHEPIN & YERMAKOV, *supra* note 5, at 63–150; Frank G. Boudreau, *International Health*, 19 AM. J. PUB. HEALTH 863 (1929).

23. Sev S. Fluss, *International Public Health Law: An Overview, in* OXFORD TEXTBOOK OF PUBLIC HEALTH 371, 379–80 (Roger Detels et al. eds. 3d ed., 1997) (discussing International Sanitary Regulations, including quarantine); DAVID P. FIDLER, INTERNATIONAL LAW AND INFECTIOUS DISEASE (1999).

24. *See generally,* WILLIAM H. MCNEILL, PLAGUES AND PEOPLES (1977); Paul Slack, *Introduction, in* EPIDEMICS AND IDEAS: ESSAYS ON THE HISTORICAL PERCEPTION OF PESTILENCE 1 (Terence Ranger & Paul Slack eds, 1992).

25. WAR AND PUBLIC HEALTH (Barry S. Levy & Victor W. Sidel eds., 1997).

26. ROSEN, *supra* note 5, at 41; *see also* SAUL N. BRODY, THE DISEASE OF THE SOUL: LEPROSY IN MEDIEVAL LITERATURE (1974).

27. Thomas B. Stoddard & Walter Rieman, *AIDS and the Rights of the Individual: Toward a More Sophisticated Analysis,* 68 (Supp. 1) MILBANK QUART. 143 (1990).

28. David Musto, *Quarantine and the Problem of AIDS,* 64 (Supp. 1) MILBANK QUART. 97, 102–04 (1986).

29. Guenter B. Risse, *Epidemics and History: Ecological Perspectives and Social Burdens, in* AIDS: THE BURDENS OF HISTORY 33 (Elizabeth Fee & Daniel M. Fox eds., 1988).

30. ALLAN M. BRANDT, NO MAGIC BULLET: A SOCIAL HISTORY OF VENEREAL DISEASE IN THE UNITED STATES SINCE 1880 (1985).

31. Guenter B. Risse, *Revolt Against Quarantine: Community Responses to the 1916 Polio Epidemic, Oyster Bay, New York,* 14 (5) TRANSACTIONS & STUD. OF THE C. OF PHYSICIANS OF PHILA. 23, 30 (1992).

32. SHEILA M. ROTHMAN, LIVING IN THE SHADOW OF DEATH: TUBERCULOSIS AND THE SOCIAL EXPERIENCE OF ILLNESS IN AMERICAN HISTORY 192–93 (1994); *see* Barron H. Lerner, *New York City's Tuberculosis Control Efforts: The Historical Limitations of War on Consumption,* 83 AM. J. PUB. HEALTH 758 (1993) (health departments have detained TB patients since 1903, principally members of socially disadvantaged groups).

33. C.-E.A. WINSLOW, LIFE OF HERMANN BIGGS 158 (1929); Charles V. Chapin, *Pleasures and Hopes of the Health Officer, in* PAPERS OF CHARLES V. CHAPIN, M.D. 6 (Frederick P. Gorham ed., 1934).

34. RENEE DUBOS & JEAN DUBOS, THE WHITE PLAGUE: TUBERCULOSIS, MAN AND SOCIETY 216–20 (attributing the decline in mortality to vastly improved social conditions); THOMAS MCKEOWN, THE ORIGINS OF HUMAN DISEASE 181 (1988). For a contemporary perspective, see Karen Brudney & Jay Dopkin, *Tuberculosis Control Laws in New York City: Human Immunodeficiency Virus, Homelessness, and the Decline of Tuberculosis Control Programs,* 144 AM. REV. RESPIR. DIS. 745 (1991).

35. RYAN WHITE, RYAN WHITE: MY OWN STORY (1991); *see also,* DAVID L. KIRP, LEARNING BY HEART: AIDS AND SCHOOL CHILDREN IN AMERICA'S COMMUNITIES (1990); Lawrence O. Gostin & David W. Webber, *The AIDS Litigation Project: HIV/AIDS in the Courts in the 1990s, Part 2,* 13 AIDS & PUB. POL'Y J. 3 (1998).

36. Robin Marantz Henig, *AIDS: A New Disease's Deadly Odyssey,* N.Y. TIMES MAG., Feb. 6, 1983, at 36 ("Innocent bystanders caught in the path of a new disease, they can make no behavioral decisions to minimize their risk: hemophiliacs cannot stop taking bloodclotting medication; surgery patients cannot stop getting transfusions; women cannot control the drug habits of their mates; babies cannot choose their mothers").

37. ALLAN M. BRANDT, *AIDS: From Social History to Social Policy,* LAW, MED., & HEALTH CARE 231, 231–32 (1986).

38. William F. Buckley, Jr., *Identify All the Carriers,* N.Y. TIMES, March 18, 1986, at A27 (recommending that persons with HIV infection be tattooed on their forearms and buttocks).

39. *See, e.g.,* Grutsch & Robertson, *The Coming of AIDS: It Didn't Start with the Homosexuals and It Won't End with Them,* 19 AM. SPECTATOR 12 (1986); *Florida Considering Locking Up Some Carriers of the AIDS Virus,* N.Y. TIMES, Jan. 27, 1988, at A15 (reporting the state's proposal "special lockup wards"); Tamar Lewin, *Rights of Citizens and Society Raise Legal Muddle on AIDS,* N.Y. TIMES, Oct. 14, 1987, at A1 (Sen. Helms and Pat Robertson suggest "quarantine may be necessary"); *see also* Eleanor Singer et al., *The Polls: A Report: AIDS,* 51 PUB. OPINION QUART. 580, 591–92 (1987) (in five national opinion polls, 28–51 percent of respondents said "people with AIDS should be put into quarantine in special places").

40. David J. Rothman, *The Single Disease Hospital: Why Tuberculosis Justifies a Departure That AIDS Does Not,* 21 J.L. MED. & ETHICS 296 (1993).

41. Francis M. Pottenger, *Is Another Chapter in Public Phthisiophobia About to be Written?,* 1 CALIF. ST. J. MED. 81 (1903).

42. *See generally* RANDY SCHILTS, AND THE BAND PLAYED ON: PEOPLE, POLITICS, AND THE AIDS EPIDEMIC (1988); DAVID ALTMAN, AIDS IN THE MIND OF AMERICA (1986).

43. While health departments have the power to confine, they may not have an affirmative duty to provide inpatient care and treatment to persons with infectious disease. The Constitution does not provide a robust set of affirmative rights (see chapter 2), nor do many public health statutes impose duties to provide services. *See* County of Cook v. City of Chicago, 593 N.E.2d 928 (Ill. App. Ct. 1st Dist. 1992) (finding that the county had no duty to provide inpatient treatment for persons with TB).

44. Cease-and-desist orders are issued on the administrative authority of the health department. An order typically specifies that the individual has failed to modify his behavior despite counseling and warns of further legal action, including criminal prosecution, if the individual persists in specified behaviors, such as unprotected sex or needle sharing. Ronald Bayer & Amy Fairchild-Carrino, *AIDS and the Limits of Control: Public Health Orders, Quarantine, and Recalcitrant Behavior,* 83 AM. J. PUB. HEALTH (1993).

45. OXFORD ENGLISH DICTIONARY 983 (2d ed. 1989).

46. *Id.* (quoting Pepys' Diary (26 November 1663), "Making of all ships coming from thence . . . to perform their quarantine for thirty days . . . contrary to the import of the word . . . it signifies now the thing, not the time spent in doing it"; and Jephson (1859), "The lepers often sought a voluntary death as the only escape from their perpetual quarantine").

47. *Id.* at 541–43 (describing two forms of quarantine: absolute and modified).

48. AMERICAN PUB. HEALTH ASS'N, CONTROL OF COMMUNICABLE DISEASES MANUAL 539–40 (Abram S. Benenson ed., 16th ed. 1995) (describing six forms of isolation: strict, contact, respiratory, tuberculosis, enteric precautions, and drainage/secretion precautions). *See also* Marguerite M. Jackson & Patricia Lynch, *Isolation Practices: A Historical Perspective,* 13 AM. J. INFECT. CONTROL 21 (1985).

49. People *ex rel.* Barmore v. Robertson, 134 N.E. 815, 819 (Ill. 1922) ("Quarantine is not a cure—it is a preventive").

50. Barron H. Lerner, *Catching Patients: Tuberculosis and Detention in the 1990s*, 115 CHEST 236 (1999); Tom Oscherwitz et al., *Detention of Persistently Nonadherent Patients with Tuberculosis*, 278 JAMA 843 (1997); George J. Annas, *Control of Tuberculosis—The Law and the Public's Health*, 328 NEW ENG. J. MED. 585 (1993).

51. Lawrence O. Gostin et al., *The Law and the Public's Health: A Study of Infectious Disease Law in the United States*, 99 COLUM. L. REV. 59, 101–18 (1999).

52. Lawrence O. Gostin, *Controlling the Resurgent Tuberculosis Epidemic: A Fifty State Survey of Tuberculosis Statutes and Proposals for Reform*, 269 JAMA 255, 256–58 (1993) (cataloguing civil commitment in the fifty states); Advisory Council for the Elimination of Tuberculosis (ACET), *Tuberculosis Control Laws—United States, 1993*, 42 MORB. MORT. WKLY. REP. 1, 7–9 (1993).

53. NATIONAL CONFERENCE OF STATE LEGISLATURES, SEXUALLY TRANSMITTED DISEASES: A POLICYMAKER'S GUIDE AND SUMMARY OF STATE LAWS 85–91 (1998) (cataloguing quarantine in the fifty states); *see* Lewis W. Petteway, *Compulsory Quarantine and Treatment of Persons Infected with Venereal Diseases*, 18 FL. L.J. 13 (1944).

54. Bayer & Fairchild-Carrino, *supra* note 44, at 1472 (in the first decade of the epidemic, twenty-five states enacted statutes for isolation of persons with HIV, usually based on risk behavior).

55. U.S. CONST. art. I, § 10, cl. 2. *See* Brown v. Maryland, 25 U.S. (12 Wheat.) 419 (1827); Cowles, *supra* note 19, 50–52 (1891).

56. Gibbons v. Ogden, 22 U.S. 1, 205 (1824).

57. Deborah Jones Merritt, *The Constitutional Balance between Health and Liberty*, 16 HASTINGS CENTER REP. 2 (Supp. Dec. 1986); Deborah Jones Merritt, *Communicable Disease and Constitutional Law: Controlling AIDS*, 61 N.Y.U. L. REV. 739, 774–83 (1986); Parmet, *supra* note 14, at 62–66.

58. *See, e.g.*, Staples v. Plymouth Co., 17 N.W. 569 (Iowa 1883); Mugler v. Kansas, 123 U.S. 623, 660–70 (1887); Haverty v. Bass, 66 Me. 71 (1876).

59. *See, e.g.*, Smith v. St. Louis & S.R. Co., 181 U.S. 248 (1901); Daniel v. Putnam County, 38 S.E. 980 (Ga. 1901); Board of Health v. Ward, 54 S.W. 725 (Ky. 1900); *Ex parte* Brown, 172 N.W. 522 (Neb. 1919); Highland v. Schlute, 82 N.W. 62 (Mich. 1900); White v. City of San Antonio, 60 S.W. 426 (Tex. 1901); People *ex rel.* Barmore v. Robertson, 134 N.E. 815 (Ill. 1922); *Ex parte* McGee, 185 P. 14 (Kan. 1919); *Ex parte* Culver, 202 P. 661 (Cal. 1921).

60. *See, e.g.*, Varholy v. Sweat, 15 So. 2d 267, 269–70 (Fla. 1943); State v. Rackowski, 86 A. 606, 608 (Conn. 1913) (and cases cited therein); Allison v. Cash, 137 S.W. 245, 247 (Ky. Ct. App. 1911); Highland v. Schulte, 82 N.W. 64 (Mich. 1900).

61. Most courts held that such delegations were constitutional and the powers exercised were not *ultra vires*. *See, e.g.*, People v. Tait, 103 N.E. 750 (Ill. 1913); Rock v. Carney, 185 N.W. 798, 801 (Mich. 1921); *but see* State *ex rel.* Adams v. Burdge, 70 N.W. 347 (Wis. 1897). The cases are collected in *General Delegation of Power to Guard Against Spread of Contagious Disease*, 8 A.L.R. 836 (1920).

62. White v. City of San Antonio, 60 S.W. 426 (Tex. 1901); Haig v. Board of Comm., 60 Ind. 511 (1878).

63. Spring v. Hyde Park, 137 Mass. 554 (1884).

64. Pinkham v. Dorothy, 55 Me. 135 (1867).

65. *In re* Martin, 188 P.2d 287 (Cal. Ct. App. 1948); State *ex rel.* Kennedy v. Head, 185 S.W.2d 530 (Tenn. 1945); Varholy v. Sweat, 15 So. 2d at 267 (Fla 1943); *Ex parte* Company, 139 N.E. 204 (Ohio 1922); *Ex parte* Arata, 198 P. 814 (Cal. Dist. Ct. App. 2d Dist. 1921); *In re application of* Shepard, 195 P. 1077 (Cal. Dist. Ct. App. 2d Dist. 1921); State *ex rel.* McBride v. Superior Court for King County, 174 P. 973 (Wash. 1918).

66. Greene v. Edwards, 263 S.E.2d 661 (W. Va. 1980); Jones v. Czapkay, 182 Cal. App. 2d 192 (1st Dist. 1960); White v. Seattle Local Union No. 81, 337 P.2d 289 (Wash. 1959).

67. Crayton v. Larrabee, 116 N.E. 355 (N.Y. 1917), *aff'g* 147 N.Y.S. 1105 (N.Y. App. Div. 1914); Allison v. Cash, 137 S.W. 245 (Ky. 1911); Hengehold v. City of Covington, 57 S.W. 495 (Ky. 1900); Henderson County Bd. of Health v. Ward, 54 S.W. 725 (Ky. 1900); Highland v. Schulte, 82 N.W. 62 (Mich. 1900); Smith v. Emery, 42 N.Y.S. 258 (N.Y. App. Div. 2d Dep't 1896); City of Richmond v. Supervisors of Henrico County, 2 S.E. 26 (Va. 1887); Spring v. Inhabitants of Hyde Park, 137 Mass. 554 (1884); Beckwith v. Sturtevant, 42 Conn. 158 (1875); Harrison v. Mayor & City Council of Baltimore, 1 Gill 264 (Md. 1843).

68. People v. Tait, 103 N.E. 750 (Ill. 1913); State v. Rackowski, 86 A. 606 (Conn. 1913).

69. Kirk v. Wyman, 65 S.E. 387 (S.C. 1909).

70. Rudolphe v. City of New Orleans, 11 La. Ann. 242 (La. 1856).

71. Jew Ho v. Williamson, 103 F. 10 (C.C.D. Cal. 1900).

72. *See, e.g.,* State *ex rel.* McBride v. Superior Court for King County, 174 P. 973 (Wash. 1918).

73. *Kirk,* 65 S.E. at 392.

74. *See, e.g., Ex parte* McGee, 185 P. 14 (Kan. 1919).

75. *See, e.g.,* Mugler v. Kansas, 123 U.S. 623, 660–61 (1887) (holding that the power to quarantine "so as to bind all, must exist somewhere; else, society will be at the mercy of the few, who, regarding only their own appetites or passions, may be willing to imperil the peace and security of the many, provided only they are permitted to do as they please"); Irwin v. Arrendale, 159 S.E.2d 719 (Ga. Ct. App. 1967) (subjecting individuals to reasonable public health measures for the common good).

76. *See, e.g.,* Huffman v. District of Columbia, 39 A.2d 558 (D.C. 1944); *In re application of* Milstead, 186 P. 170 (Cal. Dist. Ct. App. 2d 1919).

77. People v. Tait, 103 N.E. 750, 752 (Ill. 1913).

78. Viemeister v. White, 72 N.E. 97 (N. Y. 1904) (*quoted in* Jacobson v. Massachusetts, 197 U.S. 11, 34–35 (1905)).

79. Smith v. Emery, 42 N.Y.S. 258, 260 (N.Y. App. Div. 1896) ("The mere possibility that persons may have been exposed to disease is not sufficient. . . . They must have been exposed to it, and the conditions actually exist for a communication of the contagion."); *Ex parte* Shepard, 195 P. 1077 (Cal. 1921) (finding the mere suspicion of VD insufficient to uphold a quarantine order); *Ex parte* Arata, 198 P. 816 (Cal. Dist. Ct. App. 2d Dist. 1921) ("[M]ere suspicion

unsupported by facts . . . will afford no jurisdiction at all for depriving people of their liberty."); State v. Snow, 324 S.W.2d 532 (Ark. 1959) (invalidating a TB quarantine order due to meager evidentiary support).

80. *See, e.g., In re application of* Milstead, 186 P. 170 (Cal. 1919) (holding that marital status, in the absence of prostitution, cannot provide reasonable cause for suspicion of STD); *Huffman*, 39 A.2d at 558 (finding that health authorities have the burden of proof unless person is a prostitute); Wragg v. Griffin, 170 N.W. 400 (Iowa 1919) (denying that health authorities could detain a man "suspected" of having gonorrhea); *see* Parmet, *supra* note 14, at 67–68.

81. *Ex parte* Company, 139 N.E. 204, 205–06 (Ohio 1922); *see also In re application of* Johnson, 180 P. 644 (Cal. Ct. App. 1919).

82. People *ex rel.* Baker v. Strautz, 54 N.E.2d 441, 444 (Ill. 1944). As late as 1973, a federal court of appeals said, "It is not illogical or unreasonable, and on the contrary it is reasonable, to suspect that known prostitutes are a prime source of infectious venereal disease. Prostitution and venereal disease are no strangers." Reynolds v. McNichols, 488 F.2d 1378, 1382 (10th Cir. 1973); *see also* State *ex rel.* Kennedy v. Head, 185 S.W.2d 530 (Tenn. 1945); State v. Hutchinson, 18 So. 2d 723 (Ala. 1944); *In re* Caselli, 204 P. 364 (Mont. 1932).

83. The court in *Kirk v. Wyman* would not subject Mary Kirk to an unsafe environment. She was to have been isolated in a pesthouse—a "structure of four small rooms in a row, with no piazzas, used heretofore for the isolation of negroes with smallpox, situated within a hundred yards of the place where the trash of the city . . . is collected and burned." The court concluded that "even temporary isolation in such a place would be a serious affliction and peril to an elderly lady, enfeebled by disease, and accustomed to the comforts of life." 65 S.E. 387, 391 (S.C. 1909). *See* Jew Ho v. Williamson, 103 F. 10, 22 (C.C.D. Cal. 1900) (holding that confining large groups of people in an area where bubonic plague was suspected placed them at increased risk). The court was less rigorous, however, in reviewing the conditions of isolation in *Ex parte Martin*, 188 P.2d 287, 291 (Cal. 1948). The court supported giving health officers discretion as to the place of isolation. The county jail was designated as a quarantine area for people with STDs despite the uncontested evidence that it was overcrowded and had been condemned by a legislative investigating committee. The court supported the Attorney General's position that "[w]hile jails, as public institutions, were established for purposes other than confinement of diseased persons, occasions of emergency or lack of other public facilities for quarantine require that jails be used." *Id.* at 291.

84. *See* Youngberg v. Romeo, 457 U.S. 307 (1982) (holding that to effectuate the constitutional interests in "safety" and in "freedom of movement," the state must provide "minimally adequate or reasonable training to ensure safety and freedom from undue restraint").

85. *Id.* at 307, 315 (finding entitlement to such "minimally adequate or reasonable training to ensure safety and freedom from undue restraint").

86. Neimes v. Ta, 985 S.W.2d 132, 141–42 (Tex. App. 4th Dist. 1998) (reading *Youngberg* to extend to civil confinement of persons with TB).

87. Benton v. Reid, 231 F.2d 780 (D.C. Cir. 1956) (holding that persons with infectious disease are not criminals and should not be detained in jails);

State v. Hutchinson, 18 So. 2d 723 (Ala. 1944) (same); *but see Ex parte* Martin, 188 P.2d 287 (Cal. 1948) (upholding quarantine in county jail despite the fact that it was overcrowded and had been condemned).

88. 103 F. 10 (C.C.N.D. Cal. 1900). The quarantine in *Jew Ho* followed directly after another public health initiative designed to harass Chinese residents of San Francisco. In *Wong Wai v. Willliamson,* the court struck down as discriminatory an order that required all Chinese residents to be vaccinated against bubonic plague prior to leaving the city. 103 F. 1 (C.C.N.D. Cal. 1900).

89. Jew Ho v. Williamson, 103 F.10, 24 (C.C.D. Cal. 1900).

90. In addition to constitutional analysis, civil confinement could also be tested under disability discrimination law, requiring individualized assessments of significant risk. See chapter 7: Lawrence O. Gostin, *The Resurgent Tuberculosis Epidemic in the Era of AIDS: Reflections on Public Health, Law, and Society,* 54 MD. L. REV. 1, 92–96, 102–08 (1995).

91. Parmet, *supra* note 14, at 74–75; Merritt, *supra* note 57, at 778.

92. Shapiro v. Thompson, 394 U.S. 618 (1969); Korematsu v. United States, 323 U.S. 214, 218 (1944) ("[N]othing short of . . . the gravest imminent danger to the public safety can constitutionally justify" either "exclusion from the area in which one's home is located" or "constant confinement to the home" during certain hours.).

93. State v. Snow, 324 S.W.2d 532, 534 (Ark. 1959) (finding that the civil commitment law is not penal, but is to be strictly construed to protect the rights of citizens). This section will not discuss segregation of persons with infectious disease in correctional facilities. Rather than using a "strict scrutiny" approach, courts give considerable deference to prison authority decisions to isolate inmates, even where the scientific evidence of significant risk appears weak. *See, e.g.,* Onishea v. Hopper, 171 F.3d 1289 (11th Cir. 1999) (upholding segregation of HIV-infected inmates).

94. Vitek v. Jones, 445 U.S. 480, 491 (1980); *see* Addington v. Texas, 441 U.S. 418, 425 (1979) (finding that civil commitment is a "significant deprivation of liberty").

95. The intrusiveness of the detention should be taken into account in a constitutional analysis, determined by three factors: the specific purpose of confinement (e.g., purely preventive or therapeutic); the duration of confinement (e.g., a short period of curative treatment or an indefinite period of preventive detention); and the place of confinement (e.g., in a person's home, hospital, or jail). For example, scholars have uniformly rejected isolation of persons with HIV because the confinement would be preventive, indeterminate, and would require specially designated facilities. Larry Gostin, *The Politics of AIDS: Compulsory State Powers, Public Health, and Civil Liberties,* 49 OHIO L.J. 1017 (1989); Kathleen Sullivan & Martha Field, *AIDS and the Coercive Power of the State,* 23 HARV. C.R.-C.L. L. REV. 139 (1988); Parmet, *supra* note 14.

96. Greene v. Edwards, 263 S.E.2d 661, 663 (W. Va. 1980) ("[I]nvoluntary commitment for having communicable tuberculosis impinges upon the right to liberty, full and complete liberty, no less than involuntary commitment for being mentally ill.").

97. City of Cleburne v. Cleburne Living Ctr., Inc., 473 U.S. 432, 440 (1985).

98. Scott Burris, *Fear Itself: AIDS, Herpes, and Public Health Decisions,* 3 YALE L. & POL'Y REV. 479, 490–96 (1985).

99. 422 U.S. 563, 575 (1975).

100. *See, e.g.,* Suzuki v. Yuen, 617 F.2d 173, 178 (9th Cir. 1980).

101. Although courts defer to the professional judgment of health officials, they do require a finding of dangerousness. *See* State v. Snow, 324 S.W.2d 534 (Ark. 1959) (basing the rationale for commitment on "the theory that the public has an interest to be protected"); *In re* Halko, 246 Cal. App. 2d 553, 558 (2d Dist. 1966) (upholding isolation of a person with TB, which does not deprive a person of due process if the health officer has reasonable grounds to believe he is dangerous); Moore v. Draper, 57 So. 2d 648, 650 (Fla. 1952) (finding that when a person's disease is arrested to the point where she is no longer a danger, she may seek release); Moore v. Armstrong, 149 So. 2d 36, 37 (Fla. 1963) (same).

102. 614 N.Y.S.2d 8, 9 (App. Div. 1994); *see* City of New York v. Antoinette R., 630 N.Y.S.2d 1008 (Sup. Ct. 1995).

103. City of Cleburne v. Cleburne Living Ctr., Inc. 473 U.S. 432, 440 (1985).

104. City of New York City v. Doe, 614 N.Y.S.2d 8 (App. Div. 1994). The most developed expression of the right to less restrictive alternatives is in mental health cases. *See, e.g.,* Covington v. Harris, 419 F.2d 617, 623 (D.C. Cir. 1969); Lessard v. Schmidt, 349 F. Supp. 1078, 1096 (E.D. Wis. 1972).

105. Gostin, *Tuberculosis in the Era of AIDS, supra* note 90, at 108–12.

106. *But see* City of Newark v. J.S., 652 A.2d 265 (N.J. 1993) (holding that health officials usually have to show that they attempted step-by-step interventions, beginning with voluntary directly observed therapy—supplemented by incentives, such as a food or money reward for taking medication—and enablers—such as travel assistance—with commitment an absolute last resort).

107. Response to Public Comments Concerning Proposed Amendments to Section 11.47 of the Health Code 7 (March 2, 1993).

108. O'Connor v. Donaldson, 422 U.S. 563, 580 (1975) (Berger, C.J., concurring). *See* Addington v. Texas, 441 U.S. 418, 425–27 (1979); Vitek v. Jones, 445 U.S. 480, 491–92 (1980); Project Release v. Prevost, 722 F.2d 960, 971 (2d Cir. 1983).

109. Washington v. Harper, 494 U.S. 210, 229–30 (1990).

110. *See, e.g., In re* Ballay, 482 F.2d 648, 663–66 (D.C. Cir. 1973); Lessard v. Schmidt, 413 F. Supp. 1318 (E.D. Wis. 1976); *but see* Morales v. Turman, 562 F.2d 993, 998 (5th Cir. 1977) ("The state should not be required to provide the procedural safeguards of a criminal trial when imposing a quarantine to protect the public against a highly communicable disease.").

111. *Addington,* 441 U.S. at 425. *See* Jackson v. Indiana, 406 U.S. 715 (1972) (finding that due process requires that the duration of commitment bear some reasonable relation to the purpose for which the individual is committed).

112. *Addington,* 441 U.S. at 426 (requiring that the standard of proof in commitments for mental illness must be greater than the preponderance of evidence standard, but the reasonable doubt standard is not constitutionally required).

113. 263 S.E.2d 661, 663 (W. Va. 1980).

114. In this section, the term *medical treatment* includes both compulsory physical examination and compulsory treatment.

115. Riggins v. Nevada, 504 U.S. 127, 127 (1992) (requiring an "overriding justification and a determination of medical appropriateness"). For a discussion of the general justifications for regulation, see chapter 4.

116. For good discussions of informed consent, see Hales v. Pittman, 576 P.2d 493 (Ariz. 1978); Cobbs v. Grant, 502 P.2d 1 (Cal. 1972); *see also* JAY KATZ, THE SILENT WORLD OF DOCTOR AND PATIENT 48–84 (1984); RUTH R. FADEN & TOM L. BEAUCHAMP, A HISTORY AND THEORY OF INFORMED CONSENT (1986); Marjorie M. Schultz, *From Informed Consent to Patient Choice: A New Protected Interest,* 95 YALE L.J. 219 (1985); Peter H. Schuck, *Rethinking Informed Consent,* 103 YALE L.J. 899 (1994).

117. Unless there is no consent at all (e.g., a person gives permission for procedure X and the physician administers procedure Y), the doctrine of informed consent is usually based on negligence rather than on battery. PAGE KEETON ET AL., PROSSOR & KEETON ON THE LAW OF TORTS §§ 15, 30 (5th ed. 1984).

118. Approximately half the states adopt a "patient-centered" standard of disclosure—the information that a reasonable patient would want to know. *See, e.g.,* Canterbury v. Spence, 464 F.2d 772 (D.C. Cir.), *cert. denied,* 409 U.S. 1064 (1972). The remaining states adopt a "physician-centered" standard—the information a reasonable physician would disclose in the circumstances. *See, e.g.,* Chapel v. Allison, 785 P.2d 204 (Mont. 1990).

119. TOM BEAUCHAMP & JAMES CHILDRESS, PRINCIPLES OF BIOMEDICAL ETHICS 144–45, 157–59 (4th ed. 1994).

120. RESTATEMENT (SECOND) OF TORTS § 892B (consent under mistake, misrepresentation, or duress).

121. MELISSA K. HOGH, SEXUALLY TRANSMITTED DISEASES: A POLICY-MAKER'S GUIDE AND SUMMARY OF STATE LAWS (1998).

122. Advisory Council for the Elimination of Tuberculosis, *Tuberculosis Control Laws—United States, 1993,* 42 MORB. MORT. WKLY. REP. 1, 7–8 (1993); Gostin, *supra* note 52, 255, 256–58.

123. Gostin, *supra* note 52.

124. NATIONAL CONFERENCE OF STATE LEGISLATURES, *supra* note 53.

125. The right to refuse treatment is also protected under state constitutions. *See, e.g.,* Rivers v. Katz, 495 N.E.2d 337, 343 (N.Y. 1986) (finding that persons of "adult years and sound mind" have the right to "control the course of [their] medical treatment").

126. *See, e.g.,* Planned Parenthood of Southeastern Pa. v. Casey, 505 U.S. 833 (1992).

127. Cruzan v. Director, Mo. Dep't of Health, 497 U.S. 261 (1990); Washington v. Glucksberg, 521 U.S. 702 (1997); Vacco v. Quill, 521 U.S. 793 (1997); *see also* Lawrence O. Gostin, *Deciding Life and Death in the Courtroom,* 278 JAMA 1523 (1997).

128. Washington v. Harper, 494 U.S. 210, 221–22.

129. *Casey,* 505 U.S. at 851.

130. Mills v. Rogers, 457 U.S. 291, 299 (1982) ("[T]he substantive issue involves a definition of that protected constitutional [liberty] interest, as well as

identification of the conditions under which competing state interests might outweigh it.").

131. *See, e.g., Cruzan,* 497 U.S. at 261 (finding that preservation of life outweighs refusal of life-sustaining treatment); National Treasury Employees Union v. Von Raab, 489 U.S. 656 (1989) (holding that national security outweighs refusal of drug tests); *Harper,* 494 U.S. at 210 (preventing danger outweighs refusal of antipsychotic drugs).

132. The state interests that are often identified in "right to die" cases include preserving life, preventing suicide, maintaining the integrity of the medical profession, and protecting innocent third parties. *See, e.g.,* Thor v. Superior Court of Solano County, 855 P.2d 375, 383 (Cal. 1993).

133. Schloendorff v. Society of N.Y. Hosp., 105 N.E. 92, 93 (N.Y. 1914) ("Every human being of adult years and sound mind has a right to determine what shall be done with his own body.") (quoting Justice Cardozo).

134. Shine v. Vega, 709 N.E.2d 58, 62–63 (Mass. 1999) (reviewing extensive state case law upholding the right of competent adults to refuse treatment).

135. *See, e.g.,* Rogers v. Commissioner of Dep't of Mental Health, 458 N.E.2d 308 (Mass. 1983) (finding that institutionalized mental patient is competent to make treatment decisions unless adjudicated incompetent).

136. Jolly v. Coughlin, 76 F.3d 468 (2d Cir. 1996) (permitting a competent prisoner to sue for imposing a TB test over his religious objections).

137. *See, e.g.,* Public Health Trust of Dade County v. Wons, 541 So. 2d 96 (Fla. 1989) (permitting a Jehovah's Witness to refuse a blood transfusion); *but see* Application of President & Dirs. of Georgetown College, Inc., 331 F.2d 1000 (D.C. Cir. 1964) (upholding an order authorizing a hospital to administer a blood transfusion to a Jehovah's Witness).

138. A.D.H. v. State Dep't of Hum. Resources, 640 So.2d 969 (Ala. Civ. App. 1994) (ordering a parent to permit treatment of an HIV-infected child); People *ex rel.* Wallace v. Labrenz, 104 N.E.2d 769 (Ill. 1952) (authorizing a blood transfusion over the parents' religious objections).

139. The doctrine and cases are discussed in Lawrence O. Gostin & Robert F. Weir, *Life and Death Choices after Cruzan: Case Law and Standards of Professional Conduct,* 69 MILBANK QUART. 143 (1991).

140. Washington v. Harper, 494 U.S. 210, 227 (1990) (upholding forced administration of antipsychotic medication if the inmate is dangerous to himself or others and the treatment is in the inmate's medical interest); *see* McCormick v. Stalder, 105 F.3d 1059, 1061 (5th Cir. 1997) (finding that the state's compelling interest in reducing the spread of tuberculosis justifies involuntary treatment); United States v. Bechara, 935 F. Supp. 892, 894 (S.D. Tex. 1996) (upholding involuntary sedation of a deportee to ensure public safety).

141. *Harper,* 494 U.S. at 227.

142. Reynolds v. McNichols, 488 F.2d 1378 (10th Cir. 1973) (upholding mandatory physical examination, treatment, and detention of a person suspected of having venereal disease); People *ex rel.* Baker v. Strautz, 54 N.E.2d 441 (Ill. 1944) (same); Rock v. Carney, 185 N.W. 798 (Mich. 1921) (upholding physical examination, but only upon reasonable grounds).

143. City of N.Y. v. Doe, 614 N.Y.S.2d 8 (App. Div. 1994) (upholding continued detention for tuberculosis treatment based upon the fact that public health could not be protected by less restrictive means); City of N.Y. v. Antoinette R., 630 N.Y.S.2d 1008 (Sup. Ct. 1995) (finding clear and convincing evidence existed to detain women for treatment of tuberculosis based on past noncompliance).

144. Riggins v. Nevada, 504 U.S. 127, 135 (1992) (invalidating forced administration of antipsychotic medication during the course of a trial without findings that there were no less intrusive alternatives, that the medication was medically appropriate, and that it was essential for the defendant's safety or the safety of others).

145. Irwin v. Arrendale, 159 S.E.2d 719 (Ga. Ct. App. 1967) (requiring a prisoner to be X rayed had no medical reason, was wholly capricious, and done solely to exercise power).

146. See note 9 and accompanying text in chapter 7 (Alexander Fleming lecture). For a global perspective, see STEPHEN R. PALMER ET AL., THE CONTRIBUTION OF GLOBAL HEALTH POLICY TO THE CONTROL OF EMERGING INFECTIOUS DISEASES (1999).

147. See, e.g., DOUGLAS D. RICHMAN, ANTIVIRAL DRUG RESISTANCE (1996); J. Pekka Nutori et al., An Outbreak of Multidrug-Resistant Pneumococcal Pneumonia and Bacteremia among Unvaccinated Nursing Home Residents, 358 NEW ENG. J. MED. 1861 (1998); Daniel B. Jernigan et al., Minimizing the Impact of Drug-Resistant Streptococcus Pneumoniae (DRSP): A Strategy from the DRSP Working Group, 275 JAMA 206 (1996). See generally, ENRICO MIHICH, DRUG RESISTANCE AND SELECTIVITY: BIOCHEMICAL AND CELLULAR BASIS (1973).

148. See, e.g., Franz Josef Schmitz, et al., The Prevalence of Low- and High-Level Mupirocin Resistance in Staphylococci fom 19 European Hospitals, 42 J. ANTIMICROBIAL CHEMOTHERAPY 489 (1998).

149. See, e.g., Alan B. Bloch et al., Nationwide Survey of Drug-Resistant Tuberculosis in the United States, 271 JAMA 665 (1994); Barry R. Bloom et al., Tuberculosis: Commentary on a Reemergent Killer, 257 SCIENCE 1055 (1992); see also Carlos A. Ball & Mark Barnes, Public Health and Individual Rights: Tuberculosis Control and Detention Procedures in New York City, 12 YALE L. & POL'Y REV. 38 (1994); Josephine Gittler, Controlling Resurgent Tuberculosis: Public Health Agencies, Public Health Policy, and Law, 19 J. HEALTH POL., POL'Y & L. 107 (1994); Rosemary G. Reilly, Combating the Tuberculosis Epidemic: The Legality of Coercive Measures, 27 COLUM. J.L. & SOC. PROBS. 101 (1993).

150. See, e.g., Douglas L. Mayer, Prevalence and Incidence of Resistance to Zidovudine and Other Antiretroviral Drugs, 102 AM. J. MED. 70 (1997).

151. See, e.g., Michael D. Iseman, Treatment of Multidrug-Resistant Tuberculosis, 329 NEW ENG. J. MED. 784 (1993).

152. The overuse of antibiotics in animals is also thought to contribute to the problem of drug resistance. See Henrik C. Wegener, The Consequences for Food Safety of the Use of Fluoroquinolones in Food Animals, 340 NEW ENG. J. MED. 1581 (1999).

153. Ronald Bayer & David Wilkinson, Directly Observed Therapy for Tuberculosis: History of an Idea, 345 LANCET 1545 (1995).

154. OFFICE OF TECHN. ASSESSMENT, U.S. CONGRESS, THE CONTINUING CHALLENGE OF TUBERCULOSIS 27, 89 (OTA-H574, 1993).

155. *See, e.g.,* C. Patrick Chaulk & Vahe A. Kazandjian, *Directly Observed Therapy for Treatment Completion of Pulmonary Tuberculosis: Consensus Statement of the Public Health Tuberculosis Guidelines Panel,* 279 JAMA 943 (1998) (treatment completion rates for traditional self-administered therapy (SAT) ranged from 41.9–82 percent); Bruce L. Davidson, *A Controlled Comparison of Directly Observed Therapy vs. Self-Administered Therapy for Active Tuberculosis in the Urban United States,* 114 CHEST 1239 (1998) (nearly two-thirds of patients who started SAT had not completed therapy within eight months).

156. J. Volmink & Paul Garner, *Directly Observed Therapy,* 349 LANCET 1399 (1997) (evidence for the effectiveness of DOT is not reliable).

157. *See, e.g.,* Chaulk & Kazandjian, *supra* note 155 (treatment completion rates for DOT ranged from 86 to 96.5 percent); Centers for Disease Control & Prevention, *Approaches to Improving Adherence to Anti-Tuberculosis Therapy—South Carolina and New York, 1986–1991,* 42 MORB. MORT. WKLY. REP. 74 (1993) (93.9 percent completion rate).

158. Stephen E. Weiss et al., *The Effect of Directly Observed Therapy on the Rates of Drug Resistance and Relapse in Tuberculosis,* 330 NEW ENG. J. MED. 1179 (1994).

159. Kelly Morris, *WHO Sees DOTs,* 349 LANCET 855 (1997).

160. CENTERS FOR DISEASE CONTROL & PREVENTION, IMPROVING PATIENT ADHERENCE TO TUBERCULOSIS TREATMENT (rev. ed. 1994) (CDC supports DOT); Centers for Disease Control & Prevention, *Initial Therapy for Tuberculosis in the Era of Multidrug Resistance,* 42 MORB. MORT. WKLY. REP. 1 (1993) (same).

161. *See, e.g.,* American Thoracic Society, *Treatment of Tuberculosis and Tuberculosis Infection in Adults and Children,* 149 AM. J. RESPIR. CRIT. CARE MED. 1359 (1994) (supporting DOT); Chaulk & Kazandjian, *supra* note 155, (Tuberculosis Guidelines Panel supports DOT).

162. Gostin, *supra* note 90, at 1, 104–08, 124–28.

163. Ronald Bayer et al., *Directly Observed Therapy and Treatment Completion for Tuberculosis in the United States: Is Universal Supervised Therapy Necessary?,* 88 AM. J. PUB. HEALTH 1052 (1998) (many locales with high treatment completion rates do not rely on DOT).

164. Thomas R. Frieden et al., *Tuberculosis in New York City: Turning the Tide,* 333 NEW ENG. J. MED. 229 (1995); M. Rose Gasner et al., *The Use of Legal Action in New York City to Ensure Treatment of Tuberculosis,* 340 NEW ENG. J. MED. 359 (1999) (for most patients treatment completion can usually be achieved without regulatory intervention).

165. See the case study on HIV screening of pregnant women in chapter 7.

166. Pietro L. Vernazza et al., *Effect of Antiviral Treatment on Shedding of HIV-1 in Semen,* 11 AIDS 1249 (1997).

167. Samantha Catherine Halem, *At What Cost?: An Argument against Mandatory AZT Treatment of HIV-Positive Pregnant Women,* 32 HARV. C.R.-C.L. L. REV. 491 (1997).

168. *Compare In re* Fetus Brown, 689 N.E.2d 397, 405 (Ill. App. 1997) (holding that pregnant woman cannot be compelled to undergo a blood transfusion for

the benefit of her viable fetus) *and In re* A.C., 573 A.2d 1235 (D.C. 1990) (en banc) (finding that a pregnant woman cannot be forced to have a caesarian section) *with* Jefferson v. Griffin Spaulding County Hosp. Auth., 274 S.E.2d 457 (Ga. 1981) (upholding an order compelling a pregnant woman to undergo a caesarian section).

169. C.A. Hoffman et al., *Ethical Issues in the Use of Zidovudine to Reduce Vertical Transmission of HIV*, 332 NEW ENG. J. MED. 891 (1995).

170. Jennifer Frey, *Nushawn's Girls*, WASH. POST, June 1, 1999, at C2; Lynda Richardson, *Man Faces Felony Charge in HIV Case*, N.Y. TIMES, Aug. 20, 1998, at B3.

171. *HIV-Positive Woman Gets Revenge through Lengthy String of Affairs*, WASH. TIMES, Aug. 1, 1998, at A2 (an HIV-infected Tennessee woman had sex with approximately fifty men to get "revenge" for becoming infected).

172. Kristina Sauerwein, *Man's Deadly Legacy Triggers Frantic Race*, ST. LOUIS POST-DISPATCH, April 11, 1997, at A1 (a murdered Missouri man had sexual intercourse with over fifty women after learning that he was HIV positive).

173. Barnaby C. Wittels & Stephen Robert LaCheen, *The Persecution of Ed Savitz*, PHILA. INQUIRER, June 1, 1993, at A11 (an HIV-positive man had multiple sex encounters with teenage boys).

174. Lynda Richardson, *Wave of Laws Aimed at People with HIV*, N.Y. TIMES, Sept. 25, 1998, at A1; *Criminal Exposure to HIV: Evolving Laws and Court Cases*, 13 AIDS POL'Y & LAW 1 (bonus report 1998).

175. *See, e.g., Continued Sexual Risk Behavior among HIV-Seropositive, Drug-Using Men*, 45 MORB. MORT. WKLY. REP. 151 (1996) (28 percent of a sample of HIV-positive persons reported having sex without a condom in past thirty days); Carol F. Kwiatkowski & Robert E. Booth, *HIV-Seropositive Drug Users and Unprotected Sex*, 2 AIDS & BEHAVIOR 151 (1998) (47 percent of HIV-positive intraveneous drug users reported having unprotected sex in past six months); Jeffrey D. Fisher et al., *Dynamics of Sexual Risk Behavior in HIV-Infected Men Who Have Sex with Men*, 2 AIDS & BEHAVIOR 101, 106 (1998) (risk behaviors occur frequently); Christine J. De Rosa & Gary Marks, *Preventive Counseling of HIV-Positive Men and Self-Disclosure of Serostatus to Sex Partners: New Opportunities for Prevention*, 17 HEALTH PSYCHOL. 224 (1998) (77 percent of HIV-seropositive men failed to disclose to partners).

176. Michael D. Stein et al., *Sexual Ethics: Disclosure of HIV-Positive Status to Partners*, 158 ARCHIVES OF INTERNAL MED. 253 (1998).

177. Thomas A. Coburn, *Introduction of the HIV Prevention Act of 1996*, CONG. REC. E1446-E7 (1996) (more than three-quarters of Americans say that those who knowingly infect another person with HIV should face criminal charges).

178. REPORT OF THE PRESIDENTIAL COMMISSION ON THE HUMAN IMMUNODEFICIENCY VIRUS EPIDEMIC 130–131 (1988).

179. Gostin, *supra* note 95, at 1038–42.

180. *See, e.g.*, Grayned v. City of Rockford, 408 U.S. 104, 108–09 (1972).

181. There is also a separate line of cases that has been prosecuted under the military code of justice. These cases fall under two types of actions: (1) Violation of "safe-sex" orders. *See, e.g.*, United States v. Barrows, 48 M.J. 783 (A.C.C.A. 1998). (2) Criminal assault through knowing exposure to HIV. *See, e.g.*, United

States v. Schoolfield, 40 M.J. 132 (C.M.A. 1994) (upholding an aggravated assault conviction for unprotected and undisclosed sex with five partners); United States v. Joseph, 33 M.J. 960 (N-M.C.M.R. 1991) (affirming an aggravated assault conviction for one sexual encounter using a condom but not warning partner). The Supreme Court held that removing a soldier from the military after a conviction for violation of a safe-sex order does not violate constitutional proscriptions on ex post facto laws or double jeopardy. Clinton v. Goldsmith, 526 U.S. 529 (1999).

182. BLACK'S LAW DICTIONARY 370 (6th ed. 1991); see also J.C. SMITH & BRIAN HOGAN, CRIMINAL LAW 17–23 (3d ed. 1973).

183. See generally, Robert Boorstin, Criminal and Civil Litigation on Spread of AIDS Appears, N.Y. TIMES, June 19, 1987, at A1.

184. MODEL PENAL CODE § 2.02 (1998) (a person is not guilty of an offense unless he acted purposely, knowingly, recklessly, or negligently).

185. Prosecutors can also charge persons with reckless endangerment, but usually this is a lesser included offense rather than a stand-alone charge. Perhaps the reason is that reckless endangerment is considered an insufficiently serious charge. See Donald H.J. Hermann, Criminalizing Conduct Related to HIV Transmission, 9 ST. LOUIS PUB. L. REV. 351 (1990).

186. Kathleen M. Sullivan & Martha A. Field, AIDS and the Coercive Power of the State, 23 HARV. C.R.-C.L. L. REV. 139, 163 (1988).

187. Smallwood v. State, 680 A.2d 512 (Md. 1996).

188. State v. Hinkhouse, 912 P.2d 921, modified, 915 P.2d 489 (Or. Ct. App. 1996).

189. MODEL PENAL CODE § 5.01(1)(a) (1998).

190. See, e.g., State v. Smith, 621 A.2d 493 (N.J. Super. Ct. App. Div.), cert. denied, 634 A.2d 523 (N.J. 1993); Weeks v. State, 834 S.W.2d 559 (Tx. Ct. App. 1992), petition for habeas corpus denied sub nom. Weeks v. Scott, 55 F.3d 1059 (5th Cir. 1995).

191. See, e.g., Smith, 621 A.2d at 493 (inmate biting guard during an altercation).

192. See, e.g., Weeks, 834 S.W.2d at 559 (inmate spitting at guard).

193. State v. Haines, 545 N.E.2d 834 (Ind. Ct. App. 2d Dist. 1989) (throwing bloody wig at police officers after attempting suicide).

194. Jason Strait, Man Guilty of Giving Son HIV Virus, WL 23508518, Dec. 6, 1998; Michele Munz, Father Is Found Guilty of Giving His Son HIV-Tainted Injection, Jury Recommends Life in Prison on Assault Conviction, ST. LOUIS POST-DISPATCH, Dec. 6, 1998, at A1.

195. Bruce Schultz, Dr. Schmidt Found Guilty—Jury Says Physician Tried to Kill Lover with HIV Injection, BATON ROUGE ADVOCATE, Oct. 24, 1998, at B1. See also State v. Caine, 652 So. 2d 611 (La. App.1995) (upholding a second-degree murder charge against a burglar who stabbed a victim with a needle and shouted "I'll give you AIDS").

196. See, e.g., Weeks, 834 S.W.2d at 559.

197. Haines, 545 N.E.2d at 834.

198. MODEL PENAL CODE § 211.1 (1)(a)(1998).

199. See, e.g., Scroggins v. State, 401 S.E.2d 13 (Ga. Ct. App. 1990) (convicting a person of aggravated assault with intent to murder for biting a police officer dur-

ing a struggle); Brock v. State, 555 So. 2d 285 (Ala. Crim. App. 1989) (convicting an inmate of simple assault for biting a guard).

200. Newman v. State, 677 N.E.2d 590 (Ind. Ct. App. 1997) (battery conviction for shaking nasal mucus, tears, and saliva onto arresting officers); Commonwealth v. Brown, 605 A.2d 429 (Pa. Super. Ct. 1992) (affirming convictions for simple assault, aggravated assault, and recklessly endangering another person for an inmate who threw bodily waste at a guard).

201. MODEL PENAL CODE §211.1(2) (1998).

202. United States v. Sturgis, 48 F.3d 784 (4th Cir. 1995) (finding that HIV can be transmitted from a bite wound, so that the mouth and teeth are deadly weapons); United States v. Moore, 846 F.2d 1163 (8th Cir. 1988) (finding that HIV transmission is unlikely, but other infections are more likely, so that the mouth and teeth are deadly weapons).

203. MODEL PENAL CODE § 2.02(2)(b)(ii) (1998).

204. Although consent or assumption of risk are not defenses to a charge of attempted homicide, they are relevant questions in establishing whether the person's intention was to kill.

205. See, e.g., MINN. STAT. ANN. § 145.36 (1986) (prohibiting willful exposure of anyone affected with a contagious or infectious disease in any public place); UTAH CODE ANN. § 26-6-5 (prohibiting willful or knowing introduction of any communicable or infectious disease into any community).

206. See, e.g., Allan M. Brandt, AIDS in Historical Perspective: Four Lessons from the History of Sexually Transmitted Diseases, 78 AM. J. PUB. HEALTH 367 (1988); Stephen V. Kenney, Criminalizing HIV Transmission: Lessons from History and a Model for the Future, 8 CONTEMP. HEALTH L. & POL'Y 245 (1992).

207. See, e.g., In re Stoner, 73 S.E.2d 566 (N.C. 1952) (imposing criminal penalties for failing to take precautions prescribed by public health authorities).

208. Gostin, supra note 52, at 259.

209. See generally, Martha A. Field & Kathleen M. Sullivan, AIDS and the Criminal Law, 15 L. MED. & HEALTH CARE 46 (1987).

210. See generally, WILLIAM CURRAN ET AL., ACQUIRED IMMUNO-DEFICIENCY SYNDROME: LEGAL AND REGULATORY POLICY ANALYSIS i–ii, 204–07 (U.S. Dept. of Comm. 1988) (1986).

211. New York State Soc. of Surgeons v. Axelrod, 572 N.E.2d 605 (N.Y. 1991); see also Plaza v. Estate of Wisser, 626 N.Y.S.2d 446, 452 (App. Div. 1995) (finding that the public health offense in a VD statute does not apply to HIV).

212. See, e.g., FLA. STAT. ANN. § 384.24 (West 1998); IDAHO CODE § 39–601 (Michie 1988).

213. National Council of State Legislatures, Criminal Transmission and Exposure, HEALTH POLICY TRACKING SERVICE (visited May 15, 2000), <http://www.stateserv.hpts.org> (at least thirty states make it a crime to knowingly expose others to HIV); David L. McColgin & Elizabeth T. Hey, Criminal Law, in AIDS AND THE LAW 259, 287, n.134 (David W. Webber ed., 3d ed. 1997) (citing nineteen HIV-specific statutes); see also Mark H. Jackson, The Criminalization of HIV, in AIDS AGENDA: EMERGING ISSUES IN CIVIL RIGHTS 239 (Nan D. Hunter

& William B. Rubenstein eds., 1992); J. Kelly Strader, *Criminalization as a Policy Response to a Public Health Crisis*, 27 J. MARSHALL L. REV. 435 (1994).

214. 18 U.S.C. § 1118 (1994) (persons who know they are HIV infected may not "donate or sell blood, semen, tissues, organs or other bodily fluids for use by another, except as determined necessary for medical research or testing").

215. Ryan White Comprehensive AIDS Resources Emergency (CARE) Act of 1990, 42 U.S.C. § 300ff-47 (1994) (state certifying that it can prosecute knowing, and with intent to expose others to HIV, donation of blood, semen, or breast milk, sexual activity, or sharing needles). The CARE Act recommends that states use a "specific intent" standard and does not require an HIV-specific statute.

216. Although most HIV statutes require only knowledge, a few do require a specific intent. *See, e.g.,* OKLA. STAT. tit. 21 § 1192.1 (West 1991) ("with intent to infect another").

217. *See, e.g.,* CAL. HEALTH & SAFETY CODE § 1621.5 (West Supp. 2000).

218. *See, e.g.,* VA. CODE ANN. § 32.1 (Michie 1997).

219. *See, e.g.,* MICH. STAT. ANN. § 333 (West 1992) ("sexual intercourse, cunnilingus, fellatio, anal intercourse, or any other intrusion, however slight, of any part of a person's body into the genital or anal openings . . . , but emission of semen is not required").

220. *See, e.g.,* WASH. REV. CODE ANN. § 9A.36.021 (West 1988) ("exposes or transmits").

221. *See, e.g.,* ILL. COMP. ANN. STAT. Ch. 720, para. 5/12–16.2 (West Supp. 1998).

222. In North Dakota, the person must inform his partner *and* use an "appropriate prophylactic device." N.D. CENT. CODE § 12.1-20-17(3) (Michie 1997).

223. *But see* CAL. HEALTH & SAFETY CODE § 120291 (West 1999) (criminalizing only "unprotected" sex without disclosure).

224. Donald C. Ainslie, *Questioning Bioethics: AIDS, Sexual Ethics, and the Duty to Warn*, 29 HASTINGS CENTER REP. 26 (1999); *see* Ronald Bayer, *AIDS Prevention—Sexual Ethics and Responsibility*, 334 NEW ENG. J. MED. 1540 (1996).

225. *See, e.g.,* IDAHO CODE § 39-608 (Michie 1998) (intentional or knowing exposure is a felony punishable by up to fifteen years imprisonment, a fine of up to $5,000, or both); *see also* Jody B. Gabel, *Liability for "Knowing" Transmission of HIV: The Evolution of a Duty to Disclose*, 21 FLA. ST. U. L. REV. 981, 1006 n.179 (1994) (listing state laws dealing with intentional exposure of AIDS).

226. State v. Mahan, 971 S.W.2d 307, 313–14 (Mo. 1998) (upholding criminalization of "grave and unjustifiable risk" as applied to unprotected sexual intercourse); People v. Russell, 630 N.E.2d 794, 796 (Ill.), *cert. denied*, 513 U.S. 828 (1994) (statute sufficiently clear to be constitutional); People v. Dempsey, 610 N.E.2d 208, 222–24 (Ill. App. Ct. 1993) (same); State v. Gambrella, 633 So. 2d 595 (La. Ct. App. 1993) (upholding HIV-specific criminal statute).

227. *Russell,* 630 N.E.2d at 794; People v. Jensen, 586 N.W.2d 748 (Mich. Ct. App. 1998) (denying that the statute requiring infected persons to give notice of HIV status prior to sexual intercourse is overbroad).

228. Jensen, 586 N.W.2d at 752–54.

229. *See, e.g.,* State v. Stark, 832 P.2d 109, 116 (Wash. Ct. App. 1992) ("Any reasonably intelligent person would understand . . . that the term ["expose"] refers to engaging in . . . unprotected sexual intercourse."). It is certainly possible, however, that HIV statutes would be invalidated on grounds of vagueness if applied to those who are convicted of "exposure" while engaging in low-risk behavior.

230. McColgin & Hey, *supra* note 213, at 294–95.

231. Sullivan & Field, *supra* note 186, at 196.

232. *See supra* note 175, and accompanying text.

9. ECONOMIC BEHAVIOR AND THE PUBLIC'S HEALTH:
    DIRECT REGULATION

SOURCES FOR CHAPTER EPIGRAPHS: Page 237: Commonwealth v. Alger, 7 Cush. 53, 84–85 (Mass. 1851). Page 237: 1 Vanderbilt v. Adams, 7 Cow. 349, 351–52 (N.Y. 1827). Page 239: WILLIAM J. NOVAK, THE PEOPLE'S WELFARE: LAW AND REGULATION IN NINETEENTH-CENTURY AMERICA 1–2 (1996). Page 242: Public Health in New York State, *Report of the New York State Health Commission,* quoted in JAMES A. TOBEY, PUBLIC HEALTH LAW 57 (2d ed. 1939). Page 246: THE CHILDREN'S CHARTER, PRESIDENT HOOVER'S WHITE HOUSE CONFERENCE ON CHILD HEALTH AND PROTECTION RECOGNIZING THE RIGHTS OF THE CHILD AS THE FIRST RIGHTS OF CITIZENSHIP PLEDGES ITSELF TO THESE AIMS FOR THE CHILDREN OF AMERICA (1931). Page 259: JOEL BISHOP, COMMENTARIES ON NON-CONTRACT LAW § 411, n.1 (1889). Page 263: ORDER AND LAW: ARGUING THE REAGAN REVOLUTION: A FIRSTHAND ACCOUNT 183 (1991). Page 263: *The Takings Project: A Critical Analysis and Assessment of the Progress So Far,* 25 B.C. ENVTL. AFF. L. REV. 509, 510 (1998), *referring to* RICHARD A. EPSTEIN, TAKINGS, PRIVATE PROPERTY AND THE POWER OF EMINENT DOMAIN (1985). Page 265: THE ART OF MEDICINE IN EARLY ALEXANDRIA 407 (1989)

1. SOCIAL DETERMINANTS OF HEALTH (Michael Marmot & Richard G. Wilkinson eds., 1999); U.S. DEP'T OF HEALTH & HUM. SERVS., HEALTH STATUS OF MINORITIES AND LOW INCOME GROUPS (1991).

2. Perhaps the most important proponent of laissez-faire economics was the Scotsman Adam Smith. *See* ADAM SMITH, AN INQUIRY INTO THE NATURE AND CAUSES OF THE WEALTH OF NATIONS (Malcolm Graham ed., 1937) (1776) (except for limited functions such as defense, justice, and certain public works, the state should refrain from interfering with economic life).

3. *See* MILTON FRIEDMAN & ANNA J. SCHWARTZ, A MONETARY HISTORY OF THE UNITED STATES, 1867–1960 (1963).

4. *See* Ronald Bayer et al., *Trades, AIDS, and the Public's Health: The Limits of Economic Analysis,* 83 Geo. L.J. 79–107 (1995).

5. For an interesting account of the medieval town, where power was organized around protecting the economic freedoms of merchants as a class, see Gerald E. Frug, *The City as a Legal Concept,* 93 HARV. L. REV. 1059, 1083–87 (1980).

6. Elizabeth Fee, *The Origins and Development of Public Health in the United States, in* OXFORD TEXTBOOK OF PUBLIC HEALTH 35, 36 (Roger Detels et al. eds., 3d ed. 1997) ("Responding to the miasmatic theory of disease cau-

sation, city health departments attempted to regulate the filthy conditions of the docks, streets, and alleys, to inspect graveyards, tallow chandleries, tanneries, and slaughter houses, and to remove dead animals and decaying vegetable matter from the streets and public spaces.").

7. JOHN B. BLAKE, PUBLIC HEALTH IN THE TOWN OF BOSTON, 1630–1822, at 13–14 (1959).

8. JOHN DUFFY, THE SANITARIANS: A HISTORY OF AMERICAN PUBLIC HEALTH 12–13 (1990).

9. Elizabeth C. Tandy, *The Regulation of Nuisances in the American Colonies,* 13 AM. J. PUB. HEALTH 810 (1923).

10. JOHN DUFFY, PUBLIC HEALTH IN NEW YORK CITY, 1625–1866, at 10–15 (1968).

11. For a critique of the idea that early American governance embraced a laissez-faire political economy, see FRANK P. BOURGIN, THE GREAT CHALLENGE: THE MYTH OF LAISSEZ FAIRE IN THE EARLY REPUBLIC (1989).

12. Barbara Rosenkrantz, *Cart Before Horse: Theory, Practice and Professional Image in American Public Health,* 29 J. HIST. OF MED. & ALLIED SCI. 55, 57 (1974) ("[T]he field of public health exemplified a happy marriage of engineers, physicians and public spirited citizens providing a model of complementary comportment under the banner of sanitary science.").

13. See, e.g., LEMUEL SHATTUCK, REPORT OF A GENERAL PLAN FOR THE PROMOTION OF PUBLIC AND PERSONAL HEALTH, DEVISED, PREPARED, AND RECOMMENDED BY THE COMMISSIONERS APPOINTED UNDER A RESOLVE OF THE LEGISLATURE OF THE STATE (1850) (reprint Havard University Press 1948); JOHN C. GRISCOM, THE SANITARY CONDITION OF THE LABORING POPULATION OF NEW YORK WITH SUGGESTIONS FOR ITS IMPROVEMENT (1845); Benjamin W. McCready, *On the Influence of Trades, Professions, and Occupations in the United States in the Production of Disease,* 3 TRANSACTIONS OF THE MED. SOC. OF THE STATE OF N.Y. 91 (1836–37) (reprint Johns Hopkins Press 1943).

14. See GEORGE ROSEN, A HISTORY OF PUBLIC HEALTH 168–226 (expanded ed. 1993); DUFFY, *supra* note 8, at 175.

15. See SHATTUCK, *supra* note 13, at 9–10.

16. See, e.g., NORTON T. HORR & ALTON A. BEMIS, A TREATISE ON THE POWER TO ENACT, PASSAGE, AND VALIDITY AND ENFORCEMENT OF MUNICIPAL POLICE ORDINANCES §§ 211–262 (1887) (classifying ordinances according to their subject matter ranging from food, markets, and fire to care of streets, buildings, public infrastructure [e.g., sewerage and water], general nuisances, inspection, and licenses); CHRISTOPHER G. TIEDEMAN, A TREATISE ON STATE AND FEDERAL CONTROL OF PERSONS AND PROPERTY IN THE UNITED STATES, Chapters IX (regulation of trades and occupations), X–XI (regulation of real and personal property), XV (police regulation of corporations) (1900).

17. WILLIAM J. NOVAK, THE PEOPLE'S WELFARE: LAW AND REGULATION IN NINETEENTH-CENTURY AMERICA 21 (1996).

18. NANCY FRANK, FROM CRIMINAL LAW TO REGULATION: A HISTORICAL ANALYSIS OF HEALTH AND SAFETY LAW 1 (1986).

19. EDWIN SUTHERLAND, WHITE-COLLAR CRIME 42–50 (1949).

20. JAMES A. TOBEY, PUBLIC HEALTH LAW 76 (2d ed. 1939).

21. Fee, *supra* note 6, at 38.

22. ROSEN, *supra* note 14, at 210; *see* ERNEST S. GRIFFITH, HISTORY OF AMERICAN CITY GOVERNMENT: THE COLONIAL PERIOD 289–90 (1938) ("The modern health department and all save a negligible number of its several activities were completely missing.").

23. *See* DUFFY, *supra* note 8, at 148.

24. LAWS OF THE STATE OF NEW YORK, 89th Sess., I, Chap. 74 (Albany 1866). *See* CHARLES E. ROSENBERG, THE CHOLERA YEARS: THE UNITED STATES IN 1832, 1849, AND 1866, at 190–91 (1962) (The board "would be needed. New York's streets were almost impassable with a mixture of snow, ice, dirt, and garbage.").

25. HORR & BEMIS, *supra* note 16, at § 215.

26. A National Board of Health was created in 1879 principally for formulating a quarantine policy (see chapter 8.) The Board became embroiled in controversy about states' rights and was disbanded in 1883 with its powers transferred to the Marine Hospital Service. *See* FITZHUGH MULLAN, PLAGUES AND POLITICS: THE STORY OF THE UNITED STATES PUBLIC HEALTH SERVICE (1989).

27. OHIO PUB. HEALTH ASS'N, HISTORICAL DIRECTORY OF STATE HEALTH DEPARTMENTS IN THE UNITES STATES OF AMERICA (R.G. Paterson ed., 1939).

28. The first reported county health departments were in Jefferson County, Kentucky, in 1908 (*see* Jefferson v. Jefferson County Fiscal Court, 108 S.W.2d 181 (Ky. Ct. App. 1938)); Guilford County, North Carolina, and Yakima County, Washington, in 1911; and Robeson County, North Carolina, in 1912. John Atkinson Ferrell & P.A. Mead, *History of County Health Departments in the United States,* PUB. HEALTH BULL. NO. 222 (1936); *see* ALLEN WEIR FREEMAN, A STUDY OF RURAL PUBLIC HEALTH SERVICE (1933); H.S. MUSTARD, RURAL HEALTH PRACTICE (1936).

29. Charles V. Chapin, *Pleasures and Hopes of the Health Officer, in* PAPERS OF CHARLES V. CHAPIN, M.D. 11 (Frederic P. Gorham & Clarence L. Scamman eds., 1934).

30. *See, e.g.,* State Bd. of Health v. City of Greenville, 98 N.E. 1019, 1021 (Ohio 1912) ("It is now settled law that the legislature of the State possesses plenary power to deal with [health].").

31. I am grateful to one of America's most experienced health officers, Lloyd Novick, for help in developing this discussion of state and local public health agencies and for drafting Figures 16 and 17. The materials on state public health agency organization are derived from the following sources: Susan Dandoy, *The State Public Health Department, in* PRINCIPLES OF PUBLIC HEALTH PRACTICE 68 (Nancy Rawding & Martin Wasserman eds., 1997); BERNARD TURNOCK, PUBLIC HEALTH: WHAT IT IS AND HOW IT WORKS 145–56 (1997); Kristine M. Gebbie, *Steps to Changing State Public Health Structures,* 4 J. PUB. HEALTH MGMT. & PRAC. 33 (1998).

32. *See* D.J. Gossert & C. Arden Miller, *State Boards of Health, Their Members and Commitments,* 63 AM. J. PUB. HEALTH 486 (1973); J.W. Kerr & A.A. Moll, *Organization, Powers, and Duties of Health Authorities,* PUB. HEALTH BULL. NO. 54 (1912); TOBEY, *supra* note 20, Chapter IV.

33. ASSOCIATION OF STATE AND TERRITORIAL HEALTH OFFICIALS, DIRECTORY OF STATE PUBLIC HEALTH AGENCIES (1998).

34. B. Gilbert & M.K. Miller, *State Level Decision Making for Public Health: The Status of Boards of Health*, 3 J. Pub. Health Pol'y 51 (1982).

35. Centers for Disease Control & Prevention, Profile of State and Territorial Public Health Systems: United States (1999).

36. A large number of cases supporting the preeminence of public health powers in local government are presented in Eugene McQuillin, The Law of Municipal Corporations §§ 24.219–222 (3d ed. 1981) (public health and sanitation).

37. *See, e.g.,* Town of Islip v. Vollbracht's Dairy, Inc., 363 N.Y.S.2d 307 (Dist. Ct. 1975) (upholding municipal waste disposal and sanitation requirements against an equal protection challenge).

38. *See, e.g.,* Westwood Forest Estates, Inc. v. South Nyack, 244 N.E.2d 700, 702 (N.Y. 1969) (upholding a zoning law barring new construction to reduce the burden on sewers).

39. *See, e.g.,* People v. Cook, 312 N.E. 2d 452 (N.Y. 1974) (upholding a tax differential based on tar and nicotine content).

40. City of San Jose v. Department of Health Serv., 66 Cal.App. 4th 35 (Cal. App. 6th Dist. 1998) (finding that the city had state constitutional authority to enforce a smoking ban in public areas).

41. *See, e.g.,* Minnesota State Bd. of Health v. City of Brainerd, 241 N.W. 2d 624 (Minn. 1976) (requiring the city to execute the state plan for fluoridation of water).

42. *See, e.g.,* Village of Hoffman Estates v. Flipside, Hoffman Estates, Inc., 455 U.S. 489 (1982) (upholding the village enactment requiring a business to obtain a license if it sold items designed or marketed for use with illegal drugs); *see also* Lawrence O. Gostin & Zita Lazzarini, *Prevention of HIV/AIDS among Injection Drug Users: The Theory and Science of Public Health and Criminal Justice Approaches to Disease Prevention*, 46 Emory L.J. 587 (1997).

43. *See, e.g.,* City of Chicago v. Franklin, 261 N.E.2d 506 (Ill. 1970) (holding that a city ordinance requiring registration of firearms did not force the defendant to incriminate himself).

44. *See, e.g.,* Township of Chester v. Panicucci, 299 A.2d 385 (N.J. 1973) (banning possession of loaded gun within 400 feet of a school playground).

45. *See, e.g.,* Berg v. Health & Hosp. Corp. of Marion County, Ind. 865 F.2d 797 (7th. Cir. 1989) (upholding a city ordinance regulating adult bookstores to prevent HIV transmission).

46. City of Minneapolis v. Reha, 483 N.W.2d 688 (Minn. 1992) (upholding an ordinance requiring the occupant of a residential property to keep the property free from infestation).

47. *See, e.g.,* Cuz, Inc. v. Walden, 261 So. 2d 37 (Ala. 1972) (holding the minimum standards outlined by city housing codes constitutionally valid).

48. *See, e.g.,* Johnson's Market, Inc. v. New Carlisle Dept. of Health, 567 N.E.2d 1018 (Ohio 1991) (finding that the local government may regulate food and beverages).

49. *See, e.g.,* Chicago Allis Mfg. Corp. v. Metropolitan Sanitary Dist. 288 N.E.2d 436, 439 (Ill. 1972) ("A system for waste disposal and sewage treatment has long been regarded as necessary for public health.").

50. *See, e.g.,* Harkey v. deWetter, 443 F.2d 828 (5th Cir. 1971) (upholding an ordinance requiring permits, inspections, and sanitary requirements for keepers of animals).

51. *See, e.g.,* Engelsher v. Jacobs, 157 N.E.2d 626 (N.Y. 1959) (holding that city hospital regulations were not unreasonable and the city had constitutional authority to regulate hospitals).

52. *See, e.g.,* Unique Rest Haven, Inc. v. City of Chicago, 166 N.E.2d 627 (Ill. 1960); Rothner v. City of Chicago, 383 N.E.2d 1218 (Ill. 1978).

53. Zullo v. Board of Health of Woodbridge Township, 88 A.2d 625 (N.J. 1952); Fort Smith v. Roberts, 9 S.W.2d 75 (Ark. 1928); *see* C. Arden Miller et al., *Statutory Authorization for the Work of Local Health Departments,* 67 AM. J. PUB. HEALTH 940 (1977).

54. NATIONAL ASS'N OF COUNTY AND CITY HEALTH OFFICIALS, PROFILE OF LOCAL HEALTH DEPARTMENTS, 1992–1993 (1995); Nancy Rawding & Martin Wasserman, *The Local Health Department, in* PRINCIPLES OF PUBLIC HEALTH PRACTICE (Nancy Rawding & Martin Wasserman eds., 1997); Thomas B. Richards et al., *Toward a GIS Sampling Frame for Surveys of Local Health Departments and Local Boards of Health,* 5 J. PUB. HEALTH MGMT. & PRAC. 65 (1999); Glen P. Mays et al., *Assessing the Performance of Local Public Health Systems: A Survey of State Health Agency Efforts,* 4 J. PUB. HEALTH MGMT. & PRAC. 63 (1998).

55. TURNOCK, *supra* note 31, at 160–61.

56. Rawding & Wasserman, *supra* note 54, at 91–92.

57. *See, e.g.,* Zucht v. King, 260 U.S. 174 (1922) (upholding local discretion in compulsory vaccination—see chapter 7); Ellingwood v. City of Reedsburg, 64 N.W. 885 (Wis. 1895) (holding that the power to establish a water system is implied from the grant of general police power, since a good water system is important to the community's health).

58. *See* Harrison v. Baltimore, 1 Gill 264 (Md. 1843).

59. This brief discussion of local public health powers is necessarily simplified because it deals with an entire field of legal study known as local government law. *See generally,* SANDRA M. STEVENSON, ANTIEAU ON LOCAL GOVERNMENT LAW (2d ed. 1997); OSBORNE M. REYNOLDS, JR., LOCAL GOVERNMENT LAW (1982).

60. Special districts are typically created to bypass government borrowing limitations, to insulate public health activities from traditional political influence, and to ensure sufficient expertise for a specialized task.

61. Classically, states possess plenary power over local government and may create, dissolve, or deny them power, except as limited by the state constitution. Hunter v. City of Pittsburgh, 207 U.S. 161, 178–79 (1907). The federal constitution does not protect municipal corporations against state interference with its personal or economic rights. *See, e.g.,* Williams v. Mayor of Baltimore, 289 U.S. 36, 40 (1933); City of Newark v. New Jersey, 262 U.S. 192 (1923).

62. In a few states such as California, home rule charters are not thought of as grants of power, but as limitations on the reservoir of constitutionally delegated governing authority.

63. Home rule has been granted either by constitutional provision or statute in forty-three states. STEVENSON, *supra* note 59, § 21.01. *See, e.g.,* People *ex rel.* Metro. St. Ry. v. State Bd. of Tax Comm'rs, 67 N.E. 69, 70–71 (N.Y. 1903), *aff'd,* 199 U.S. 1 (1905) ("The principle of home rule, or the right of self-government as to local affairs, existed before we had a constitution.").

64. ILL. CONST. art. VII, § 6.

65. JOHN FORREST DILLON, MUNICIPAL CORPORATIONS § 55 (1st ed. 1872).

66. *See* HENDRIK HARTOG, PUBLIC PROPERTY AND PRIVATE POWER: THE CORPORATION OF THE CITY OF NEW YORK IN AMERICAN LAW, 1730–1870, 235 (1983) (the strict construction of delegations to local governments "provided an [important] technique for justifying judicial intervention" to block actions judges regarded as unwarranted).

67. *See* STEVENSON, *supra* note 59, at §§ 24.01–24.04.

68. James G. Hodge, Jr., *The Role of New Federalism and Public Health Law,* 12 J. LAW & HEALTH 309 (1998).

69. CONTRA COSTA COUNTY HEALTH SERVS. DEP'T PREVENTION PROGRAM, TAKING AIM AT GUN DEALERS: CONTRA COSTA'S PUBLIC HEALTH APPROACH TO REDUCING FIREARMS IN THE COMMUNITY 1 (March 1995) (forty-one states preempt local regulation of gun sales).

70. Suter v. City of Lafayette, 57 Cal. App. 4th 1109 (Cal. App. 1st Dist. 1997) (upholding against preemption challenge a city ordinance requiring firearm dealers to obtain land use and police permits in addition to licenses already required by state and federal law); *see also* Jon S. Vernick & Stephen P. Teret, *New Courtroom Strategies Regarding Firearms: Tort Litigation against Firearm Manufacturers and Constitutional Challenges to Gun Laws,* 36 HOUST. L. REV. 1713 (1999); LEGAL COMMUNITY AGAINST VIOLENCE, ADDRESSING GUN VIOLENCE THROUGH LOCAL ORDINANCES (San Francisco Foundation 1997).

71. *See generally,* KENNETH R. WING, THE LAW AND THE PUBLIC'S HEALTH 177–82 (4th ed. 1995).

72. Some agencies, particularly at the federal level, are placed within the legislative or even the judicial branch, and some are so-called independent agencies that are insulated from executive control (e.g., quasi-autonomous commissions and boards sometimes referred to as the "fourth branch" of government). The Supreme Court has upheld the constitutionality of independent agencies. *See, e.g.,* Morrison v. Olson, 487 U.S. 654 (1988) (upholding the constitutionality of independent counsel).

73. For a more detailed review of administrative law principles, see, e.g., KENNETH CULP DAVIS & RICHARD J. PIERCE, JR., ADMINISTRATIVE LAW TREATISE (3d ed. 1994); ALFRED C. AMAN, JR. & WILLIAM T. MAYTON, ADMINISTRATIVE LAW (1993); ERNEST GELLHORN & RONALD M. LEVIN, ADMINISTRATIVE LAW AND PROCESS (4th ed. 1997).

74. *See* Jerry L. Mashaw, *Prodelegation: Why Administrators Should Make Political Decisions,* 1 J.L. ECON. & ORG. 81 (1985).

75. Chief Justice Rehnquist in the *Benzene* case (discussed below) observed that Congress had "simply avoided a choice which was both fundamental . . . and yet politically so divisive that the necessary decision or compromise was difficult,

if not impossible, to hammer out in the legislative forge." Industrial Union Dep't. v. American Petroleum Inst., 448 U.S. 607, 687 (1980) (plurality opinion).

76. Since 1935, the Supreme Court has rarely, if ever, invalidated health and safety regulation as an impermissible delegation of lawmaking power to the executive. For the early twentieth-century view, see *A.L.A. Schechter Poultry Corp. v. United States*, 295 U.S. 495 (1935) (invalidating agency rules regarding maximum hour and minimum wage because the legislature did not provide clear standards). For the modern view, see, e.g., *Touby v. United States*, 500 U.S. 160 (1991) (rejecting a nondelegation doctrine challenge to congressional authorization of the Attorney General to criminalize distribution of any drug that posed a risk to public health). *But see,* American Trucking Ass'ns v. EPA, 195 F.3d 4 (D.C. Cir. 1999) (invalidating the EPA Clear Air Act rules that significantly tightened air quality standards for ozone and particulate matters under the nondelegation doctrine).

77. See ARTHUR E. BONFELD & MICHAEL ASIMOW, STATE AND FEDERAL ADMINISTRATIVE LAW 451–61 (1988).

78. *See, e.g.,* Howe v. City of St. Louis, 512 S.W.2d 127, 133 (Mo. 1974) (noting a modern tendency toward greater liberality in permitting grants of discretion to administrative officials as the complexity of government increases).

79. *See, e.g.,* People v. Tibbitts, 305 N.E.2d 152 (Ill. 1973) (striking down a statute allowing absolute and unguided discretion to an administrative agency as an unlawful delegation of power).

80. Boreali v. Axelrod, 517 N.E.2d 1350, 1356 (N.Y. 1987).

81. Industrial Union Dep't v. American Petroleum Inst., 448 U.S. 607 (1980) (plurality opinion) (narrowing the authority of OSHA to regulate toxic substances in the workplace).

82. *Id.* (construing the congressional grant of authority as requiring OSHA to find a significant risk of harm to workers, which the agency had not found in issuing the rule).

83. Unless specified by statute, state administrative procedure acts generally have been held not to apply to local government agencies. *See, e.g.,* Arthur D. Little, Inc. v. Commissioner of Health & Hosps., 481 N.E.2d 441 (Mass. 1985); *but see, e.g.,* Justewicz v. Hamtramck Civil Serv. Comm'n, 237 N.W.2d 555 (Mich. 1975).

84. In rulemaking, agencies set general standards that apply to classes of people, whereas in adjudication, agencies adjudicate the claims of individuals, which may involve a deprivation of liberty or property. *Compare* Londoner v. Denver, 210 U.S. 373 (1908) (requiring an evidentiary hearing for assessment of an individual owner's property) *with* Bi-Metallic Inv. Co. v. State Bd. of Equalization, 239 U.S. 441 (1915) (finding no due process was required when agency regulation increases the valuation of all taxable property).

85. The exemptions are for interpretive rules, policy statements, procedural rules, certain substantive rules (e.g., pertaining to the military, foreign affairs, agency management, loans, grants, benefits, or contracts), and where notice and comment procedures are "impracticable, unnecessary, or contrary to the public interest." 5 U.S.C. § 553(a) (1997).

86. *Id.* at § 553.

87. Automotive Parts & Accessories Ass'n v. Boyd, 407 F.2d 330, 338 (D.C. Cir. 1968) (holding that a standard requiring installation of seat belts in cars is a "concise general statement" under the Administrative Procedure Act).

88. 5 U.S.C. §§ 553(c), 556, 557 (1997).

89. National Nutritional Foods Ass'n v. FDA, 504 F.2d 761, 792–99 (2d Cir. 1974), cert. den., 420 U.S. 946 (1975); see Robert W. Hamilton, Rulemaking on a Record by the Food and Drug Administration, 50 TEX. L. REV. 1132 (1972) (discussing the FDA hearings where experts were cross-examined on whether peanut butter should contain 87 percent or 90 percent peanuts).

90. Philip J. Harter, Negotiated Regulations: A Cure for Malaise, 71 GEO. L.J. 1 (1982).

91. CORNELIUS M. KERWIN, RULEMAKING: HOW GOVERNMENT AGENCIES WRITE LAW AND MAKE POLICY 185–91 (1994).

92. DAVID M. PRITZKER & DEBORAH S. DALTON, NEGOTIATED RULEMAKING SOURCEBOOK 3–5 (1990).

93. 5 U.S.C. § 553(c) (1997).

94. Id. at §§ 554, 556, 557.

95. Steven P. Croley, See Theories of Regulation: Incorporating the Administrative Process, 98 COLUM. L. REV. 1, 101 (1998).

96. Although the terms license and permit are often used interchangeably, Professor Grad explains that they are historically different. A license was thought of as a special privilege, granted by the sovereign, to do what otherwise would be unlawful, such as selling liquor or running a lottery; a permit was thought of as official leave to carry on an activity or to perform an act that, although not morally questionable, was not allowable without such authority, such as practicing medicine or driving a car. FRANK GRAD, PUBLIC HEALTH LAW MANUAL 97, n.3 (2d ed. 1990). In this section the term "license" is used to refer to both licenses and permits.

97. See Dent v. West Virginia, 129 U.S. 114 (1889) (upholding the licensing of physicians on public health grounds, thus becoming one of the most important licensing precedents).

98. Local government has no inherent power to require permits or licenses. Accordingly, permits or licenses are void if the local government does not have the power under state law to impose them. See, e.g., Arnold v. City of Chicago, 56 N.E. 2d 795 (Ill. 1944); Nugent v. City of E. Providence, 238 A.2d 758, 761 (R.I. 1968).

99. Individuals may be required to record information as a condition of engaging in certain conduct but, unlike licenses and permits, registration does not impose standards or qualifications for pursuing the occupation. Through registration, public health officials are informed of the persons engaging in activities, but the agency does not actively supervise the conduct.

100. GRAD, supra note 96, at 97.

101. See, e.g., National Bank v. East Whiteland Township, 27 Pa. D. & C.2d 384 (Pa. Comm. Ct. 1962).

102. See, e.g., Gaudiya Vaishnava Soc'y v. San Francisco, 952 F.2d 1059 (9th Cir. 1991) (granting of the power to license without providing public servants

with standards is an unconstitutional delegation of legislative power); State *ex rel.* Bennett v. Stow, 399 P.2d 221, 231 (Mont. 1965) (allowing an administrative officer to ascertain whether qualifications, facts, or conditions exist for a license).

103. *See, e.g.,* State *ex rel.* Sims v. Eckhardt, 322 S.W.2d 903 (Mo. 1959) (finding unconstitutional the denial of building permits violating private restrictive covenants).

104. Thomas Cusack Co. v. City of Chicago, 242 U.S. 526 (1917) (finding that the Constitution does not prevent the city from lifting a prohibition based on consents of private individuals). However, even in those states permitting the use of consents to make permissible what is otherwise forbidden, the need to obtain too many consents from owners can be unreasonable. *See* Starin v. Village Brd. of Zoning Appeals, 101 N.Y.S.2d 80 (Sup. Ct. 1950).

105. *See* Dolan v. City of Tigard, 512 U.S. 374 (1994) (holding that the city's conditions on issuance of a permit must be reasonably related to legitimate state interest). Licenses can also be denied under a quota system if quotas are reasonably necessary to protect the public's health. *See* Strub v. Village of Deerfield, 167 N.E.2d 178 (Ill. 1960).

106. *See, e.g.,* CATHERINE M. BIDESE, U.S. MEDICAL LICENSURE STATISTICS AND CURRENT LICENSURE REQUIREMENTS (1995).

107. *See, e.g.,* Restivo v. City of Shreveport, 566 So. 2d 669 (La. 1990) (licensing plumbers is the duty of the state).

108. *See* Clark Havighurst & Nancy M.P. King, *Private Credentialing of Health Care Personnel: An Antitrust Perspective, Parts One & Two,* 9 AM. J.L. & MED. 131, 264 (1983).

109. *See, e.g.,* Florida v. Mathews, 526 F.2d 219 (5th Cir. 1976) (affirming that regulation of public health institutions is within state agency jurisdiction); *see generally,* AMERICAN HOSP. ASS'N, HOSPITAL REGULATION: REPORT OF THE SPECIAL COMMITTEE ON THE REGULATORY PROCESS (1977).

110. *See generally* United Beverage Co. v. Indiana Alcoholic Beverage Comm'n, 760 F.2d 155 (7th Cir. 1985) ("A state has power to delegate licensing authority to agencies independent of federal constraint.").

111. *See, e.g.,* Belleville Chamber of Commerce v. Town of Belleville, 238 A.2d 181 (N.J. 1968).

112. City of Laconia v. Gordon, 219 A.2d 701, 703 (N.H. 1966) ("To be valid charges made as license fees must bear a relation to and approximate the expense of issuing the licenses and of inspecting and regulating the business licensed.").

113. City of Prichard v. Richardson, 17 So. 2d 451, 454 (Ala. 1944) ("It seems well settled by authority that the power to license if granted as a police power, must be exercised as a means of regulation only, and cannot be used as a source of revenue.").

114. Lewis v. City of Grand Rapids, 356 F.2d 276, 296 (6th Cir.), *cert. denied,* 385 U.S. 838 (1966) (finding racial discrimination in licensing to be unconstitutional).

115. People *ex rel.* Nechamcus v. Warden, 39 N.E. 686 (N.Y. 1895) (alleging that Jews, immigrants, and those who did not belong to a union were discriminated against in obtaining a plumber's license).

116. *See* Steele v. FCC, 770 F.2d 1192 (D.C. Cir. 1985); *see also* Baehr v. Lewin, 852 P.2d 44 (Haw. 1993).

117. Yick Wo v. Hopkins, 118 U.S. 356 (1886). The white owners of steam laundries who competed with Chinese hand laundries provided the motivating force behind the laundry ordinance. *See In re* Wo Lee, 26 F. 471, 474 (C.C.D. Cal.), *rev'd sub nom.* Yick Wo v. Hopkins, 118 S. Ct. 356 (1886).

118. *See* David E. Bernstein, *Licensing Laws: A Historical Example of the Use of Government Regulatory Power against African Americans,* 31 SAN DIEGO L. REV. 89, 90 (1994) (because unions did not admit certain minorities or women into their apprenticeship training programs and because the public education system offered little formal training, certain groups could not satisfy licensing standards despite their practical experience).

119. *Id.* at 98–99 (as late as 1972, only one black plumber was licensed in Montgomery County, Alabama, and he was only able to get his license after a ferocious struggle with the local plumbers' union).

120. *See* Reuben A. Kessel, *The A.M.A. and the Supply of Physicians,* 35 LAW & CONTEMP. PROBS. 267 (1970); Todd L. Savitt, *The Education of Black Physicians at Shaw University, 1882–1918, in* BLACK AMERICANS IN NORTH CAROLINA AND THE SOUTH 160, 181–85 (Jeffrey J. Crow & Flora J. Hatley eds., 1984).

121. *See* Lawrence M. Friedman, *Freedom of Contract and Occupational Licensing 1890–1910: A Legal and Social Study,* 53 CAL. L. REV. 487, 496–97 (1965) (even if the licensing system originated in the public interest, the licensed group quickly gained control of the process and used it to benefit its members by limiting the number of new entrants, thus assuring those already in the field of higher incomes).

122. *See generally,* RICHARD A. EPSTEIN, FORBIDDEN GROUNDS: THE CASE AGAINST EMPLOYMENT DISCRIMINATION LAWS 91–129 (1992).

123. *See* Timothy S. Jost et al., *Consumers, Complaints, and Professional Discipline: A Look at Medical Licensure Boards,* 3 HEALTH MATRIX 309 (1993).

124. *See, e.g.,* STANLEY J. GROSS, OF FOXES AND HEN HOUSES: LICENSING AND THE HEALTH PROFESSIONS (1977).

125. *See, e.g.,* Bird v. State of Minn. Dep't of Public Safety, 375 N.W.2d 36 (Minn. Ct. App. 1985); *see also* Perry v. Sindermann, 408 U.S. 593 (1972).

126. *See, e.g.,* Cox v. New Hampshire, 312 U.S. 569 (1941) (finding that a license for a religious parade is constitutional only where no censorship or prohibitory fee is imposed and the license is necessary for public safety).

127. *See, e.g.,* FW/PBS, Inc. v. City of Dallas, 493 U.S. 215 (1990) (finding a licensing provision unconstitutional due to lack of procedural safeguards).

128. New York v. New St. Mark's Baths, 497 N.Y.S.2d 979 (Sup. Ct. 1986).

129. City of Lakewood v. Plain Dealer Publ'g Co., 486 U.S. 750 (1988) (finding the portion of an ordinance giving the mayor unfettered discretion to deny a permit and unbounded authority to condition a permit on any additional terms unconstitutional).

130. U.S. CONST. art. I, § 10, cl. 2 (permitting states to lay imposts or duties on imports or exports, without the consent of Congress, where "absolutely necessary for executing its inspections Laws").

131. *See, e.g.*, City of Smyrna v. Parks, 242 S.E.2d 73 (Ga. 1978) (upholding an ordinance regulating fence design and construction to minimize injury is a valid exercise of police powers).

132. *See, e.g.*, Food, Drug, and Cosmetic Act, 21 U.S.C. § 374(a) (1994) (authorizing FDA inspectors to enter and inspect a food, drug, or cosmetic factory or warehouse).

133. *See, e.g.*, Patapsco Guano Co. v. North Carolina Bd. of Agri., 171 U.S. 345 (1898) (allowing tax to be spent to appoint officials to enforce agricultural inspection laws).

134. Johnson's Markets Inc. v. New Carlisle Dep't of Health, 567 N.E.2d 1018 (Utah 1991) (commenting on the constitutionality of inspection of food service establishments).

135. *See, e.g.*, Occupational Safety and Health Act, 29 U.S.C. §§ 651–678 (1997) (describing inspection of workplace).

136. Federal Environmental Pesticide Control Act, 42 U.S.C. §§ 136 (e)–(q) (1997) (establishing an investigation program for pesticide manufacture and use).

137. Resource Conservation and Recovery Act, 42 U.S.C. §§ 6900–07 (1997) (describing inspection programs for generators of hazardous waste).

138. The Fourth Amendment safeguards an individual's "reasonable expectation of privacy." Wilson v. Health & Hosp. Corp., 620 F.2d 1201, 1210 (7th Cir. 1980) (finding that health officials' warrantless, consentless searches violated a reasonable expectation of privacy).

139. Frank v. Maryland, 359 U.S. 360 (1959) (upholding conviction of a home owner who refused to permit a health inspector to enter and inspect his residence without a warrant); Ohio *ex rel.* Eaton v. Price, 364 U.S. 263 (1960) (similar holding).

140. 387 U.S. 523 (1967) (finding that the Fourth Amendment was violated when a housing inspector entered an apartment to make a routine inspection without consent or a warrant).

141. *Id.* at 543 (finding that the Fourth Amendment was violated when a fire inspector sought to inspect a business without consent or warrant: "The businessman, like the occupant of a residence, has a constitutional right to go about his business free from unreasonable official entries upon his private commercial property").

142. The cases are collected in the Criminal Procedure Project, *Twenty-Eighth Annual Review of Criminal Procedure*, 87 GEO. L.J. 1095, 1189–93 (1999); Judy E. Zelin, *Propriety of State or Local Government Health Officer's Warrantless Search-Post-Camera Cases*, 53 A.L.R. 1168 (1998); *see also* GRAD, *supra* note 96, at 123–45.

143. Michigan v. Clifford, 464 U.S. 287, 291–95 (1984) (requiring a warrant for administrative search of a residence to investigate the cause of a fire).

144. *In re* Establishment Insp. of Caterpillar, Inc., 55 F.3d 334, 339 (7th Cir. 1995) (requiring a warrant for an administrative search of a business for occupational safety inspection).

145. J.L. Foti Constr. Co. v. Donovan, 786 F.2d 714, 717 (6th Cir. 1986) (finding that consent by general contractor with "common authority" over

work site conferred valid third-party consent to OSHA inspection); Lenz v. Winburn, 51 F.3d 1540 (11th Cir. 1995) (finding that a minor's consent conferred valid third-party consent to the entry of a social worker); Pollard v. Cockrell, 578 F.2d 1002, 1006 (5th Cir. 1978) (finding the administrative search of a massage parlor valid with consent).

146. Camara v. Municipal Court, 387 U.S. 523, 539 (1967) ("[W]arrants should normally be sought only after entry is refused."). See People v. Cacciola, 315 N.Y.S.2d 586 (Dist Ct. 1970) (upholding a search as an implied consent when a baker did not explicitly refuse to allow inspection). Consent should normally be given by the person who has the greatest privacy interest, such as a tenant. Village of Palatine v. Reinke, 454 N.E.2d 1099 (Ill. App. Ct. 1st Dist. 1983).

147. Clifford, 464 U.S. at 293 (justifying entry without a warrant by the immediate threat that a fire might rekindle); North Am. Cold Storage Co. v. City of Chicago, 211 U.S. 306 (1908) (justifying entry to seize unwholesome food intended for human consumption); McCabe v. Life-Line Ambulance Serv., 77 F.3d 540 545 (1st Cir. 1996) (justifying entry to protect a suicidal mentally ill resident).

148. See generally Katz v. United States, 389 U.S. 347, 361 (1967) (describing reasonable expectation of privacy).

149. Donovan v. Lone Steer, Inc., 464 U.S. 498 (1984) (finding that entry to the public lobby of a motel-restaurant does not violate the Fourth Amendment).

150. Air Pollution Variance Bd. v. Western Alfalfa Corp., 416 U.S. 861 (1974), on remand, 534 P.2d 796 (Colo. Ct. App. 1975), aff'd, 553 P. 811 (Colo. 1976) (upholding visual pollution tests of smoke being emitted from a business' chimney); Ehlers v. Bogue, 626 F.2d 1314 (5th Cir. 1980) (upholding visual inspection by a county health officer of the exterior of an apartment and a refuse dumpster); Department of Transp. v. Armacost, 474 A.2d 191 (Md. 1984), rev'd on other grounds, 532 A.2d 1056 (Md. 1987) (testing automobile exhaust for pollutants held valid).

151. See, e.g., Coolidge v. New Hampshire, 403 U.S. 443 (1971).

152. Marshall v. Barlow's, Inc., 436 U.S. 307, 320–21 (1978) (holding that an OSHA inspector's entitlement to search does not depend on his demonstrating probable cause); Tri-State Steel Const., Inc. v. Occupational Safety & Health Review Comm'n, 26 F.3d 173, 177 (D.C. Cir. 1994) (holding that the court may issue a warrant on showing specific evidence of an existing OSHA violation).

153. Barlow's, Inc., 436 U.S. at 320–21; Camara v. Municipal Court, 387 U.S. 523, 535–39 (1967); Martin v. International Matex Tank Terminals-Bayonne, 928 F.2d 614, 624–25 (3d Cir. 1991) (finding that written complaints from employees and an investigation to confirm the complaint provided OSHA with specific evidence); United States v. Two Units, 49 F.3d 479, 481 (9th Cir. 1995) (finding a report that the company was selling a fraudulent cure for AIDS sufficient for FDA inspection).

154. Barlow's, Inc., 436 U.S. at 320–21; In re Trinity Indus., Inc., 876 F.2d 1485, 1490 (11th Cir. 1989) (finding an OSHA search reasonable when based on neutral criteria and a detailed inspection plan); City of Chicago v. Pudlo, 462 N.E.2d 494 (Ill. App. Ct. 1983) (inspection of food facility); Commonwealth v.

Frodyma, 436 N.E.2d 925 (Mass. 1982) (inspection of pharmacy); Board of County Comm'r of Johnson County v. Grant, 954 P.2d 695 (Kan. 1998) (finding that valid public interest justifies a warrant for inspection of drains connected to sewer line).

155. Michigan v. Clifford, 464 U.S. 287, 294–95 (1984); Abel v. United States, 362 U.S. 217 (1960) (holding that an inspection warrant may not be used as a pretext for obtaining criminal evidence); Swint v. City of Wadley, 51 F.3d 988, 996, 998–99 (11th Cir. 1995) (finding an inspection unlawful when directed at finding illicit drugs rather than violation of liquor laws).

156. *Clifford,* 464 U.S. at 294.

157. New York v. Burger, 482 U.S. 691, 716 (1987) (holding that the discovery of criminal evidence during an otherwise lawful inspection did not render the search illegal). As to the role of police in an administrative search, *compare United States v. Nechy,* 827 F.2d 1161, 1167–68 (7th Cir. 1987) (holding that police participation does not invalidate a search) *with Alexander v. City & County of San Francisco,* 29 F.3d 1355, 1360 (9th Cir. 1994) (plurality opinion) (holding that police participation invalidates an inspection if their primary purpose was to arrest the house owner, not assist the health department).

158. *See Clifford,* 464 U.S. at 294 (holding that criminal evidence revealed during valid inspection may be seized under "plain view" doctrine; United States v. Doe, 61 F.3d 107, 110–11 (1st Cir. 1995) (finding that authorities properly seized contraband inadvertently discovered during a routine airline security search) contra United States v. Bulacan, 156 F.3d 963, 971 (9th Cir. 1998) (drug paraphernalia improperly seized in Social Security offices following Oklahoma City bombing because search for items other than weapons was unconstitutional expansion of administrative search).

159. *See Burger,* 482 U.S. at 708 (permitting warrantless inspection of a junkyard, which was extensively regulated under New York law); United States *ex rel.* Terraciano v. Montanye, 493 F.2d 682, 685 (2d Cir. 1974) (permitting the health department to audit pharmacy narcotic records).

160. *Burger,* 482 U.S. at 702–03; Contreras v. City of Chicago, 119 F.3d 1286, 1290–91 (7th Cir. 1997) (requiring no warrant to inspect a restaurant where necessary to further a regulatory scheme); Hroch v. City of Omaha, 4 F.3d 693, 697 (8th Cir. 1993) (requiring no warrant to implement an order to condemn buildings).

161. Donovan v. Dewey, 452 U.S. 594, 602 (1981) (permitting a warrantless administrative search of mining facilities as required by the Mine Safety and Health Act).

162. United States v. Biswell, 406 U.S. 311, 316–17 (1972).

163. Colonnade Catering Corp. v. United States, 397 U.S. 72, 76–77 (1970).

164. United States v. V-1 Oil Co., 63 F.3d 909, 911 (9th Cir. 1995).

165. United States v. Albers, 136 F.3d 670, 673 (9th Cir. 1998) (houseboat); United States v. Cardona-Sandoval, 6 F.3d 15, 23 (1st Cir. 1993) (vessels on high seas); Condon v. Reno, 155 F.3d 453, 465 (4th Cir. 1998) rev'd on other grounds, Reno v. Condon 120 S. Ct. 660 (2000) (motor vehicle records).

166. Blue v. Koren, 72 F. 3d 1075, 1080–81 (2d Cir. 1995) (justifying extensive warrantless inspections by a strong state interest in the highly regulated

nursing industry); Uzzillia v. Commissioner of Health, 367 N.Y.S.2d 795 (App. Div. 2d Dep't 1975).

167. People v. Firstenberg, 155 Cal. Rptr. 80 (Cal. App. 2d Dist. 1979). In theory, operators of licensed businesses give their implied consent to searches. People v. White, 65 Cal. Rptr. 923 (Cal. App. Dep't Super. Ct. 1968) (finding that the license to operate a hospital provided implied consent to inspection).

168. People v. Curco Drugs, Inc., 350 N.Y.S.2d 74, 77 (Crim. Ct. 1973).

169. See New York v. Burger, 482 U.S. 691, 710 (1987); Donovan v. Dewey, 452 U.S. 594, 603 (1981); Marshall v. Texoline Co., 612 F.2d 935, 938 (5th Cir. 1980).

170. See Burger, 482 U.S. at 704–07; Dewey, 452 U.S. at 598–600.

171. United States v. Biswell, 406 U.S. 311, 315 (1972) (holding that a search must be "carefully limited in time, place and scope"); United States ex rel. Terraciano, 493 F.2d 682 (2d Cir. 1974) (permitting a search during normal business hours); People v. Hedges, 447 N.Y.S.2d 1007 (Dist. Ct. 1982).

172. Finn's Liquor Shop Inc. v. State Liquor Authority, 294 N.Y.S.2d 592, 596 (App. Div. 1st Dep't 1968) (applying the exclusionary rule in a license suspension proceeding). Courts that apply the exclusionary rule in administrative proceedings also apply a "good faith" exception that permits use of illegal evidence if the agency acted in good faith. See Donovan v. Federal Clearing Die Casting Co., 695 F.2d 1020 (7th Cir. 1982) (admitting evidence obtained pursuant to an OSHA warrant subsequently declared invalid).

173. United States v. Article of Food Consisting of Twelve Barrels, 477 F. Supp. 1185, 1191 (S.D.N.Y. 1979) (FDA condemnation proceedings).

174. Nuisance originated with the common law action of the assize of nuisance, dealing with interferences with rights in enjoyment of land, including private easements like a neighbor's right of way. By a natural process, interference with a public easement, like a public right of way over private land, also came to be known as a nuisance. F.H Newark, The Boundaries of Nuisance, 65 L.Q. REV. 480, 482 (1949); see also John R. Spencer, Public Nuisance: A Critical Examination, 48 CAMB. L.J. 55 (1989).

175. The cases on public nuisance are collected in W. PAGE KEETON ET AL., PROSSER AND KEETON ON TORTS § 90 (5th ed. 1984); J.D. LEE, MODERN TORT LAW: LIABILITY & LITIGATION § 35.03 (1988); STEVENSON, supra note 59, at § 29.02.

176. Louise A. Halper, Untangling the Nuisance Knot, 26 B.C. ENVTL. AFF. L. REV. 89, 96–97 (1998).

177. See, e.g., Kitsap County v. Kev, Inc., 720 P.2d 818, 821 (Wash. 1986) (declaring an erotic dance studio sufficiently offensive to be deemed a public nuisance).

178. RESTATEMENT (SECOND) OF TORTS § 821C (1965).

179. JAMES STEPHEN, A GENERAL VIEW OF THE CRIMINAL LAW OF ENGLAND 105 (1890); see McKee v. City of Mt. Pleasant, 328 S.W.2d 224, 229 (Tex. Civ. App. 1959) ("[a]nything that worketh hurt, inconvenience or damage to the subjects of the Crown").

180. State v. Excelsior Powder Mfg. Co, 169 S.W. 267 (Mo. 1914) (gunpowder); Landau v. City of N.Y., 72 N.E. 631 (N.Y. 1904) (fireworks).

181. Seacord v. People, 13 N.E. 194 (Ill. 1887); Board of Health v. Vink, 151 N.W. 672 (Mich. 1915).

182. Durand v. Dyson, 111 N.E. 143 (Ill. 1915).

183. Bearcreek Township. v. De Hoff, 49 N.E.2d 391 (Ind. 1943).

184. Gay v. State, 18 S.W. 260 (Tenn. 1891); Kays v. City of Versailles, 22 S.W.2d 182 (Mo. 1929).

185. 65 ILL. COMP. Stat. § 5/11-20-5 (West 1999); see TEX. LOCAL GOV'T CODE ANN. § 217.042 (West 1999) ("Each city shall have the power to define all nuisances and prohibit the same within the city and outside the city limits for a distance of 5000 feet."); Board of Comm'rs v. Elm Grove Mining Co., 9 S.E.2d 813 (W.Va. 1940) ("The health officer shall inquire into all nuisances affecting public's health.").

186. CAL. CIV. CODE § 3479 (West 1999); see GA. CODE ANN. § 41-1-1 (1999) (anything that "causes hurt, inconvenience, or damage to another"); Pottawattamie County v. Iowa Dep't of Envtl. Quality, Air Quality Comm'n, 272 N.W.2d 448, 453 (Iowa 1978) ("anti-social conduct that injures a substantial number of people"); New York Trap Rock Corp. v. Town of Clarkstown, 85 N.E.2d 873 (N.Y. 1949) (defining a public nuisance as an act or omission that obstructs or causes damage to the public in exercise of rights common to all).

187. ARIZ. REV. STAT. § 36-601(A)(1)(1999); Spur Indus., Inc. v. Del E. Webb Dev. Co., 494 P.2d 700, 705 (Ariz. 1972) (entitling a developer to enjoin a cattle feeding operation as a nuisance).

188. N.Y. COMP. CODES R. & REGS. tit. 10, § 24-2.2 (1999).

189. See, e.g., Mitchell v. Commission on Adult Entertainment Establishments, 10 F.3d 123 (3d Cir. 1993) (finding that the constitutional rights of an adult video store were not infringed by "open booth" regulation that sought to reduce high-risk sexual activity).

190. City of Nokomis v. Sullivan, 153 N.E.2d 48, 51 (Ill. 1958) ("[T]he cases have turned, in the last analysis, upon the court's appraisal of the reasonableness of the municipal action.").

191. City of Corsicana v. Wilson, 249 S.W.2d 290, 293 (Tex. Civ. App. 1952).

192. Ozark Poultry Prods., Inc. v. Garman, 472 S.W.2d 714 (Ark. 1971) (odors that prevented neighbors from sleeping or eating meals without nausea).

193. Skinner v. Coy, 90 P.2d 296 (Cal. 1939) (peach trees).

194. New Hampshire v. Charpentier, 489 A.2d 594 (N.H. 1985); Craig v. City of Macon, 543 S.W.2d 772 (Mo. 1976); Commonwealth ex rel. Shumaker v. New York & Penn. Co., 79 A.2d 439 (Pa. 1951).

195. Shaw v. Salt Lake County, 224 P.2d 1037 (Utah 1950); Department of Pub. Health v. Cumberland Cattle Co., 282 N.E.2d 895 (Mass. 1972).

196. Polsgrove v. Moss, 157 S.W. 1133 (Ky. 1913); City of Honolulu v. Cavness, 364 P.2d 646 (Haw. 1961).

197. Springfield v. City of Little Rock, 290 S.W.2d 620 (Ark. 1956).

198. Ritholz v. Arkansas State Bd. of Optometry, 177 S.W.2d 410 (Ark. 1944) (optometry); Attorney Gen. ex rel. Mich. Bd. of Optometry v. Peterson, 164 N.W.2d 43 (Mich. 1969) (same); Minnesota v. Red Owl Stores, 115 N.W.2d 643 (Minn. 1962) (pharmacy); State ex rel. Marron v. Compere, 103 P.2d 273 (N.M. 1940) (medicine).

199. *See, e.g.,* Doe v. City of Minneapolis, 898 F.2d 612 (8th Cir. 1990).

200. Hirsh v. City of Atlanta, 401 S.E.2d 530 (Ga. 1991).

201. *See* Ralph Bolton et al., *Gay Baths Revisited: An Empirical Analysis,* 1 GLQ: J. LESBIAN & GAY STUD. 255 (1994) (arguing that bathhouses could serve as a focal point in which gay men could be educated about AIDS).

202. New York v. New St. Mark's Baths, 497 N.Y.S.2d 979 (Sup. Ct. 1986).

203. State Fire Marshal v. Schaneman, 279 N.W.2d 101 (Neb. 1979).

204. City of Philadelphia v. Watt, 57 A.2d 591, 594 (Pa. 1948).

205. The Fifth and Fourteenth Amendments, respectively, provide that neither the federal government nor the states shall deprive any person of "life, liberty, or property without due process of law."

206. U.S. CONST., art. I, § 10: "No State shall . . . pass any . . . law impairing the obligations of Contracts."

207. *Id.* at amend. V: "nor shall private property be taken for public use without just compensation."

208. For early conservative scholarship see HERBERT SPENCER, SOCIAL STATICS (1851) (advocating a laissez-faire, unregulated economy); CHRISTOPHER TIEDEMAN, A TREATISE ON THE LIMITATIONS OF THE POLICE POWER IN THE UNITED STATES (1886) (government regulations unduly interfere with the natural rights of people to own and use property). For more recent accounts, see RICHARD A. EPSTEIN, TAKINGS: PRIVATE PROPERTY AND THE POWER OF EMINENT DOMAIN (1985); BERNARD SIEGAN, ECONOMIC LIBERTIES AND THE CONSTITUTION (1980).

209. Calder v. Bull, 3 U.S. 386 (1798); Fletcher v. Peck, 10 U.S. 87 (1810); Terrett v. Taylor, 13 U.S. 43 (1815).

210. Slaughter-House Cases, 83 U.S. 36, 81 (1873) ("[U]nder no construction of [due process] . . . can the restraint . . . upon the exercise of their trade be held to be a deprivation of property."). *See also* Wendy E. Parmet, *From Slaughter-House to Lochner: The Rise and Fall of the Constitutionalization of Public Health,* 40 AM. J. LEGAL HIST. 476 (1996).

211. Mugler v. Kansas, 123 U.S. 623 (1887) (upholding a state prohibition on the sale of alcoholic beverages).

212. Jacobson v. Massachusetts, 197 U.S. 11 (1905).

213. See further chapter 3.

214. Ogden v. Saunders, 25 U.S. 213 (1827).

215. Manigault v. Springs, 199 U.S. 473, 480 (1905).

216. A more stringent test is used for interference with government contracts. United States Trust Co. v. New Jersey, 431 U.S. 1 (1977).

217. Energy Reserves Group, Inc. v. Kansas Power & Light Co. 459 U.S. 400, 411–413 (1983).

218. *See generally,* Jed Rubenfeld, *Usings,* 102 YALE L.J. 1077 (1993); ROBERT MELTZ ET AL., THE TAKINGS ISSUE: CONSTITUTIONAL LIMITS ON LAND-USE CONTROL AND ENVIRONMENTAL REGULATION (1999); STEVEN J. EAGLE, REGULATORY TAKINGS (1996).

219. Eastern Enters. v. Apfel, 424 U.S. 498 (1998) (per O'Connor J., with three justices concurring and one justice concurring in the judgment); *see also* Frank I. Michelman, *Property, Utility and Fairness: Comments on the*

Ethical Foundations of "Just Compensation Law," 80 HARV. L. REV. 1165 (1967).

220. *See* EPSTEIN, *supra* note 208.

221. Pennsylvania Coal Co. v. Mahon, 260 U.S. 393 (1922).

222. *Id.* at 413 ("As long recognized, some values are enjoyed under an implied limitation and must yield to the police power."); *see* Catherine Connors, *Back to the Future: The "Nuisance Exception" to the Just Compensation Clause,* 19 CAP. U.L. REV. 139 (1990); Joseph Sax, *Takings and the Police Power,* 74 YALE L.J. 36 (1964).

223. 505 U.S. 1003 (1992); *see* Richard J. Lazarus, *Putting the Correct "Spin" on Lucas,* 45 STAN. L. REV. 1411 (1993).

224. Regulatory takings doctrine applies to real property (real estate or land) and not to personal property (e.g., commercial activities such as manufacture or sale): "[B]y reason of the State's traditionally high degree of control over commercial dealings, he [the regulatory subject] ought to be aware of the possibility that new regulation might even render his property worthless." Lucas v. South Carolina Coastal Council, 505 U.S. 1003, 1029 (1992).

225. *Id.* at 1029. The Court has also said that police power regulation becomes a taking if the burden imposed is not roughly proportionate to the government's justification for regulating. Dolan v. City of Tigard, 512 U.S. 374 (1994).

226. *See, e.g., Lucas,* 505 U.S. at 1055 (Blackman, J., dissenting) ("[O]ne searches in vain . . . for anything resembling a principle in the common law of nuisance."); William Prosser, *Nuisance without Fault,* 20 TEX. L. REV. 399, 410 (1942) (describing common law nuisance as "an "impenetrable jungle," "legal garbage," and full of "vagueness, uncertainty and confusion").

227. *See, e.g.,* Gazza v. New York State Dep't of Envtl. Conservation, 679 N.E.2d 1035 (N.Y. 1997) (protecting wetlands); Anello v. Zoning Board of Appeals, 678 N.E.2d 870 (N.Y. 1997) (preventing development on steep slopes).

228. Loveladies Harbor v. United States, 28 F.3d 1171 (Fed. Cir. 1994); Preseault v. United States, 100 F.3d 1525 (Fed. Cir. 1996).

229. Florida Rock Indus. v. United States, 18 F.3d 1560, 1570–71 (Fed. Cir. 1994).

230. Philip Morris v. Harshbarger, 159 F.3d 670 (1st Cir. 1998); *see* Ruckelshaus v. Monsanto Co., 467 U.S. 986 (1984) (upholding, in part, a pesticide manufacturer's claim that compelled disclosure of trade secrets constituted a regulatory taking).

231. The four consistent votes favoring an expansive reading of the Takings Clause are Chief Justice Rehnquist and Justices Scalia, Thomas, and O'Connor. *See* Lazarus, *supra* note 223, at 109–21; Douglas T. Kendall & Charles P. Lord, *The Takings Project: A Critical Analysis and Assessment of the Progress So Far,* 25 B.C. ENVTL. AFF. L. REV. 583–84 (1998).

232. Eastern Enterprises v. Apfel, 524 U.S. 498, 523–24 (1998).

233. *See, e.g.,* Miller v. Schone, 276 U.S. 272, 279 (1928) ("[W]hen forced to make a choice the state does not exceed its constitutional powers by deciding upon the destruction of one class of property to save another which, in the judgment of the legislature, is the greater value to the public.").

10.   TORT LAW AND THE PUBLIC'S HEALTH:
      INDIRECT REGULATION

SOURCES FOR CHAPTER EPIGRAPHS: Page 269: *Tort Law in the Regulatory State,* in TORT LAW AND THE PUBLIC INTEREST 80, 81 (Peter H. Schuck ed., 1991). Page 271: Donoghue v. Stevenson [1932] A.C. 562, 580. Page 277: Rylands v. Fletcher, L.R. 3 H.L. 330 (1868). Page 282: GEORGE BERKELEY, A TREATISE OF HUMAN NATURE (2d ed. with text revised and notes by P.H. Nidditch, 1978) (1935). Page 288: San Diego Building Trades Council v. Garmon, 359 U.S. 236, 247 (1959). Page 290: Haines v. Liggett 975 F.2d 81 (3rd Cir. 1992). Page 293: William E. Townsley and Dale K. Hanks, *The Trial Court's Responsibility to Make Cigarette Disease Litigation Affordable and Fair,* 25 Cal. W.L. Rev. 275, 277 (1989). Page 293: Haines v. Liggett Group, Inc., 814 F. Supp. 414, 421 (D.N.J. 1993) (quoting J. Michael Jordan, defending R.J. Reynolds tobacco). Page 297: McLaughlin v. United States, 476 U.S. 17, 17 (1986).

1. For an excellent illustration in the context of tobacco litigation see, Peter D. Jacobson & Kenneth E. Warner, *Litigation and Public Health Policy: The Case of Tobacco Control,* 24 J. HEALTH POL., POL'Y & L. 769 (1999); *see also* Richard A. Posner, *A Theory of Negligence,* 1 J. LEGAL STUD. 29, 30–31 (1972).

2. Private rights of action are also created by statutes such as the Clean Air Act, 42 U.S.C. §§ 7401–7671q (1994) and the Clean Water Act, 33 U.S.C. §§ 1251–1387 (1994), which authorize citizen suits to abate pollution.

3. K-Mart Corp. v. Ponsock, 732 P.2d 1364, 1368 (Nev. 1987). Note that this is an imperfect definition because some civil actions for monetary damages are not torts, such as remedies afforded in environmental statutes; some torts have elements of contract, such as breach of warranty; and some torts provide nonmonetary damages, such as an injunction to cease the continuation of a nuisance.

4. Controversy remains over just what the goals of the tort system should be. *See* Heidi L. Feldman, *Science and Uncertainty in Mass Exposure Litigation,* 74 TEX. L. REV. 1, 34–35 (1995); STEVEN SHAVELL, ECONOMIC ANALYSIS OF ACCIDENT LAW 7 (1987); GUIDO CALABRESI, THE COSTS OF ACCIDENTS: A LEGAL AND ECONOMIC ANALYSIS 16 (1970).

5. Stephen P. Teret, *Litigating for the Public's Health,* 76 AM. J. PUB. HEALTH 1027 (1986); *see also* TOM CHRISTOFFEL & STEPHEN P. TERET, PROTECTING THE PUBLIC: LEGAL ISSUES IN INJURY PREVENTION (1993).

6. *See, e.g.,* Reserve Mining Co. v. EPA, 514 F.2d 492 (8th Cir. 1975) (emissions from mining operations).

7. *See, e.g.,* Anderson v. Cryovac, Inc., 862 F.2d 910 (1st Cir. 1988) (phenol contamination of wells).

8. *See, e.g.,* Villari v. Terminix Int'l, Inc., 692 F. Supp 568 (E.D. Pa. 1988) (pesticide contamination of home).

9. *See, e.g.,* Allen v. United States, 588 F. Supp. 247 (D. Utah 1984), *rev'd,* 816 F.2d 1417 (10th Cir. 1987) (radiation exposure from atmospheric testing of nuclear devices).

10. *See, e.g.,* In re Agent Orange Prod. Liab. Litig., 597 F. Supp. 740 (E.D.N.Y. 1984), *aff'd,* 818 F.2d 145 (2d Cir. 1987) (dioxin spraying in Vietnam); *see also* PETER H. SCHUCK, AGENT ORANGE ON TRIAL (Harvard, 1986).

11. Sindell v. Abbott Laboratories, 607 P.2d 924 (Cal. 1980) (market share liability for DES); Bichler v. Eli Lilly & Co., 436 N.E.2d 182 (N.Y. 1988) (liability for cancer caused by DES).

12. See, e.g., Reyes v. Wyeth Lab., 498 F.2d 1264 (5th Cir.), cert. denied sub nom. Wyeth Lab. v. Reyes, 419 U.S. 1096 (1974) (holding the manufacturer liable for marketing polio vaccine with insufficient warnings); Fraley v. American Cyanamid Co., 570 F. Supp. 497 (D. Colo. 1983) (manufacturer liable for inadequate warnings when vaccinated child contracted polio).

13. See, e.g., Wooderson v. Ortho Pharm. Corp., 681 P.2d 1038 (Cal. 1984) (finding the manufacturer had a duty to warn a physician of the inherent dangers of oral contraceptives); In re A.H. Robins Co., 88 B.R. 742 (E.D. Va. 1988), aff'd, 880 F.2d 694 (4th Cir. 1989) (establishing a manufacturer's trust fund to settle 300,000 claims of women who had been injured by the Dalkon Shield, an intrauterine contraceptive device); see also Kenneth R. Feinberg, The Dalkon Shield Claimants Trust, 53 L. & CONTEMP. PROBS. 79 (1990).

14. See, e.g., Batten v. Bobo, 528 A.2d 572 (N.J. 1986) (holding that an intoxicated minor guest involved in a car accident can bring a cause of action against his or her social host); Estate of Hernandez v. Arizona Bd. of Regents, 866 P.2d 1330 (Ariz. 1994) (finding that the fraternity and university had a duty of care to avoid serving alcohol to minors). The courts have refused to hold alcoholic beverage manufacturers liable for failing to warn consumers about the adverse effects of alcohol. See, e.g., Maguire v. Pabst Brewing Co., 387 N.W.2d 565 (Iowa 1986) (finding the brewing company not liable for alcohol-related pancreatitis).

15. See, e.g., Moning v. Alfono, 254 N.W.2d 759 (Mich. 1977) (pogo sticks); Cunningham v. Quaker Oats Co., 639 F. Supp. 234 (W.D.N.Y. 1986) (toy figurines); Moning v. Playskool Inc., 30 F.3d 459 (3d Cir. 1994) (building blocks).

16. See, e.g., Fiske v. MacGregor, Div. of Brunswick, 464 A.2d 719 (R.I. 1983) (football helmets); AMF v. Victor J. Andrew High School, 526 N.E. 2d 584 (Ill. App. Ct. 1988) (trampolines).

17. See, e.g., Parsons v. Honeywell, Inc., 929 F.2d 901 (2d Cir. 1991) (water heater); Bean et al. v. Bic Corp., 597 So. 2d 1350 (Ala. 1992) (cigarette lighter); Tafoya v. Sears Roebuck & Co., 884 F.2d 1330 (10th Cir. 1989) (lawnmower).

18. Losee v. Buchanan, 51 N.Y. 476, (N.Y. 1873).

19. Percy H. Winfield, The History of Negligence in the Law of Torts, 42 L.Q. REV. 184 (1926); Charles O. Gregory, Trespass to Negligence to Absolute Liability, 37 VA. L. REV. 359 (1951). But see Robert L. Rabin, The Historical Development of the Fault Principle: A Reinterpretation, 15 GA. L. REV. 925, 927 (1981) ("I view it as a serious mistake to characterize the pre-industrial era as one of strict liability.").

20. Chief Justice Lemuel Shaw is often credited with first imposing fault-based liability for unintentionally caused harm. Brown v. Kendall, 60 Mass. 292, 296 (1850) (articulating a standard of "ordinary care": "that kind and degree of care, which prudent and cautious men would use, such as is required by the exigency of the case, and such as is necessary to guard against probable danger").

21. W. PAGE KEETON ET AL., PROSSER AND KEETON ON THE LAW OF TORTS §
30 (5th ed. 1984) [hereinafter PROSSER AND KEETON ON TORTS]; 57A AM. JUR.
2d *Negligence* § 78 (1989); RESTATEMENT (SECOND) OF TORTS § 281 (1965).

22. Barry R. Furrow, *Forcing Rescue: The Landscape of Health Care
Provider Obligations to Treat Patients*, 3 HEALTH MATRIX 31 (1993).

23. PROSSER AND KEETON ON TORTS, *supra* note 21, at §56.

24. *See, e.g.*, The Nitro-Glycerine Case, 82 U.S. 524, 536–37 (1872) (The
law does "not charge culpable negligence upon anyone who takes the usual
precautions against accident, which careful and prudent men are accustomed to
take under similar circumstances.").

25. MARSHALL S. SHAPO, BASIC PRINCIPLES OF TORT LAW § 19.01 (1999).

26. OLIVER WENDELL HOLMES, THE COMMON LAW (rev. ed. 1963) (1881).

27. Troyen A. Brennan, *Environmental Torts*, 46 VAND. L. REV. 1, 56
(1993).

28. PROSSER AND KEETON ON TORTS, *supra* note 21, at § 41. If two causes
concur to bring about an injury and either one of them, operating alone, would
have been sufficient to cause the same result, the courts ask whether the defendant's conduct was a "substantial factor" in causing the injury.

29. Lawrence O. Gostin & David W. Webber, *The AIDS Litigation Project:
HIV/AIDS in the Courts in the 1990s, Part I*, 12 AIDS & PUB. POL'Y J. 105,
111 (1997).

30. For a more detailed discussion of "risk," see chapter 4.

31. United States v. Carroll Towing Co., 159 F.2d 169 (2d Cir. 1947).

32. A private nuisance is different from, but not inconsistent with, the concept of trespass. Trespass protects an interest in the exclusive possession of
land, while a private nuisance protects an interest in the use and enjoyment of
land; trespass requires a physical entry, while private nuisance does not. JAMES
A. HENDERSON ET AL., THE TORTS PROCESS 501 (5th ed. 1994).

33. Scholars often associate nuisances with the full spectrum of tort culpability, ranging from "intentional" conduct and negligence to strict liability for
abnormally dangerous activity. *See, e.g.*, 58 RESTATEMENT (SECOND) OF TORTS
§ 822 (1965); SHAPO, *supra* note 25, at § 36.01. Conceptually, it may be better to think of these as independent sources of liability.

34. PROSSER AND KEETON ON TORTS, *supra* note 21, at § 88.

35. *Id.*

36. Guido Calabresi & Douglas A. Melamed, *Property Rules, Liability
Rules, and Inalienability: One View of the Cathedral*, 85 HARV. L. REV. 1089
(1972); A. Mitchell Polinsky, *Resolving Nuisance Disputes: The Simple
Economics of Injunctive and Damage Remedies*, 32 STAN. L. REV. 1075 (1980).

37. One way of thinking about nuisance actions is that they require the payment of compensation to those injured in exchange for the right to pollute. *See,
e.g.*, Boomer v. Atlantic Cement Co., 257 N.E.2d 870 (N.Y. 1970) (awarding damages despite the company's positive effect on local employment); RESTATEMENT
(SECOND) OF TORTS § 826 (1965) (industry may have to compensate for unreasonable interferences even if a favorable balance of benefits and burdens exists).

38. United States v. Reserve Mining Co., 380 F. Supp. 11, 55–56 (D. Minn.
1974). Ecological morality is a theme among environmentalists, with advocates

arguing that pollution is morally offensive; polluters should not be permitted to pay for the privilege of harming the ecosystem. *See, e.g.,* Christopher Stone, Earth and Other Ethics: The Case for Moral Pluralism (1987).

39. Laird v. Nelms, 406 U.S. 797 (1972) (sonic boom generated by aircraft).

40. Rylands v. Fletcher, L.R. 3 H.L. 330, 339–40 (1868), (per Lord Cairns).

41. *Id.* at 340, (per Lord Cairns).

42. Restatement (Second) of Torts §§ 519–520 (1965).

43. *Id.* at § 520, comment i.

44. T & E Indus. v. Safety Light Corp., 587 A.2d 1249 (N.J. 1991) (disposal of radium tailings); Prospect Indus. Corp. v. Singer Co., 569 A.2d 908 (N.J. Super. Ct. Law Div. 1989) (leaking of PCBs); Department of Envtl. Protection v. Ventron Corp., 468 A.2d 150 (N.J. 1982) (disposal of mercury); *see also* Andrew Allen Lemmon, *The Developing Doctrine of* Rylands v. Fletcher: *Hazardous Waste Remediation Contractors Beware,* 42 Loy. L. Rev. 287 (1996).

45. Prosser and Keeton on Torts, *supra* note 21, at § 78.

46. Shapo, *supra* note 25, at 166–67.

47. 111 N.E. 1050 (N.Y. 1916).

48. *See, e.g.,* Henningsen v. Bloomfield Motors, 161 A.2d 69 (N.J. Sup. Ct. 1960) (finding implied warranty liability against a nonprivity car manufacturer that ran off the road, causing personal injuries).

49. Greenman v. Yuba Power Prods., 377 P.2d 897 (Cal. 1963) (finding strict tort liability for manufacturer that places a product on the market "knowing that it is to be used without inspection for defects, [which] then proves to have a defect that causes injury").

50. Restatement (Second) of Torts § 402A (1965) (a seller of a product "in a defective condition unreasonably dangerous to the consumer is liable for physical harm thereby caused to the ultimate user or consumer if . . . it is expected to and does reach the user or consumer without substantial change in the condition in which it is sold").

51. Products liability has extended to include intangibles such as electricity. *See* Houston Lighting & Power Co. v. Reynolds, 765 S.W.2d 784 (Tex. 1988) (finding that electricity is a product once it is delivered to the consumer).

52. *See, e.g.,* Richardson v. Volkswagenwerk, A.G., 552 F. Supp. 73 (W.D. Mo. 1982) (finding a Volkswagen model to be defectively designed).

53. *See, e.g.,* Ferdig v. Melitta, Inc., 320 N.W.2d 369 (Mich. Ct. App. 1981) (finding a coffee-filtering apparatus defective based on express warranty and negligence theories when hot water spilled on the plaintiff's legs).

54. *See, e.g.,* Roe v. Deere & Co., 855 F.2d 151 (3d Cir. 1988) (allowing the plaintiff to present a theory of liability based upon the lack of crashworthiness of a tractor).

55. *See, e.g.,* Everett v. Bucky Warren, Inc., 380 N.E.2d 653 (Mass. 1978) (finding a hockey helmet to be defectively designed).

56. *See, e.g.,* Shanks v. Upjohn Co., 835 P.2d 1189 (Alaska 1992) (refusing to exempt prescription drugs from strict liability design defect claims).

57. *See, e.g.,* Jones v. Lederle Lab., 695 F. Supp. 700 (E.D.N.Y. 1988) (holding that the claim of defective design of whole-cell pertussis vaccine was not preempted by federal law).

58. *See, e.g.,* Medtronic, Inc. v. Lohr, 518 U.S. 470 (1996) (finding that FDA approval of an allegedly defective heart pacemaker did not preempt product liability claims); Goodlin v. Medtronic, Inc., 167 F.3d 1367 (11th Cir. 1999) (same); Haudrich v. Howmedica, Inc., 662 N.E.2d 1248 (Ill. 1996) (finding a knee prosthesis could be found defective when it failed three years after it had been implanted).

59. Cavan v. General Motors Corp., 571 P.2d 1249, 1251–52 (Or. 1977).

60. *See, e.g.,* Weishorn v. Miles-Cutter, 721 A.2d 811 (Pa. Super. Ct. 1998) (holding that the blood shield statute precludes strict liability and breach of warranty claims); *see also* Timothy P. Blanchard, *Strict Liability for Blood Derivative Manufacturers: Statutory Shield Incompatible with Public Health Responsibility,* 28 ST. LOUIS L.J. 443 (1984); BLOOD FEUDS: AIDS, BLOOD, AND THE POLITICS OF MEDICAL DISASTER (Eric A. Feldman & Ronald Bayer, eds., 1999).

61. Barker v. Lull Eng'g Co., 573 P.2d 443, 545 (Cal. 1978).

62. The factors in the risk-utility calculation are product utility for the consumer and the public; likelihood of risk and severity of harm; alternative products with the same function; manufacturer's ability to reduce the risk without impairing usefulness or creating inordinate expense; the user's awareness of the risk and ability to avoid it by exercising care; and feasibility of the manufacturer to spread the loss through price increases or liability insurance. John Wade, *On the Nature of Strict Tort Liability for Products,* 44 MISS. L.J. 825, 837–38 (1973).

63. RESTATEMENT (THIRD) OF TORTS: PRODUCTS LIABILITY § 2 (1998).

64. *Id.* § 2(a) ("the product departs from its intended design").

65. *But see* American Tobacco Co., Inc. v. Grinnell, 951 S.W.2d 420 (Tex. 1977) (finding that pesticide residue, unintentionally but "normally" found in the defendant's tobacco after fumigation, was a manufacturing rather than a design defect).

66. RESTATEMENT (THIRD) OF TORTS: PRODUCTS LIABILITY, *supra* note 63, at § 2(b).

67. The "reasonable design alternative standard may not be required if the product has low social utility with high risk." Potter v. Chicago Pneumatic Tool Co., 694 A.2d 1319, 1331 (Conn. 1997).

68. Pharmaceutical companies and others sometimes use the "learned intermediary defense," arguing that parties with superior knowledge, notably the physician, had the responsibility to warn the user of the product's hazards. *See, e.g.,* Swayze v. McNeil Lab., Inc., 807 F.2d 464 (5th Cir. 1987) (applying the learned intermediary defense where a drug manufacturer only warned the prescribing physician); Mazur v. Merck & Co., 964 F.2d 1348 14157 (3d Cir. 1992) (finding that the CDC was a learned intermediary when Merck sold the MMRII vaccine to the CDC for a mass immunization program).

69. RESTATEMENT (THIRD) OF TORTS: PRODUCTS LIABILITY *supra* note 63, at § 2(c).

70. Beshada v. Johns-Manville Prods. Corp., 447 A.2d 539, 546–49 (N.J. 1982) (danger of asbestos).

71. PROSSER AND KEETON ON TORTS, *supra* note 21, at § 106.

72. Restatement (Second) of Torts § 402B (1965) (A seller who "makes to the public a misrepresentation of a material fact . . . is subject to liability for physical harm to a consumer . . . caused by justifiable reliance upon the misrepresentation").

73. *See, e.g.,* Ladd v. Honda Motor Co., 939 S.W.2d 83 (Tenn. Ct. App. 1996) (holding that a plaintiff may recover based on advertisements for an entire product line).

74. Wilkinson v. Bay Shore Lumber Co., 227 Cal. Rptr. 327 (Cal. App. 2d. 1986) (comment k cases overwhelmingly involve "prescription drugs, vaccines, blood, and medical devices such as intrauterine devices and breast implants"). The courts are divided, however, over whether comment k bars strict liability for all prescription drugs or whether the determination should be made on an individual basis by balancing utility and risk. *Compare* Grundberg v. Upjohn Co., 813 P.2d 89 (Utah 1991) (favoring an across-the-board rule for all FDA-approved drugs) *with* Hill v. Searle Lab., 884 F.2d 1064 (8th Cir. 1989) (adopting a case-by-case approach to deny comment k immunity for the CU-7 intrauterine device). In an attempt to narrow prescription drug and medical device liability, the revised restatement elaborates on comment k. Restatement (Third) of Torts: Products Liability *supra* note 63, at § 6, holds manufacturers of drugs and medical devices strictly liable only if a reasonable health care provider, informed of the risks and benefits of the therapy, would not prescribe it to any class of patient.

75. Borel v. Fibreboard Paper Prods. Corp., 493 F.2d 1076 (5th Cir. 1973).

76. Purvis v. PPG Indust., Inc., 502 So. 2d 714 (Ala. 1987).

77. Brown v. Superior Court, 751 P.2d 470, 482 (Cal. S. Ct. 1988).

78. Restatement (Second) of Torts § 402A, comment i (1965).

79. Restatement (Third) of Torts: Products Liability, *supra* note 63, at § 2, comment d.

80. Learned Hand, *Historical and Practical Considerations Regarding Expert Testimony,* 15 Harv. L. Rev. 40 (1901). *See* John Monahan and Laurens Walker, *Judicial Use of Social Science Research,* 15 Law & Hum. Behav. 571 (1991).

81. *Developments in the Law: Confronting the New Challenges of Scientific Evidence,* 108 Harv. L. Rev. 1481, 1484 (1995); *see also* Sheila Jasanoff, Science at the Bar: Law, Science and Technology in America (1995); Peter H. Schuck, *Multi-Culturalism Redux: Science, Law, and Politics,* 11 Yale L. & Pol'y Rev. 1 (1993); Margaret G. Farrell, Daubert v. Merrell Dow Pharmaceuticals, Inc.: *Epistemology and Legal Process,* 15 Cardozo L. Rev. 2183 (1994); Bert Black, *A Unified Theory of Scientific Evidence,* 56 Fordham L. Rev. 595 (1988).

82. For an insightful explanation, *see* Tom Cristoffel & Stephen P. Teret, *Epidemiology and the Law: Courts and Confidence Intervals,* 81 Am. J. Pub. Health 1661, 1665 (1991) ("The scientist's conclusion is achieved when truth is illuminated, and the level of certainty or proof required is very high. The court's conclusion is achieved when the best decision, given the weight of the evidence, is made for that case . . . [and the resolution] is socially acceptable.").

83. *In re* Union Carbide Gas Plant Disaster at Bhopal, India in Dec. 1984, 809 F.2d 195 (2d Cir. 1987).

84. Causality is easier to prove with "signature" diseases that are rare in the absence of specific exposures. Kenneth S. Abraham, *Individual Action and Collective Responsibility: The Dilemma of Mass Tort Reform*, 73 VA. L. REV. 845 (1987). For example, vaginal adenocarcinoma of the cervix was thought to be a rare condition except in women exposed to diethylstilbestrol (DES).

85. Allen v. United States, 588 F. Supp. 247 (D. Utah 1984), *rev'd*, 816 F.2d 1417 (10th Cir. 1987).

86. Mancuso v. Consolidated Edison Co. of N.Y., 967 F. Supp. 1437, 1445–46 (S.D.N.Y. 1997) ("Numerous courts have followed this method": (1) determine the dosage of the toxin to which the plaintiff was exposed; (2) establish general causation by demonstrating that the level of the toxin comparable to those received by the plaintiff can cause the specific types of injuries; and (3) establish specific causation by demonstrating that, more likely than not, the toxin caused the plaintiff's actual injuries).

87. Wright v. Willamette Indus. Inc., 91 F.3d 1105, 1107–08 (8th Cir. 1996) (holding that the dose is necessary to address the issue of general causation).

88. Christopher H. Buckley Jr. & Charles H. Haake, *Separating the Scientist's Wheat from the Charlatan's Chaff: Daubert's Role in Toxic Tort Litigation*, 28 ENVTL. L. REP. 10293, 10298 (1998).

89. CHRISTOFFEL & TERET, *supra* note 5, at 1662–63.

90. Troyen Brennan, *Causal Chains and Statistical Links: The Role of Scientific Uncertainty in Hazardous-Substance Litigation*, 73 CORNELL L. REV. 1 (1989).

91. For an account of the salience of probabilistic thinking, see Daniel M. Fox, *Epidemiology and the New Political Economy of Medicine*, 89 AM. J. PUB. HEALTH 493, 495 (1999).

92. Kenneth J. Rothman & Sander Greenland, *Causation and Causal Inference, in* OXFORD TEXTBOOK OF PUBLIC HEALTH 617 (Roger Detels et al. eds., vol. 2 1997) [hereinafter OXFORD TEXTBOOK OF PUBLIC HEALTH]; Laurens Walker & John Monahan, *Sampling Liability*, 85 VA. L. REV. 329 (1999).

93. If the study is based on a random sample, confidence intervals may be calculated to obtain an interval that has a high probability of containing the true value of the measure in the total target population. Joseph Herbert Abramson, *Cross-Sectional Studies, in* OXFORD TEXTBOOK OF PUBLIC HEALTH, *supra* note 92, at 517, 522.

94. 293 F. 1013 (D.C. Cir. 1923).

95. *Id.* at 1014.

96. FED. R. EVID. § 702.

97. The Supreme Court in 1983 endorsed this idea in *Barefoot v. Estelle*, 463 U.S. 880, 901 (1983) ("We are unconvinced . . . that the adversary process cannot be trusted to sort out the reliable from the unreliable evidence."); *see also* Michael H. Gottesman, *From* Barefoot *to* Daubert *to* Joiner: *Triple Play or Double Error?*, 40 ARIZ. L. REV. 753 (1998).

98. PETER W. HUBER, GALILEO'S REVENGE: JUNK SCIENCE IN THE COURTROOM (1991).

99. MARCIA ANGELL, SCIENCE ON TRIAL: THE CLASH OF MEDICAL EVIDENCE AND LAW IN THE BREAST IMPLANT CASE (1997); *see* INSTITUTE OF MEDICINE, SAFETY OF SILICONE BREAST IMPLANTS (1999) (no evidence of association of

implants with adverse health outcomes); Zena A. Stein, *Silicone Breast Implants: Epidemiological Evidence of Sequelae*, 89 AM. J. PUB. HEALTH 484 (1999) (reviewing epidemiologic evidence); Doug Bandow, *Many Torts Later, the Case against Implants Collapses*, WALL ST. J., Nov. 30, 1998, at A23 (independent U.K. committee found no histo-pathological, immunological, or epidemiological evidence of implant-related disease). The independent expert panel created by the trial court overseeing the breast implant litigation came to a similar result, perhaps vindicating the judicial process. Thomas M. Burton, *Implant Makers Get a Boost from a Report*, WALL ST. J., Dec. 2, 1998, at B1.

100. 509 U.S. 579 (1993).

101. *See* FEDERAL JUDICIAL CENTER, REFERENCE MANUAL ON SCIENTIFIC EVIDENCE (1994); *see also* John M. Conley & David W. Paterson, *The Science of Gatekeeping: The Federal Judicial Center's New Reference Manual on Scientific Evidence*, 74 N.C. L. REV. 1183 (1996).

102. Consider Prof. Feldman's critique of the Court's "shift to science": "The more closely legal standards hew to scientific ones for selecting information worth considering, the more often it will be apparent that science is severely uncertain about the causal effects of [toxic] substances. . . . When scientists are severely uncertain, . . . legal factfinders will lack a basis [for decision-making]." Feldman, *supra* note 4, at 2–3.

103. Daubert v. Merrell Dow Pharmaceuticals, Inc., 509 U.S. 579, 589. For post-*Daubert* cases, *see, e.g., Allen v. Pennsylvania Eng'g Corp.*, 102 F.3d 194 (5th Cir. 1996) (finding expert testimony that exposure to ethylene oxide caused cancer not scientifically valid under *Daubert*).

104. *Daubert*, 509 U.S., at 592–94. On remand, the Ninth Circuit added an additional factor—whether the expert has conducted research independent of the litigation. The court reasoned that research conducted for the purpose of the litigation was more likely to be biased. Daubert v. Merrell Dow Pharm., Inc. 43 F.3d 1311, 1317 (9th Cir. 1995) (*"Daubert II"*).

105. Kumho Tire Co. v. Carmichael, 526 U.S. 137 (1999) (holding that *Daubert* factors do not constitute a definitive checklist or test).

106. *Daubert*, 509 U.S. at 591.

107. *Daubert II*, 43 F.3d at 1315.

108. *In re* Paoli R.R. Yard PCB Litig., 35 F.3d 717, 745 (3d Cir. 1994) (finding an expert's extrapolation from animal studies to humans inadmissible).

109. Schudel v. General Elec. Co., 120 F.3d 991, 997 (9th Cir. 1997).

110. Buckley & Haake, *supra* note 88, at 10297.

111. 522 U.S. 136 (1997).

112. *Id.* at 146.

113. 526 U.S. 137 (1999).

114. *Id.* at 152.

115. Gottesman, *supra* note 97, at 759; Adina Schwartz, *A "Dogma of Empiricism" Revisited: Daubert v. Merrell Dow Pharmaceuticals, Inc. and the Need to Resurrect the Philosophy of Insight of Frye v. United States*, 10 HARV. J.L. & TECH. 149, 151 (1995).

116. G. EDWARD WHITE, TORT LAW IN AMERICA: AN INTELLECTUAL HISTORY 220–23, 230 (1980); Scott Burris, *Law and the Social Risk of Health Care: Lessons from HIV Testing*, 61 ALB. L. REV. 831 (1998).

117. My appreciation goes to my colleague Lisa Heinzerling for the idea that limitations of traditional tort doctrines can sometimes be helpful to public health advocates.

118. Jon Hanson, *Taking Behavioralism Seriously: Some Evidence of Market Manipulation,* 112 HARV. L. REV. 1420 (1999).

119. Edward Hammond & Daniel Horn, *Smoking and Death Rates: Report on 44 Months of Follow-up on 187,783 Men, I & II,* 166 JAMA 1159, 1294 (1958); Richard Doll & A. Bradford Hill, *A Study of the Aetiology of Carcinoma of the Lung,* 2 BRIT. MED. J. 1271 (1952); Ernest L. Wynder & Evarts A. Graham, *Tobacco Smoking as a Possible Etiologic Factor in Bronchiogenic Carcinoma: A Study of Six Hundred and Eighty-Four Proved Cases,* 143 JAMA 329 (1950).

120. Roy Norr, *Cancer by the Carton,* READER's DIG., Dec. 1952, at 7; Lois Mattox Miller & James Monahan, *The Facts Behind the Cigarette Controversy,* READER's DIG., July 1954, at 1.

121. Lowe v. R.J. Reynolds Tobacco Co., No. 9673(C) (E.D. Mo. filed March 10, 1954) (case subsequently dropped).

122. Robert Rabin, *A Socio-Legal History of the Tobacco Tort Litigation,* 44 STAN. L. REV. 853, 857 (1992). See Wendy E. Parmet, *Tobacco, HIV, and the Courtroom: The Role of Affirmative Litigation in the Formation of Public Health Policy,* 36 HOUS. L. REV. 1663 (1999).

123. *See, e.g.,* Lartigue v. R.J. Reynolds Tobacco Co., 317 F.2d 19 (5th Cir.), *cert. denied,* 375 U.S. 865 (1963); Green v. American Tobacco Co., 304 F.2d 70 (5th Cir. 1962), *aff'd,* 409 F.2d 1166 (5th Cir. 1969) (en banc), *cert. denied,* 397 U.S. 911 (1970).

124. Graham E. Kelder, Jr. & Richard A. Daynard, *The Role of Litigation in the Effective Control of the Sale and Use of Tobacco,* 8 STAN. L. & POL'Y REV. 63, 71 (1997).

125. SMOKING AND HEALTH: REPORT OF THE ADVISORY COMMITTEE TO THE SURGEON GENERAL OF THE PUBLIC HEALTH SERVICE (1964) (marshaling scientific data on the health risks posed by tobacco).

126. RESTATEMENT (SECOND) OF TORTS § 402A, comment i (1965).

127. 15 U.S.C. § 1333 (1994).

128. Linda Greenhouse, *Court to Say if Cigarette Makers Can Be Sued for Smokers' Cancer,* N.Y. TIMES, March 26, 1991, at A1.

129. Larry O. Gostin, et al., *Tobacco Liability and Public Health Policy,* 266 JAMA 3178, 3179 (1991).

130. Thayer v. Liggett & Meyers Tobacco Co., No. 5314 (W.D. Mich., Feb. 20, 1970) (cataloguing in detail how the industry wore down plaintiffs). The industry was also strident in its opposition to direct regulation. *See* Peter S. Arno, et al., *Tobacco Industry Strategies to Oppose Federal Regulation,* 275 JAMA 1258 (1996).

131. Richard A. Daynard & Graham E. Kelder, Jr., *The Many Virtues of Tobacco Litigation,* 34 TRIAL 34, 36 (1998).

132. Donald Janson, *Data on Smoking Revealed at Trial,* N.Y. TIMES, March 13, 1988, at A34.

133. 79 Stat. 282 (1965), *as amended,* 15 U.S.C. §§ 1331–1340 (1965) ("No statement relating to smoking and health [other than the congressionally mandated warnings] shall be required on any cigarette package.").

134. Public Health Cigarette Smoking Act, 84 Stat. 88 (1970), *as amended*, 15 U.S.C. §§ 1331–1340 (1969) ("No requirement or prohibition based on smoking and health shall be imposed [by a state] with respect to the advertising or promotion of any cigarettes.").

135. 505 U.S. 504 (1992).

136. *Id.* at 530–531.

137. Stanton A. Glantz et al., *Looking through a Keyhole at the Tobacco Industry: The Brown and Williamson Documents*, 274 JAMA 219 (1995); Peter Slade et al., *Nicotine and Addiction: The Brown and Williamson Documents*, 274 JAMA 225 (1995). The Brown and Williamson documents are available at <http://www.library.ucsf.edu/tobacco> (visited on May 22, 2000).

138. *See, e.g.,* Philip J. Hilts, *Tobacco Company Was Silent on Hazards,* N.Y. TIMES, May 7, 1994, at A1; Philip J. Hilts & Glenn Collins, *Records Show Philip Morris Studies Influence of Nicotine,* N.Y. TIMES, June 8, 1995, at A1.

139. *See, e.g.,* Richard D. Hurt & Channing R. Robertson, *Prying Open the Door to the Tobacco Industry's Secrets About Nicotine,* 280 JAMA 1173 (1998) (reviewing more than 39,000 internal documents disclosed in Minnesota's Medicaid recoupment suit).

140. *In re* Mike Moore, Attorney General *Ex. Rel.,* State of Mississippi Tobacco Litigation, No 94-1429 (Miss. Chanc., Jackson Co. 1994).

141. S. 1415 (105th Cong.) (1998). *See also* John Schwartz & Saundra Torry, *Tobacco Targets the McCain Bill,* WASH. POST, April 11, 1998, at A6.

142. The text of these settlements is available at <http://www.tobaccoresolution.com> (visited on May 22, 2000). Minnesota settled on perhaps the most favorable terms. *See* Minnesota v. Philip Morris et al., 551 N.W.2d 490 (Minn. 1996) (en banc). The Minnesota settlement is available at 1998 WL 394331.

143. Master Settlement Agreement (visited on May 22, 2000), <http://www.naag.org/tobac/cigmsa.rtf> .

144. United States v. Philip Morris, No. 1: 99 CVO2496 (D.D.C. 2000) (motion to dismiss filed Mar. 10, 2000). *See* Marc Lacey, *Tobacco Industry Accused of Fraud in Lawsuit by U.S.,* N.Y. TIMES, Sept. 23, 1999, at A1; Barry Meir, *2 Strategies at Work and Stiff Challenges Ahead in Federal Lawsuit,* N.Y. TIMES, *id.,* at A18 (U.S. seeking recovery for money spent on treating smoking-related diseases of elderly, military, and federal employees and also using racketeering statutes against manufacturers).

145. Thus far, medical reimbursement claims by trade unions have not been successful. *See, e.g.,* Massachusetts Laborers' Health and Welfare Fund v. Philip Morris, 62 F. Supp.2d 236 (D. Mass. 1999); Milwaukee Carpenter's District Council Health Fund v. Philip Morris, 70 F. Supp.2d 888 (E.D. Wisc. 1999); Saundra Torry, *Tobacco Firms Win Suit Filed by Unions,* WASH. POST, March 19, 1999, at A2 (Ohio jury ruling against 114 union health funds).

146. Republic of Guatemala v. Tobacco Institute et al., 83 F. Supp.2d 125 (D.D.C. 1999); Republic of Panama v. American Tobacco Co. et al. (No. 98-3279 E.D. La. 1999); Republic of Venezuela v. Philip Morris Co. et al. (No. 99-586 S.D. Fla. 1999).

147. Falise v. American Tobacco Co., 2000 U.S. Dist. LEXIS 5758 (E.D.N.Y. 2000).

148. Broin v. Philip Morris Co., 641 So. 2d 888 (Fla. App. 3d Dist. 1994), *rev. denied*, 654 So. 2d 919 (Fla. 1995) (certifying a class defined as all non-smoking flight attendants employed by U.S.–based airlines and suffering from diseases caused by exposure to second-hand smoke).

149. Ramos v. Philip Morris Co., No. 98–389, 1999 WL 157370 (Mar. 24, 1999).

150. Engle v. R.J. Reynolds Co., No. 94–08273 CA-22 (Fla. Cir. Ct. 11th Jud. Cir., April 7, 2000).

151. 84 F.3d 734 (5th Cir. 1996).

152. Daynard & Kelder, *supra* note 131, at 72–73.

153. *See, e.g.,* Barnes v. American Tobacco Co., 161 F.3d 127 (3rd Cir. 1998) (decertifying a class of Pennsylvania residents who began smoking before age nineteen), *cert. denied*, 526 U.S. 1760 (1999).

154. Brown & Williamson Tobacco Corp. v. Carter, No. 96-4831, 1998 Fla. App. LEXIS 7477 (Fla. Dist. Ct. App. June 22, 1998) (the jury awarded a verdict of $750,000, but the verdict was overturned and further appeals are planned).

155. Estate of Jesse D. Williams v. Philip Morris Inc., No. 9705 03957 (Ore. Cir. Multnomah Co. Mar. 30, 1999) (the jury awarded the family of a smoker $80 million, but the damages are expected to be reduced by the court). *See* Milo Geyelin, *Philip Morris Hit with Record Damages*, WALL ST. J., March 31, 1999, at A3.

156. Barry Meir, *Punitive Damages Added in Smoking Case Verdict*, N.Y. TIMES, March 28, 2000, at A11 (San Francisco jury ordering two cigarette manufacturers to pay $20 million in punitive damages in the first case decided in favor of a person who started smoking after government-imposed warning labels); Patricia Henley v. Philip Morris Inc., No. 995172, Calif. Super., San Francisco Co. (April 7, 1999) (the trial judge reduced the punitive damages award from $50 to $25 million).

157. Some individual actions are being dismissed because of the "common knowledge" that tobacco is harmful. *See, e.g.,* Tompkins v. R.J. Reynolds Tobacco Co., 2000 U.S. Dist. LEXIS 4451 (N.D.N.Y. 2000).

158. Work-product discovery allows plaintiffs to request materials from other plaintiffs or previous cases that would normally be protected.

159. Milo Geyelin, *Behind Giant Tobacco Verdicts, A Legal SWAT Team*, WALL ST. J., April 12, 1999, at B1.

160. Danny David, *Three Paths to Justice: New Approaches to Minority Instituted Tobacco Litigation*, 15 HARV. BLACKLETTER L.J. 185 (1999).

161. Saundra Torry, *Anti-Smoking Efforts Getting Little from Deal*, WASH. POST, April 28, 1999, at A3.

162. The two leading mechanisms causing fatal injury in the United States are motor vehicles and firearms. INSTITUTE OF MEDICINE, REDUCING THE BURDEN OF INJURY: ADVANCING PREVENTION AND TREATMENT 124–25 (Richard J. Bonnie, et al. eds., 1999).

163. Robert J. Blendon et al., *The American Public and the Gun Control Debate*, 275 JAMA 1719 (1996).

164. Centers for Disease Control & Prevention, *Nonfatal and Fatal Firearm-Related Injuries—United States*, 48 MORBID. & MORTAL. WKLY. REP. 1029 (1999). *See* Jon S. Vernick and Stephen P. Teret, *New Courtroom Strategies*

Regarding Firearms: Tort Litigation against Firearm Manufacturers and Constitutional Challenges to Gun Laws, 36 Hous. L. Rev. 1713, 1714–1716 (1999); Kimberley D. Peters et al., *Deaths: Final Data for 1996,* 47 Nat'l Vital Stat. Rep. 67 (1998); Joseph L. Annest et al., *National Estimates of Nonfatal Firearm-Related Injures: Beyond the Tip of the Iceberg,* 273 JAMA 1749, 1751 (1995); Nancy Sinauer et al., *Unintentional, Nonfatal Firearm-Related Injuries: A Preventable Public Health Burden,* 275 JAMA 1740 (1996).

165. *See, e.g.,* Lois A. Fingerhut & Margy Warner, National Ctr. for Health Statistics, Injury Chartbook: Health, United States, 1996–1997 (1997); National Ctr. for Injury Prevention and Control, Fatal Firearm Injuries in the United States, 1962–1994 (1997); D. Cherry et al., *Trends in Nonfatal and Fatal Firearm-Related Injury Rates in the United States, 1985–1995,* 32 Ann. Emerg. Med. 51 (1998).

166. National Ctr. for Health Statistics, Health, United States, 1998 with Socioeconomic Status and Health Chartbook (1998) (black male firearm deaths per 100,000 population is 57.5, compared with a rate of 14 for the general population).

167. *See, e.g.,* Centers for Disease Control & Prevention, *Rates of Homicide, Suicide, and Firearm-Related Death among Children—26 Industrialized Countries,* 46 Morb. Mort. Wkly. Rep. 101 (1997); Etienne G. Krug et al., *Firearm-Related Deaths in the United States and 35 Other High and Upper-Middle-Income Countries,* 27 Int. J. Epidemiol. 214 (1998).

168. *See, e.g.,* McAndrew v. Mularchuk, 162 A.2d 820 (N.J. 1960) (finding that the potential of a loaded revolver to inflict serious injury is such that the law imposes a duty to employ extraordinary care in its handling and use). *But see* Miller v. Kennedy, 196 Cal. App. 3d 141 (Cal. App. 2d Dist. 1987) (finding that, in an action against a police officer by a man accidentally shot, the standard is ordinary care); Shaw v. Lord, 137 P. 885 (Okla. 1914) (requiring ordinary negligence for liability for firearm use in self-defense).

169. Mark D. Polston & Douglas S. Weil, *Unsafe By Design: Using Tort Actions to Reduce Firearm-Related Injuries,* 8 Stan. L. & Pol'y Rev. 13, 16 (1997).

170. Restatement (Second) of Torts § 308 (App. 1986) (duty on the person who controls a dangerous instrument to refrain from entrusting it to any person the controller has reason to know is likely to create an unreasonable risk of harm).

171. *See, e.g.,* Kitchen v. K-Mart Corp., 697 So. 2d 1200 (Fla. 1997) (holding the seller of a firearm to an intoxicated buyer liable to an injured person under the theory of negligent entrustment); 16 Verdicts, Settlements & Tactics 112 (a gun show was found liable for the criminal acts of juveniles who stole weapons from the gun show).

172. Richard C. Miller, *A Call to Arms: Trends in Firearms Litigation,* 29 Trial 24 (1993).

173. Polston & Weil, *supra* note 169, at 14.

174. American Acad. of Pediatrics & Am. Psychol. Ass'n, Raising Children to Resist Violence: What You Can Do (1995).

175. Yvonne D. Senturia et al., *Gun Storage Patterns in U.S. Homes with Children,* 150 Archives Pediatrics & Adolescent Med. 265 (1996).

176. *See, e.g,* National Inst. of Justice, Guns in America: Results of a Comprehensive National Survey on Firearms Ownership and Use (1997) (34 percent of owners keep their handguns loaded and unlocked); Douglas Weil & David Hemenway, *Loaded Guns in the Home: Analysis of a National Random Survey of Gun Owners,* 267 JAMA 3033 (1992); David Hemenway et al., *Firearm Training and Storage,* 273 JAMA 46 (1995).

177. *See, e.g.,* Cal. Penal Code § 12035 (West 1991).

178 Restatement (Second) of Torts § 308, comment b (1965) (using a child's access to a firearm as an illustration of negligent entrustment).

179. *See, e.g.,* Butcher v. Cordova, 728 P.2d 388 (Colo. Ct. App. 1986) (applying § 308 to child access to a firearm); Reida v. Lund, 18 Cal. App. 3d 698 (1971) (imposing liability even though the rifle was kept locked, since the son knew the location of the key). *But see* Robertson v. Wentz, 187 Cal. App. 3d 1281 (Cal. Ct. App. 1986) (failing to impose liability when the parent had no ability to restrain a minor's access to firearms kept in the house).

180. Centers for Disease Control & Prevention, *Motor-Vehicle Safety: A 20th Century Public Health Achievement,* 48 Morb. Mort. Wkly. Rep. 369 (1999) (reduction of the rate of death from motor vehicle crashes due to technology changes represents one of the great public health achievements of the century); David Hemenway, *Regulation of Firearms,* 339 New Eng. J. Med. 843, 844 (1998) ("[I]njury control experts recognized that to increase the safety of driving, it would be more cost effective to try to change the vehicle and the highway environment than to try to change human behavior.").

181. General Accounting Office, Accidental Shootings: Many Deaths and Injuries Caused By Firearms Could Be Prevented 2 (1991) (31 percent of deaths occurred either because a child was able to fire the gun or because it was fired by a person unaware that the gun was loaded).

182. Stephen P. Teret et al., *Making Guns Safer,* 14 Issues Sci. Technol. 37 (1998); Garen J. Wintemute, *The Relationship between Firearm Design and Firearm Violence,* 275 JAMA 1749 (1996).

183. A gun can be personalized with electronic technologies (e.g., "fingerprint" recognition or radio frequencies) or "self-locking" devices so the firearm can only be discharged with a key or combination. K.D. Robinson et al., Personalized Guns: Reducing Gun Deaths through Design Changes (2d ed. 1997); Jon S. Vernick, *I Didn't Know the Gun Was Loaded: An Examination of Two Safety Devices That Can Reduce the Risk of Unintentional Firearm Injuries,* 20 J. Pub. Health Pol'y 427 (1999).

184. John P. McNicholas & Matthew McNicholas, *Ultrahazardous Products Liability: Providing Victims of Well-Made Firearms Ammunition to Fire Back at Gun Manufacturers,* 30 Loy. L.A. L. Rev. 1599, 1601 (1997) ("There is no other reason [but mass killing] to allow the gun to swivel from the hip in a spray-fire fashion, to . . . permit the user to fire thirty-two rounds without reloading, or to adjust the trigger so that the product can empty its hail of fire.").

185. *See, e.g.,* Johnson v. Colt Indus. Operating Corp., 797 F.2d 1530 (10th Cir. 1986) (holding the manufacturer, as one engaged in a dangerous enterprise, to a higher standard of care to avoid negligence in a products liability action where a revolver discharged when dropped, injuring the plaintiff).

186. Herman v. Markham Air Rifle Co., 258 F. 475 (D.C. Cir. 1918) (failure to test and inspect rifle before selling it, loaded, to a consumer who subsequently accidentally shot the plaintiff).

187. The following cases involving failure to provide a loaded chamber indicator or a magazine safety were not allowed to proceed to trial: Bolduc v. Colt's Mfg. Co., Inc., 968 F. Supp. 16 (D. Mass. 1997); Wasylow v. Glock, 975 F. Supp. 370 (D. Mass. 1996); Raines v. Colt Indus., 757 F. Supp 819 (E.D. Mich. 1991); Crawford v. Navegar, 554 N.W.2d 311 (Mich. 1996).

188. See Richman v. Charter Arms Corp., 571 F. Supp 192 (E.D. La. 1983) (holding that criminal use of a handgun was a "normal" use and marketing to the public was not an "unreasonably dangerous activity").

189. See, e.g., Perkins v. F.I.E. Corp., 762 F.2d 1250 (5th Cir.), reh'g. denied en banc, 768 F.2d 1350 (1985) (denying strict liability as an available remedy where guns functioned as designed and dangers were obvious and well known); Raines, 757 F. Supp. at 819 (manufacturer absolved from liability because risks of firearms are known and expected).

190. See, e.g., Moore v. R.G. Indus., 789 F.2d 1326 (9th Cir. 1986) (refusing to impose strict liability on the manufacturer of a .25 caliber automatic handgun for injuries to a woman shot by her husband since the product "performed as intended"); Shipman v. Jennings Firearms, Inc., 791 F.2d 1532 (11th Cir. 1986) (refusing to impose liability on the manufacturer of a .22 caliber pistol that was used by a husband to kill his wife where the handgun "performed exactly as intended"). But see Kelly v. R.G. Indus., 497 A.2d 1143 (Md. 1985) (holding the manufacturer of the "Saturday Night Special" handgun strictly liable, but the court's reasoning was later rejected by the legislature, Md. Ann. Code, Art. 27 § 36-I(h) (1992)).

191. See, e.g., Mavilia v. Stoeger Indus., 574 F. Supp 107 (D. Mass. 1983) (finding that, in the death of a bystander, an automatic pistol was not inherently defective based on the claim that the risk outweighed the social utility); Patterson v. Rohm Gesellschaft, 608 F. Supp 1206, 1211 (N.D. Tex. 1985) (finding that strict liability against the manufacturer of a .38 caliber revolver for death during robbery based on risk-utility theory was "nonsense"); Moore, 789 F.2d at 1326 (Cal. Civ. Code § 1714.4 (1999) provides that no firearm is defective in design on the basis that its risks outweigh its benefits).

192. See Decker v. Gibson Prods. Co. of Albany, 679 F.2d 212, 215–16 (11th Cir. 1982) (holding that the foreseeability of an ex-convict murdering his former wife with a handgun was a jury question).

193. Merrill v. Navegar Inc., 75 Cal. App. 4th 500 (Cal. Ct. App., 1st App. Dist., Div. 2 filed Sept. 1999) (allowing jury determination on alleged negligence in manufacturing, marketing, and distributing a semiautomatic assault weapon used to kill eight people in a law firm).

194. See, e.g., Hurst v. Glock, Inc., 684 A.2d 970 (N.J. Super. Ct. App. Div. 1996) (finding that, even though guns present "obvious" danger, a gun could be defective because it did not have a device that prevents discharge when the ammunition magazine is removed).

195. Joseph Sugarmann & Kristen Rand, Violence Policy Center, Cease Fire: A Comprehensive Strategy to Reduce Firearms Violence (1997).

196. Bubalo et al. v. Navegar, No. 96-C-3664, 1997 U.S. Dist. LEXIS 855 (N.D. Ill. June 11, 1997), *reconsidered*, 1998 U.S. Dist. LEXIS 3598 (March 30, 1998); *In re* 101 California Street, Master File No. 959-316 (Cal. Super. Ct., May 6, 1997).

197. Jon S. Vernick et al., *Regulating Firearm Advertisements That Promise Home Protection: A Public Health Intervention*, 277 JAMA 1391 (1997).

198. Garen J. Wintemute, et al., *Mortality among Recent Purchasers of Handguns*, 341 NEW ENG. J. MED. 1583 (1999); Arthur L. Kellermann et al., *Gun Ownership as a Risk Factor for Homicide in the Home*, 329 NEW ENG. J. MED. 1084 (1993); Arthur L. Kellermann et al., *Suicide in the Home in Relation to Gun Ownership*, 327 NEW ENG. J. MED. 467 (1992); *but see* John R. Lott & David B. Mustard, *Crime, Deterrence and Right-to-Carry Concealed Handguns*, 26 J. LEGAL STUD. 1 (1997).

199. Hamilton v. ACCU-Tek, 62 F. Supp. 2d 802 (E.D.N.Y. 1996) (allowing a jury to decide the claim that manufacturers negligently created a nationwide market in handguns and, foreseeably, these guns were obtained by criminals in N.Y. City).

200. *See* Andrew O. Smith, *The Manufacture and Distribution of Handguns as an Abnormally Dangerous Activity*, 54 U. CHI. L. REV. 369 (1987); McNicholas & McNicholas, *supra* note 184.

201. *See, e.g.,* Copier v. Smith & Wesson, 138 F.3d 833 (10th Cir. 1998); Martin v. Harrington & Richardson, Inc., 743 F.2d 1200 (7th Cir. 1984); Armijo v. Ex Cam, Inc., 656 F. Supp 771 (D.N.M. 1987); Riordan v. International Armament Corp., 477 N.E.2d 1293 (Ill. App. Ct. 1985); Burkett v. Freedom Arms, Inc., 704 P.2d 118 (Or. 1985).

202. Wendy Max & Dorothy P. Rice, *Shooting in the Dark: Estimating the Cost of Firearm Injuries*, 12 HEALTH AFFS. 171 (1993); Ted R. Miller & Mark A. Cohen, *Costs of Gunshot and Cut/Stab Wounds in the United States, with Some Canadian Comparisons*, 29 ACCID. ANAL. & PREV. 329 (1997) (total costs estimated at $126 billion annually).

203. U.S. DEP'T OF JUSTICE, FEDERAL BUREAU OF INVESTIGATION, CRIME IN THE UNITED STATES, 1996 (1997).

204. Fox Butterfield, *Safety and Crime at Heart of Talks on Gun Lawsuits*, N.Y. TIMES, Oct. 2, 1999, at A1 (twenty eight cities and counties are in the discovery phase of gun litigation); Stephanie Stapleton, *Cities Take Aim at Gun Industry*, AMA NEWS (Jan. 25, 1999), at 1, 30 (50–100 local governments could litigate); *see* Brian J. Siebel, *City Lawsuits against the Gun Industry: A Roadmap for Reforming Another Deadly Industry*, 18 ST. LOUIS U. PUB. L. REV. 247 (1999); David Kairys, *Legal Claims of Cities against the Manufacturers of Handguns*, 71 TEMP. L. REV. 1 (1998). Thus far, the city lawsuits have been unsuccessful. *See* City of Cincinnati v. Beretta, 1999 Ohio Misc. LEXIS 27 (1999) (finding that absent statutory authorization, plaintiff was not permitted to recover for expenditures for ordinary public services it had a duty to provide); Ganim v. Smith & Wesson Corp., 1999 Conn. Super. LEXIS 3330 (1999) (finding that plaintiffs lacked standing and granting motion to dismiss).

205. Civ. Action No. 98-18578 (Civ. Dist. Parish of New Orleans, filed Oct. 30, 1998).

206. No. 98 CH 15596 (Cook County Cir. Ct., Ill., filed Nov. 12, 1998).
207. Public nuisance theory is discussed, in chapter 9.
208. Siebel, *supra* note 204 (a substantial proportion of the 2.5–3.9 million handguns sold end up being used in crime).
209. *Id.*
210. James Dao, *Under Legal Siege, Gunmaker Agrees to Accept Curbs,* N.Y. TIMES, March 18, 2000, at A1.
211. Polston & Weil, *supra* note 169, at 17.
212. Jon S. Vernick, *New Courtroom Strategies Regarding Firearms: Tort Litigation against Firearm Manufactures and Constitutional Challenges to Gun Laws,* 36 HOUS. L. REV. 1713 (1999).
213. Stephen P. Teret et al., *Support for New Policies to Regulate Firearms,* 339 NEW ENG. J. MED. 813 (1998).
214. 15 U.S.C. § 2052(a)(1)(E) (1994).
215. American Shooting Sports Council Inc. v. Attorney General, 429 Mass. 871 (1999) (upholding regulations on the sale of defective or unsafe handguns).
216. *See, e.g.,* H.B. 189, 145th Gen. Assem., Reg. Sess., Ga. (1999).
217. SOCIAL DETERMINANTS OF HEALTH (Michael Marmot and Richard G. Wilkinson eds., 1999); Rich Hahn et al., *Poverty and Death in U.S.—1973 and 1991,* 6 EPIDEMIOLOGY 490–97 (1995), Department of Health & Hum. Servs., *Missed Opportunities in Monitoring SES,* 112 PUBLIC HEALTH REPORTS 492–94 (Nov. 1997).
218. Tort costs may be viewed as much higher than they actually are, but if companies have inflated views of these costs, they may respond in the same way as if the costs were real.
219. Tort costs have had profound effects on company decisions and national policy, as illustrated with vaccine litigation. In response to industry concerns about the tort costs of vaccine-induced injuries, Congress enacted the National Childhood Vaccine Injury Act, 42 U.S.C. §§ 300aa–1 (1997) (providing "no fault" compensation for vaccine-induced injury to children). *See* Derry Ridgway, *No-Fault Vaccine Insurance: Lessons from the National Vaccine Injury Compensation Program,* 24 J. HEALTH POL., POL'Y & L. 59 (1999).
220. For example, Merrell Dow withdrew the morning sickness drug Bendectin from the market due to escalating insurance and litigation costs even though there was no scientific evidence of a causal relationship between the drug and birth defects. *See* JOSEPH SANDERS, BENDECTIN ON TRIAL: A STUDY OF MASS TORT LITIGATION (1998); KENNETH R. FOSTER & PETER W. HUBER, JUDGING SCIENCE: SCIENTIFIC KNOWLEDGE AND THE FEDERAL COURTS 1–7 (1997).
221. For example, each year the tort system generates one suit for every 2.5 obstetricians, neurosurgeons, and orthopedists and nearly one suit for every 5 physicians overall.
222. Think about the silicone breast implant litigation discussed above, where Dow Corning filed for bankruptcy as part of a $3.2 billion settlement; the jury verdicts appeared to fly in the face of the scientific evidence. Does the deterrent signal in this litigation teach corporations to engage in reasonable safety checks before putting a product on the market or does it simply retard innovation? In the face of scientific uncertainty, what out-

come would be more unjust: failure to compensate women if implants did, in fact, cause systemic disease or corporate bankruptcy for unwarranted product liability? For an exposition of this dilemma, see Ruth Macklin, *Ethics, Epidemiology, and Law: The Case of Silicone Breast Implants*, 89 Am. J. Pub. Health 487 (1999); George J. Annas, *Burden of Proof: Judging Science and Protecting Public Health in (and out of) the Courtroom*, 89 Am. J. Pub. Health 490, 492 (1999) (arguing that Dow Corning was wrong for failing to conduct pre- and post-marketing safety studies or to warn surgeons and potential users).

11. PUBLIC HEALTH LAW REFORM

SOURCES FOR CHAPTER EPIGRAPHS: Page 309: *The Untilled Fields of Public Health*, 51 Science 23, 30 (1920). Page 311: William Roper, *Why the Problem of Leadership in Public Health?, in* Leadership in Public Health 20, 21 (C.-E.A. Winslow, Ed., 1994) (Roper was first head of the Health Care Financing Administration [HCFA] and then head of the Centers for Disease Control and Prevention [CDC]). Page 315: Isaiah Berlin, Two Concepts of Liberty, Inaugural Lecture Before the University of Oxford (Oct. 31, 1958) (transcript available in the Georgetown University Law Center Library).

1. Frank P. Grad, Public Health Law Manual 4 (2d ed. 1990).

2. Institute of Medicine, The Future of Public Health 19 (1988).

3. *Id.* at 10.

4. *See* Lawrence O. Gostin, Scott Burris, & Zita Lazzarini, Improving State Law to Prevent and Treat Infectious Disease (1998); Lawrence O. Gostin, Scott Burris, & Zita Lazzarini, *The Law and the Public's Health: A Study of Infectious Disease Law in the United States*, 99 Colum. L. Rev. 59 (1999); Lawrence O. Gostin, *The Future of Public Health Law*, 12 Am. J.L. & Med. 461 (1986).

5. Barbara Gutmann Rosenkrantz, Public Health and the State: Changing Views in Massachusetts, 1842–1936, at 5 n.10 (citing N.Y. City Health Dep't, Monthly Bull., October 1911).

6. *See, e.g.,* Daniel M. Fox, *Accretion, Reform, and Crisis: A Theory of Public Health Politics in New York City*, 64 Yale J. Bio. & Med. 455 (1991) (describing the politics of public health in New York City and proposing three descriptive models: accretion, reform, and crisis).

7. See discussion of "lay" and "expert" perceptions of risk in chapter 4.

8. Under Geoffrey Rose's "prevention paradox," measures that have the greatest potential for improving public health (such as seat belt use) offer little absolute benefit to any individual, while measures that heroically save individual lives (such as heart transplants) make no significant contribution to the population's health. Public health, in other words, has as its chief duty the unenviable tasks of providing common goods and controlling negative externalities, both difficult at best. Telling individuals and businesses to change what they do (and profit by) in order to achieve the absence of illness in others is a hard sell in the marketplace for social resources. Geoffrey Rose, *Sick Individuals and Sick Populations*, 14 Int. J. Epidemiol. 32, 38 (1985).

9. *See* Kay W. Eilbert et al., Measuring Expenditures for Essential Public Health Services 17 (1996). Eilbert and her colleagues base their figures on a survey of nine states. These results are consistent with other research findings indicating a declining trend in expenditures for public health. During the past two decades, public health funding has declined from 1.2 cents of the national health dollar to 0.9 cents. *See* Edward L. Baker et al., *Health Reform and the Health of the Public: Forging Community Health Partnerships*, 272 JAMA 1277 (1994). *See also* Centers for Disease Control, *Estimated National Spending on Prevention: United States, 1988*, 41 Morb. Mort. Wkly. Rep. 529, 531 (1992); Philip R. Lee, *Reinventing Public Health*, 270 JAMA 2670, 2670 (1993).

10. Richard H. Morrow & John H. Bryant, *Health Policy Approaches to Measuring and Valuing Human Life: Conceptual and Ethical Issues*, 85 Am. J. Pub. Health 1356, 1356 (1995).

11. Institute of Medicine, *supra* note 2, at 17–18 (stressing the need for public health agencies to find ways to build political support).

12. *Id.* at 119–22. The crisis is reflected in the fact that the average tenure of a state health director in the United States is less than two years. *See* William Roper, *Why the Problem of Leadership in Public Health?*, in Leadership in Public Health 21–27 (Paul D. Cleary ed., 1994). Roper makes two recommendations to overcome barriers to leadership: Public health authorities should integrate leadership training into preparation for a public health career, and they should improve working conditions and reduce the impact of job insecurity on professionals.

13. *See* Arthur P. Liang et al., *Survey of Leadership Skills Needed for State and Territorial Health Officers, United States, 1988*, 108 Pub. Health Rep. 116, 119 (1993) (concluding that development of effective public health leaders requires recognition that they need political skills; knowledge of the legislative, administrative, and legal systems; and a familiarity with strategic planning in facing political and financial constraints).

14. *See* Baker et al., *supra* note 9, at 1276, 1280–82.

15. *See* Institute of Medicine, Improving Health in the Community: A Role for Performance Monitoring 77–125 (1997).

16. *Id.* at 77–85.

17. *See* U.S. Dep't of Health & Hum. Servs., Public Health Serv., Healthy People 2000: National Health Promotion and Disease Prevention Objectives 85–88 (1990). *See also* U.S. Dep't of Health & Hum. Servs., Healthy People 2010 (2000). The extensive literature on the problems of regulating health risks has repeatedly emphasized the problems that arise because of bureaucratic borders, which include not simply competing or overlapping jurisdiction over various threats, but even conflicting approaches to defining, measuring, and assessing risks. *See, e.g.*, Cass R. Sunstein, *Health-Health Tradeoffs*, 63 U. Chi. L. Rev. 1533, 1539–42 (1996).

18. *See, e.g.*, Elizabeth Fee, *History and Development of Public Health*, in Principles of Public Health Practice 10 (F. Douglas Scutchfield & C. William Keck eds., 1996).

19. Joel Feinberg, The Moral Limits of the Criminal Law: Harm to Self 27 (vol. 3, 1986).

20. There is a pervasive scholarly discussion of "positive" rights, and their justification, in the human rights literature. *See, e.g.*, LAWRENCE O. GOSTIN & ZITA LAZZARINI, HUMAN RIGHTS AND PUBLIC HEALTH IN THE AIDS PANDEMIC 12–32 (1997); Steven D. Jamar, *The International Human Right to Health*, 22 S. U. L. REV. 1 (1994); Michael Kirby, *The Right to Health Fifty Years On: Still Skeptical*, 4 HEALTH HUM. RTS. 7 (1999).

21. A few states have largely eliminated these distinctions by revising their statutes to apply a unified disease control system. *See, e.g.*, TEX. HEALTH & SAFETY CODE ANN. § 81 (West 1992 & Supp. 1998); MINN. STAT. §§ 144. 989–.993 (1996). Of course, consolidation may only be temporary. Texas consolidated its statute in 1989, but since then has enacted several provisions dealing solely with HIV. *See* TEX. HEALTH & SAFETY CODE ANN. §§ 81.050–.052, .090, .102–.103, .109 (West 1992 & Supp. 1998).

22. Legislatures, understandably, may be wary of imposing affirmative duties on agencies because of resource constraints. Government normally does not want to promise services that in the future it may be unable to deliver. Affording a right to services, moreover, can lead to political disputes about which departmental entity is responsible for incurring the expense. *See* County of Cook v. City of Chicago, 593 N.E. 2d 928 (Ill. 1992) (finding that the county, not the city, was responsible for expenses for treating city residents with TB at county hospital after the city closed a sanitarium). Some legislatures, however, may deem public health so important that they would create enforceable duties. Others could adopt creative mechanisms for setting expectations without promising unlimited resources. This could be achieved by legislative language making clear that individuals could not enforce these duties in court and/or that the duties are bounded by resource constraints (e.g., "the highest level of disease prevention and health promotion that the health department can achieve within the limits of its resources").

23. Kristine M. Gebbie & Inseon Hwang, *Identification of Health Paradigms in Use in State Public Health Agencies*, COLUM. U. SCH. OF NURSING 5 (Oct. 28, 1997) ("Study of organization or reorganization in state government illustrates the importance of the understood goal or paradigm in decisions regarding the structure of state health agencies, a structure which is only partially within the control of the agency and partially decided by the state's governor and legislature.").

24. SUTHERLAND STAT. CONST. § 47.04 (4th ed.) (while the preamble cannot control the enacting part of the statute, it may illuminate the intent of the legislature).

25. This is the model recommended by experts in the field of public health. *See* INSTITUTE OF MEDICINE, *supra* note 15.

26. Gebbie & Hwang, *supra* note 23.

27. *See, e.g.*, Scott Burris, *Law and the Social Risk of Health Care: Lessons from HIV Testing*, 61 ALB. L. REV. 831, 841–42 (1998) (discussing problems of stigma and social hostility in HIV control).

28. Lawrence O. Gostin et. al., *The Public Health Information Infrastructure: A National Review of the Law on Health Information Privacy*, 275 JAMA 1921–1927 (1996).

29. *See, e.g.*, Sutton v. United Air Lines, Inc., 527 U.S. 471 (1999).

30. *See, e.g.,* Alsbrook v. City of Maumelle, 184 F.3d 999 (8th Cir. 1999) (finding that Title II of the ADA did not validly abrogate Eleventh Amendment immunity from private suit in federal court).

31. 42 U.S.C. 12201 (b) (1994).

32. 42 U.S.C. 12113 (d) (1994).

33. Lawrence O. Gostin & James G. Hodge, Jr., *Model State Public Health Information Privacy Act* (last visited May 22, 2000), <http://www.critpath.org/msphpa/privacy.htm>.

34. *See* Baker et al., *supra* note 9, at 1277.

35. Scott Burris, *The Invisibility of Public Health: Population-Level Measures in a Politics of Market Individualism,* 87 AM. J. PUB. HEALTH 1607, 1609 (1997).

Selected Bibliography

This is a selective listing of books and articles on public health, ethics, and the law arranged by topic and listed in reverse chronological order. Each work is listed only once, even if it covers more than one topic.

TABLE OF CONTENTS

I.   PUBLIC HEALTH LAW IN THE UNITED STATES

Gostin, Lawrence O., Scott Burris, and Zita Lazzarini. "The Law and the Public's Health: A Study of Infectious Disease Law in the United States." *Columbia Law Review* 99 (1999): 59–128.

Gostin, Lawrence O., Scott Burris, Zita Lazzarini, and Kathleen Maguire. *Improving State Law to Prevent and Treat Infectious Disease.* New York: Milbank Memorial Fund, 1998.

Parmet, Wendy E. "From Slaughter-House to Lochner: The Rise and Fall of the Constitutionalization of Public Health." *American Journal of Legal History* 40 (1996): 476–505.

Wing, Kenneth R. *The Law and the Public's Health.* 4th ed. Ann Arbor, MI: Health Administration Press, 1995.

Christoffel, Tom, and Stephen P. Teret. *Protecting the Public: Legal Issues in Injury Prevention.* New York: Oxford University Press, 1993.

Grad, Frank P. *The Public Health Law Manual.* 2nd ed. Washington, DC: American Public Health Association, 1990.

Burris, Scott. "Rationality Review and the Politics of Public Health." *Villanova Law Review* 34 (1989): 933–982.

Gostin, Lawrence O. "The Future of Public Health Law." *American Journal of Law and Medicine* 12 (1986): 461–490.

Merritt, Deborah Jones. "Communicable Disease and Constitutional Law: Controlling AIDS." *New York University Law Review* 61 (1986): 739–799.

Merritt, Deborah Jones. "The Constitutional Balance between Health and Liberty." *Hastings Center Report* 16 Supp. (Dec. 1986): 2–10.

Tobey, James A. *Public Health Law: A Manual of Law for Sanitarians.* 2nd ed. New York: Commonwealth Press, 1939.

Parker, Leroy, and Robert H. Worthington. *The Law of Public Health and Safety, and the Powers and Duties of Boards of Health.* Albany, NY: Bender, 1892.

II.   INTERNATIONAL AND COMPARATIVE PUBLIC HEALTH LAW

Fidler, David P. *International Law and Infectious Diseases.* Oxford: Clarendon Press, 1999.

Bidmeade, Ian, and Chris Reynolds. *Public Health Law in Australia: Its Current State and Future Directions.* Canberra; ACT: Australian Government Publishing Service, 1997.

Fluss, Sev S. "International Public Health Law: An Overview." In *Oxford Textbook of Public Health.* Edited by Roger Detels, Walter W. Holland,

James McEwen, and Gilbert S. Omenn, 3rd ed., 371–390. New York: Oxford University Press, 1997.

Roemer, Ruth. "Comparative National Public Health Legislation." In *Oxford Textbook of Public Health*. Edited by Roger Detels, Walter W. Holland, James McEwen, and Gilbert S. Omenn, 3rd ed., 351–370. New York: Oxford University Press, 1997.

III. PUBLIC HEALTH HISTORY

Porter, Dorothy. *Health, Civilization and the State: A History of Public Health from Ancient to Modern Times*. New York: Routledge, 1999.

Hays, J.N. *The Burdens of Disease: Epidemics and Human Response in Western History*. Brunswick, NJ: Rutgers University Press, 1998.

McNeill, William H. *Plagues and Peoples*. New York: Anchor Books, 1998.

Henig, Robin Marantz. *The People's Health: A Memoir of Public Health and Its Evolution at Harvard*. Washington, DC: Joseph Henry Press, 1997.

Watts, Sheldon. *Epidemics and History: Disease, Power and Imperialism*. New Haven, CT: Yale University Press, 1997.

Novak, William J. *The People's Welfare: Law and Regulation in Nineteenth-Century America*. Chapel Hill: University of North Carolina Press, 1996.

Porter, Dorothy, ed. *The History of Public Health and the Modern State*. Amsterdam: Rodopi, 1994.

Rosen, George. *A History of Public Health*. Expanded ed. Baltimore: Johns Hopkins University Press, 1993.

Duffy, John. *The Sanitarians: A History of American Public Health*. Urbana: University of Illinois Press, 1990.

Bayer, Ronald. *Private Acts, Social Consequences: AIDS and the Politics of Public Health*. New York: Free Press, 1989.

Dubos, Rene, and Jean Dubos. *The White Plague: Tuberculosis, Man and Society*. New Brunswick, NJ: Rutgers University Press, 1987.

Fee, Elizabeth. *Disease and Discovery: A History of the Johns Hopkins School of Hygiene and Public Health 1916–1939*. Baltimore: Johns Hopkins University Press, 1987.

Rosenberg, Charles. *The Cholera Years: The United States in 1832, 1849, and 1866*. Chicago: University of Chicago Press, 1987.

Rosenkrantz, Barbara G. *Public Health and the State: Changing Views in Massachusetts, 1842–1936*. Cambridge, MA: Harvard University Press, 1972.

Duffy, John. *A History of Public Health in New York City 1625–1866*. New York: Russell Sage Foundation, 1968.

Blake, John B. *Public Health in the Town of Boston 1630–1822*. Cambridge, MA: Harvard University Press, 1959.

Duffy, John. *Epidemics in Colonial America*. Baton Rouge: Louisiana State University Press, 1953.

Williams, R.C. *The United States Public Health Service, 1798–1950*. Washington, DC: Commissioned Officers Association of the United States Public Health Service, 1951.

Shattuck, Lemuel. *Report of a General Plan for the Promotion of Public and Personal Health, Devised, Prepared, and Recommended by the Commissioners*

Appointed under a Resolve of the Legislature of Massachusetts, Relating to a Sanitary Survey of the State. Boston: Dutton & Wentworth, 1850. Reprint, Cambridge, MA: Harvard University Press, 1948.

Winslow, Charles-Edward A. *Life of Hermann Biggs.* Philadelphia: Lea & Febiger, 1929.

Farr, William. *Vital Statistics: A Memorial Volume of Selections from the Reports and Writing, with a Biographical Sketch.* Edited by Noel A. Humphreys. London: Sanitary Institute, 1885.

IV. PUBLIC HEALTH THEORY AND POLITICS

Daniels, Norman. "Justice Is Good for Our Health." *Boston Review* (Feb/March 2000) 6–15.

Malmot, Micheal, and Richard G Wilkinson, eds. *Social Determinants of Health.* New York: Oxford University Press, 1999.

Burris, Scott. "The Invisibility of Public Health: Population-Level Measures in a Politics of Market Individualism." *American Journal of Public Health* 87 (1997): 1607–1610.

Fox, Daniel M. "The Politics of Public Health in New York City: Contrasting Styles since 1920." In *Hives of Sickness: Public Health and Epidemics in New York City,* edited by David Rosner, 197–210. New Brunswick, NJ: Rutgers University Press, 1995.

Lessig, Lawrence. "The Regulation of Social Meaning." *University of Chicago Law Review* 62 (1995): 943–1045.

McGinnis, J. Michael, and William H. Foege. "Actual Causes of Death in the United States." *Journal of the American Medical Association* 270 (Nov. 10, 1993): 2207–2212.

Turshen, Meredith. *The Politics of Public Health.* New Brunswick, NJ: Rutgers University Press, 1989.

Beauchamp, Dan E. *The Health of the Republic: Epidemics, Medicine, and Moralism as Challenges to Democracy.* Philadelphia: Temple University Press, 1988.

Beauchamp, Dan E. "Community: The Neglected Tradition of Public Health." *Hastings Center Report* 15 (1985): 28–36.

Rose, Geoffrey. "Sick Individuals and Sick Populations." *International Journal of Epidemiology* 14 (1985): 32–38.

Walzer, Michael. *Spheres of Justice: A Defense of Pluralism and Equality.* New York: Basic Books, 1983.

Beauchamp, Dan E. "What Is Public about Public Health?" *Health Affairs* 2 (1983): 76–87.

Beauchamp, Dan E. "Public Health as Social Justice." *Inquiry* (1976): 123–125.

V. PUBLIC HEALTH SYSTEMS AND PRACTICE

Mays, Glen P., C. Arden Miller, and Paul K. Halverson, eds. *Local Public Health Practice: Trends and Models.* Washington, DC: American Public Health Association, 2000.

Novick, Lloyd F., and Glen P. Mays, eds. *Public Health Administration: Principles of Population-Based Management.* Gaithersburg, MD: Aspen Publishers, 2000.

McKinlay, John B., and Lisa D. Marceau. "Public Health Matters." *American Journal of Public Health* 90 (2000): 25–33.

Gebbie, Kristine M. "State Public Health Laws: An Expression of Constituency Expectations." Journal of Public Health Management Practice 6 (2000): 46–54.

Centers for Disease Control and Prevention. "Ten Great Public Health Achievements—United States, 1900–1999 (series)." *Morbidity & Mortality Weekly Report* 48 (1999): 241–248.

Breslow, Lester. "From Disease Prevention to Health Promotion." *Journal of the American Medical Association* 281 (Mar. 17, 1999): 1030–1033.

Wall, Susan. "Transformations in Public Health Systems." *Health Affairs* 17, no. 3 (1998): 64–80.

Durch, Jane S., Linda A. Bailey, and Michael A. Stoto. *Improving Health in the Community: A Role for Performance Monitoring.* Washington, DC: National Academy Press, 1997.

Gebbie, Kristine M., and Inseon Hwang. *Identification of Health Paradigms in Use in State Public Health Agencies.* New York: Columbia University School of Nursing, 1997.

Holland, Walter W., and Susie Stewart. *Public Health: The Vision and the Challenge.* London: Nuffield Trust, 1997.

Lasker, Roz D. *Medicine & Public Health: The Power of Collaboration.* Chicago: Health Administration Press, 1997.

Lee, Philip R., and Carroll L. Estes, eds. *The Nation's Health.* 5th ed. Sudbury, MA: Jones & Bartlett Publishers, 1997.

Scutchfield, F. Douglas, and C. William Keck, eds. *Principles of Public Health Practice.* Albany, NY: Delmar, 1997.

Turnock, Bernard J. *Public Health: What It Is and How It Works.* Gaithersburg, MD: Aspen, 1997.

Stoto, Michael A., Cynthia Abel, and Anne Dievler, eds. *Healthy Communities: New Partnerships for the Future of Public Health.* Washington, DC: National Academy Press, 1996.

Roper, William. "Why the Problem of Leadership in Public Health?" In *Leadership in Public Health.* New York: Milbank Memorial Fund, 1994.

Baker, Edward L., Robert J. Melton, P.V. Stange, et al. "Health Reform and the Health of the Public: Forging Community Health Partnerships." *Journal of the American Medical Association* 272 (Oct. 26, 1994): 1276–1282.

Hanlon, John J., and George E. Pickett. *Public Health: Administration and Practice.* 9th. ed. St. Louis: Times Mirror/Mosby College Publishers, 1990.

Institute of Medicine. *The Future of Public Health.* Washington, DC: National Academy Press, 1988.

Smillie, Wilson G. *Public Health: Its Promise for the Future.* New York: Macmillan, 1955.

Winslow, Charles-Edward A. *The Evolution and Significance of the Modern Public Health Campaign.* New Haven, CT: Yale University Press, 1923.

Winslow, Charles Edward A. "The Untilled Fields of Public Health." *Science* 51 (Jan. 1920): 23–33.

VI. PUBLIC HEALTH ETHICS AND HUMAN RIGHTS

Kahn, Jeffery, and Anna Mastroianni. "Bioethics and Public Health: Trends for the New Millennium." *Annual Review of Public Health* (forthcoming).

Bradley, Peter, and Amanda Burls, eds. *Ethics in Public and Community Health*. New York: Routledge, 2000.

Beauchamp, Dan E, and Bonnie Steinbock, eds. *New Ethics for the Public's Health*. New York: Oxford University Press, 1999.

Dworkin, Gerald. "Paternalism." In *Philosophy of Law*. Edited by Joel Feinberg and Jules L. Coleman, 6th ed.271. Belmont, CA: Wadsworth, 1999.

Kirby, Michael. "The Right to Health Fifty Years On." *Health and Human Rights* 4 (1999) 7–25.

Mann, Jonathan M., Sofia Gruskin, and Michael A. Grodin et al. , eds. *Health and Human Rights: A Reader*. New York: Routledge, 1999.

Morone, James A. "Enemies of the People: The Moral Dimensions of Public Health." *Journal of Health Politics, Policy and Law* 22 (August 1997): 993–1020.

Coughlin, Steven S., ed. *Ethics in Epidemiology and Public Health Practice: Collected Works*. Columbus, GA: Quill Publications, 1997.

Gostin, Lawrence O., and Zita Lazzarini. *Human Rights and Public Health in the AIDS Pandemic*. New York: Oxford University Press, 1997.

Mann, Jonathan M. "Medicine and Public Health, Ethics and Human Rights." *Hastings Center Report* 27 (May 15, 1997): 6–13.

Coughlin, Steven S., and Tom L. Beauchamp. *Ethics and Epidemiology*. New York: Oxford University Press, 1996.

Cook, Rebecca J. *Women's Health and Human Rights: The Promotion and Protection of Women's Health through International Human Rights Law*. Geneva: World Health Organization, 1994.

Mann, Jonathan M., Lawrence O. Gostin, Sofia Gruskin, et al. "Health and Human Rights." *Journal of Health and Human Rights* 1 (1994): 6–22.

Gostin, Lawrence O., and Jonathan M. Mann. "Towards the Development of a Human Rights Impact Assessment for the Formulation and Evaluation of Health Policies." *Journal of Health and Human Rights* 1 (1994): 58–81.

Bonnie, Richard J. "The Efficacy of Law as a Paternalistic Instrument." In *Nebraska Symposium on Motivation*, 131–211. Lincoln: University of Nebraska Press, 1985.

VII. PUBLIC HEALTH POWERS: CONSTITUTIONAL STRUCTURE AND PRINCIPLES

Bowser, René, and Lawrence O. Gostin. "Managed Care and the Health of the Nation." *University of Southern California Law Review* 72 (1999): 1209–1295.

Hodge, James G. Jr. "The Role of New Federalism and Public Health Law." *Journal of Law and Health* 12 (1998): 309–357.

Parmet, Wendy E. "Health Care and the Constitution: Public Health and the Role of the State in the Framing Era." *Hastings Constitutional Law Quarterly* 20 (Winter 1992): 267–334.
Roettinger, Ruth Locke. *The Supreme Court and State Police Power: A Study in Federalism*. Washington, DC: Public Affairs Press, 1957.
Mustard, Harry. *Government in Public Health*. New York: Commonwealth Fund, 1945.
Tobey, James A. "Public Health and the Police Power." *New York University Law Review* 4 (1927): 126–133.
Freund, Ernst. *The Police Power: Public Policy and Constitutional Rights*. Chicago: Callaghan & Co., 1904.
Prentice, William Packer *Police Powers Arising under the Law of Overruling Necessity*. Albany, NY: Banks & Brothers, 1894.
Tiedeman, Christopher. *A Treatise on the Limitations of the Police Power in the United States*. New York: Da Capo Press, 1886.

VIII. LAW AND ECONOMICS: RISKS, BENEFITS, AND COSTS

Bennett, Peter, and Kenneth Calman, eds. *Risk Communication and Public Health*. New York: Oxford University Press, 1999.
Burris, Scott. "Law and the Social Risk of Health Care: Lessons from HIV Testing." *Albany Law Review* 61 (1998): 831–895.
Heinzerling, Lisa. "Regulatory Costs of Mythic Proportions." *Yale Law Journal* 107 (1998): 1981–2070.
Jolls, Christine, Cass R. Sunstein, and Richard Thaler. "A Behavioral Approach to Law and Economics." *Stanford Law Review* 50 (1998): 1471–1550.
Sunstein, Cass R. "A Note on 'Voluntary' versus 'Involuntary' Risks." *Duke Environmental Law and Policy Forum* 8 (1997): 173–180.
Arrow, Kenneth J. *Benefit-Cost Analysis in Environmental, Health, and Safety Regulations: A Statement of Principles*. Washington, DC: AEI, 1996.
Margolis, Howard. *Dealing with Risk: Why the Public and the Experts Disagree on Environmental Issues*. Chicago: University of Chicago Press, 1996.
Edited by Paul C. Stern, and Harvey V. Fineberg. Institute of Medicine *Understanding Risk: Informing Decisions in a Democratic Society*. Washington, DC: National Academy Press, 1996.
Arrow, Kenneth J., Maureen L. Cropper, George C. Eads, et al. "Is There a Role for Benefit-Cost Analysis in Environmental, Health, and Safety Regulation?" *Science* 272 (1996): 221–222.
Sunstein, Cass R. "Health-Health Tradeoffs." *University of Chicago Law Review* 63 (1996): 1533–1571.
Bayer, Ronald, Lawrence O. Gostin, and Devon C. McGraw. "Trades, AIDS, and the Public's Health: The Limits of Economic Analysis." *Georgetown Law Journal* 83 (1994): 79–107.
Breyer, Stephen. *Breaking the Vicious Circle: Toward Effective Risk Regulation*. Cambridge, MA: Harvard University Press, 1993.

Philipson, Thomas J., and Richard A. Posner. *Private Choices and Public Health: The AIDS Epidemic in an Economic Perspective.* Cambridge, MA: Harvard University Press, 1993.

Viscusi, W. Kip. *Fatal Tradeoffs: Public and Private Responsibilities for Risk.* New York: Oxford University Press, 1992.

Jasanoff, Sheila. *Risk Management and Political Culture: A Comparative Study of Science in the Policy Context.* New York: Russell Sage Foundation, 1986.

IX. SURVEILLANCE AND PRIVACY

Etzioni, Amitai. *The Limits of Privacy.* New York: Basic Books, 1999.

Edited by the Institute of Medicine. *For the Record: Protecting Electronic Health Information.* National Research Council. Washington, DC: National Academy Press, 1997.

Gostin, Lawrence O., Zita Lazzarini, Verla S. Neslund, et al. "The Public Health Information Infrastructure: A National Review of the Law on Health Information Privacy." *Journal of the American Medical Association* 275 (June 26, 1996): 1921–1927.

Gostin, Lawrence O. "Health Information Privacy." *Cornell Law Review* 80 (1995): 451–528.

Teutsch, Steven M., and R. Elliott Churchill. *Principles and Practice of Public Health Surveillance.* New York: Oxford University Press, 1994.

Berkelman, Ruth L., Ralph T. Bryon, Michael T. Osterholm, et al. "Infectious Disease Surveillance: A Crumbling Foundation." *Science* 264 (1994): 368–370.

Thacker, Stephen B., R.L. Berkelman and D.F. Stroup, et al. "The Science of Public Health Surveillance." *Journal of Public Health Policy* 10 (1989): 187–203.

Langmuir, Alexander D. "The Surveillance of Communicable Diseases of National Importance." *New England Journal of Medicine* 268 (Jan. 24, 1963): 182–192.

X. HEALTH PROMOTION AND HEALTH COMMUNICATION: FREE EXPRESSION

Buchanan, David R. *An Ethic for Health Promotion: Rethinking the Sources of Human Well-Being.* New York: Oxford University Press, 2000.

Callahan, Daniel, ed. *Promoting Health Behavior: How Much Freedom? Whose Responsibility?* Washington, DC: Georgetown University Press, 2000.

Sage, William M. "Regulating through Information: Disclosure Laws and American Health Care." *Columbia Law Review* 99 (1999): 1701–1829.

Law, Sylvia. "Addiction, Autonomy and Advertising." *Iowa Law Review* 77 (1992): 909–955.

Strauss, David A. "Persuasion, Autonomy and Freedom of Expression." *Columbia Law Review* 91 (1991): 334–371.

Rice, Ronald E., and Charles K. Atkin. *Public Communication Campaigns.* 2nd ed. Newbury Park, CA: Sage Publications, 1990.

Faden, Ruth R. "Ethical Issues in Government Sponsored Public Health Campaigns." *Health Education Quarterly* 14 (Spring 1987): 27–37.

Bayer, Ronald, and Johnathan Moreno. "Health Promotion: Ethical and Social Dimensions of Government Policy." *Health Affairs* (Summer 1986): 72–85.
Yudof, Mark G. *When Government Speaks: Politics, Law, and Government Expression in America.* Berkeley: University of California Press, 1983.

XI. PUBLIC HEALTH POWERS: LIBERTY INTERESTS

A. CIVIL CONFINEMENT: ISOLATION, QUARANTINE, AND COMPULSORY HOSPITALIZATION

Bayer, Ronald, and Amy Fairchild-Carrino. "AIDS and the Limits of Control: Public Health Orders, Quarantine, and Recalcitrant Behavior." *American Journal of Public Health* 83 (Oct. 1993): 1471–1476.
Schepin, Oleg P., and Waldemar V. Yermakov. *International Quarantine.* Translated by Boris Meerovich and Vladimir Bobrov. Madison, CT: International Universities Press, 1991.
Gostin, Lawrence O. "The Politics of AIDS: Compulsory State Powers, Public Health, and Civil Liberties." *Ohio State Law Journal* 49 (1989): 1017–1058.
Sullivan, Kathleen M., and Martha A. Field. "AIDS and the Coercive Power of the State." *Harvard Civil Rights-Civil Liberties Law Review* 23 (1988): 139–197.
Musto, David. "Quarantine and the Problem of AIDS." *Milbank Quarterly* 64 Supp. 1 (1986): 97–117.
Parmet, Wendy. "AIDS and Quarantine: The Revival of an Archaic Doctrine." *Hofstra Law Review* 14 (1985): 53–90.
Clemons, F.G. "Origin of Quarantine." *British Medical Journal* (Jan. 19, 1929): 122–123.
Tandy, Elizabeth C. "Local Quarantine and Inoculation for Smallpox in the American Colonies (1620–1775)." *American Journal of Public Health* 13 (Mar. 1923): 203–207.
Eager, John M. *The Early History of Quarantine: Origin of Sanitary Measures Directed against Yellow Fever.* Washington, DC: US Government Printing Office, 1903.

B. IMMUNIZATION

Salmon, Daniel A., Michael Harbor, Eugene J. Gangarosa, et al. "Health Consequenses of Religious and Philosophical Exemptions from Immunization Laws." *Journal of the American Medical Association* 282 (July 7, 1999): 47–53.
Gostin, Lawrence O., and Zita Lazzarini. "Childhood Immunization Registries: A National Review of Public Health Information Systems and the Protection of Privacy." *Journal of the American Medical Association* 274 (Dec. 13, 1995): 1793–1799.
National Vaccine Advisory Committee. *Developing a National Childhood Immunization System: Registries, Reminders, and Recall.* Washington, DC: U.S. Department of Health and Human Services, 1994.

Mariner, Wendy. "The National Vaccine Injury Compensation Program." *Health Affairs* 11 (Spring 1992): 255–265.

Neustadt, Richard E., and Harvey Fineberg. *The Epidemic That Never Was: Policy-Making and the Swine Flu Affair.* New York: Vintage Books, 1983.

Jackson, Charles L. "State Laws on Compulsory Immunization in the United States." *Public Health Report* 84 (Sept. 1969): 787–795.

Fowler, William. "Principal Provisions of Smallpox Vaccination Law and Regulations in the United States." *Public Health Report* 56 (Mar. 1942): 325–366.

C. TESTING AND SCREENING

Faden, Ruth R., Gail Geller, and Madison Powers. "Warrants for Screening Programs: Public Health, Legal and Ethical Frameworks." In *AIDS, Women, and the Next Generation: Towards a Morally Acceptable Public Policy for HIV Testing of Pregnant Women and Newborns,* edited by Ruth R. Faden, Gail Geller, and Madison Powers, 3–26. New York: Oxford University Press, 1991.

Gostin, Lawrence O., and William J. Curran. "The Case against Compulsory Casefinding in Controlling AIDS: Testing, Screening and Reporting." *American Journal of Law and Medicine* 12 (1987): 1–47.

Bayer, Ronald, Carol Levine, and Susan Wolf. "HIV Antibody Screening: An Ethical Framework for Evaluating Proposed Programs." *Journal of the American Medical Association* 256 (Oct. 3, 1986): 1768–1774.

D. REPORTING

Roush, Sandra, Guthrie Birkhead, Denise Koo, et al. "Mandatory Reporting of Diseases and Conditions by Health Care Providers and Laboratories." *Journal of the American Medical Association* 282 (July 14, 1999): 164–170.

American Civil Liberties Union. *HIV Surveillance and Name Reporting.* New York: ACLU, 1998.

Gostin, Lawrence O., and James G. Hodge, Jr. "The 'Names Debate': The Case for National HIV Reporting in the United States." *Albany Law Review* 61 (1998): 679–743.

Gostin, Lawrence O., John W. Ward, and A. Cornelius Baker. "National HIV Case Reporting for the United States: A Defining Moment in the History of the Epidemic." *New England Journal of Medicine* 337 (Oct. 16, 1997): 1162–1167.

Chorba, Terence L., R.L. Berkelman, S.K. Safford, et al. "Mandatory Reporting of Infectious Diseases by Clinicians." *Journal of the American Medical Association* 262 (Dec. 1, 1989): 3018–3026.

Fox, Daniel M. "From TB to AIDS: Value Conflicts in Reporting Disease." *Hastings Center Report* 11 (Dec., 1986): 11–16.

E. PARTNER NOTIFICATION

Gostin, Lawrence O., and James G. Hodge, Jr. "Piercing the Veil of Secrecy in HIV/AIDS and Other Sexually Transmitted Diseases: Theories of Privacy and Disclosure in Partner Notification." *Duke Journal on Gender Law and Policy* 5 (1998): 14–51.

Rothenberg, Karen H., and Stephen J. Paskey. "The Risk of Domestic Violence and Women with HIV Infection: Implications for Partner Notification, Public Policy, and the Law." *American Journal of Public Health* 85 (1995): 1569–1576.

Bayer, Ronald, and Kathleen E. Toomey. "HIV Prevention and the Two Faces of Partner Notification." *American Journal of Public Health* 82 (1992): 1158–1164.

F. PHYSICAL EXAMINATION AND TREATMENT

Bayer, Ronald; "Directly Observed Therapy and Treatment Completion for Tuberculosis in the United States: Is Universal Supervised Therapy Necessary?" *American Journal of Public Health* 88 (1998): 1052–1058.

Bayer, Ronald, and David Wilkinson. "Directly Observed Therapy for Tuberculosis: History of an Idea." *Lancet* 345 (June 17, 1995): 1545–1548.

XII. PUBLIC HEALTH POWERS: PROPERTY INTERESTS

Lazarus, Richard. "Putting the Correct 'Spin' on Lucas." *Stanford Law Review* 45 (1993): 1411–1432

Epstein, Richard. *Takings: Private Property and the Power of Eminent Domain.* Cambridge, MA: Harvard University Press, 1985.

Tandy, Elizabeth C. "The Regulation of Nuisances in the American Colonies." *American Journal of Public Health* 13 (Oct. 1923): 810–813.

XIII. TORT LAW AND THE PUBLIC'S HEALTH

*Reducing the Burden of Injury: Advancing Prevention and Treatment.*Edited by Richard J. Bonnie, Carolyn E. Fulco, and Catharyn T. Liverman. Washington, DC: National Academy Press, 1999.

Jacobson, Peter, and Kenneth E. Warner. "Litigation and Public Health Policy Making: The Case of Tobacco Control." *Journal of Health Politics, Policy & Law* 24 (1999): 769–804.

Farrell, Margaret G. "*Daubert v. Merrell Dow Pharmaceuticals, Inc.*: Epistemology and Legal Process." *Cardozo Law Review* 15 (1994): 2183–2217.

Brennan, Troyen A. "Environmental Torts." *Vanderbilt Law Review* 46 (1993): 1–73.

Huber, Peter W. *Galileo's Revenge: Junk Science in the Courtroom.* New York: Basic Books, 1991.

Cristoffel, Tom, and Stephen P. Teret. "Epidemiology and the Law: Courts and Confidence Intervals." *American Journal of Public Health* 81 (1991): 1661–1666.

XIV. PUBLIC HEALTH: ISSUES AND CONCERNS

A. EMERGING INFECTIOUS DISEASES

Gostin, Lawrence O. "The Law and Commmunicable Diseases: The Role of Law in an Era of Microbial Threats." *International Digest of Health Legislation* 49 (1998): 221–233.

Fidler, David P. "Return of the Fourth Horseman: Emerging Infectious Diseases and International Law." *Minnesota Law Review* 81 (1997): 771–868.

Lederberg, Joshua. "Infectious Diseases as an Evolutionary Paradigm." *Emerging Infectious Diseases* 3 (Oct.-Dec., 1997): 417–423.

Centers for Disease Control and Prevention. *Addressing Emerging Infectious Disease Threats: A Prevention Strategy for the United States.* Washington, DC: U.S. Department of Health and Human Services, 1994.

Garrett, Laurie. *The Coming Plague: Newly Emerging Diseases in a World Out of Balance.* New York: Farrar, Straus & Giroux, 1994.

Berkelman, Ruth L. "Emerging Infectious Diseases in the United States, 1993." *Journal of Infectious Disease* 170 (Aug. 1994): 272–277.

Institute of Medicine. *Emerging Infections: Microbial Threats in the United States.* Edited by Joshua Lederberg, Robert E. Shope, and Stanley C. Oaks, Jr. Washington, DC: National Academy Press, 1992.

B. BIOTERRORISM

Inglesby, Thomas V., David T. Dennis, Donald A. Henderson, et al. "Plague as a Biological Weapon: Medical and Public Health Management." *Journal of the American Medical Association* 283 (May 3, 2000): 2281–2290.

Macintyre, Anthony G., George W. Christopher, Edward Eitzen, Jr., et al. "Weapons of Mass Destruction: Events with Contaminated Casualties." *Journal of the American Medical Association* 283 (Jan. 12, 2000): 242–249.

Henderson, Donald A., Thomas V. Inglesby, John G. Bartlett, et al. "Smallpox as a Biological Weapon: Medical and Public Health Management." *Journal of the American Medical Association* 281 (June 9, 1999): 2127–2137.

Inglesby, Thomas V., Donald A. Henderson, John G. Bartlett, et al. "Anthrax as a Biological Weapon: Medical and Public Health Management." *Journal of the American Medical Association* 281 (May 12, 1999): 1735–1745.

Henderson, Donald A. "The Looming Threat of Bioterrorism." *Science* 283 (Feb. 26, 1999): 1279–1282.

C. HIV/AIDS

Feldman, Eric, and Ronald Bayer, eds. *Blood Feuds: AIDS, Blood, and the Politics of Medical Disaster.* New York: Oxford University Press, 1999.

Institute of Medicine. *Reducing the Odds: Preventing Perinatal Transmission of HIV in the United States.* Edited by Michael A. Stoto, Donna A. Almario, and Marie C. McCormick. Washington, DC: National Academy Press, 1999.

National Conference of State Legislatures. *HIV/AIDS: Facts to Consider.* Denver, Co: National Conference of State Legislatures, 1999.

Gostin, Lawrence O., and David W. Webber. "The AIDS Litigation Project: HIV/AIDS in the Courts in the 1990s, Part 2." *AIDS and Public Policy Journal* 13 (1998): 3–19.

Gostin, Lawrence O., and David W. Webber. "The AIDS Litigation Project: HIV/AIDS in the Courts in the 1990s, Part 1." *AIDS and Public Policy Journal* 12 (1997): 105–121.

Webber, David W., ed. *AIDS and the Law*. 4th ed. New York: Wiley Law Publications, 1997.

Bayer, Ronald "AIDS Prevention—Sexual Ethics and Responsibility." *New England Journal of Medicine* (June 6, 1996) 334: 1540–1542.

Gostin, Lawrence O., Zita Lazzarini, and Diane Alexander, et al. "HIV Testing, Counseling, and Prophylaxis after Sexual Assault." *Journal of the American Medical Association* 271 (May 11, 1994): 1436–1444.

Burris, Scott, Harlon L. Dalton, and Judith Leonie Miller, eds. *AIDS Law Today: A New Guide for the Public*. New Haven, CT: Yale University Press, 1993.

Burris, Scott. "Prisons, Law and Public Health: The Case for a Coordinated Response to Epidemic Disease behind Bars." *University of Miami Law Review* 47 (1992): 291–335.

Stoddard, Thomas B., and Walter Rieman. "AIDS and the Rights of the Individual: Toward a More Sophisticated Understanding of Discrimination." *Milbank Quarterly* 8 Supp. 1 (1990): 143–174.

Gostin, Lawrence O., Paul Cleary, Kenneth Mayer, et al. "Screening and Exclusion of International Travelers and Immigrants for Public Health Purposes: An Evaluation of United States Policy." *New England Journal of Medicine* 332 (June 14, 1990): 1743–1746.

Curran, William, Lawrence O. Gostin, and Mary Clark. *AIDS: Legal, Regulatory, and Policy Analysis*. Washington, DC: U.S. Department of Health and Human Services (1986; republished, Frederick, MD: University Publishing Group, 1988).

Burris, Scott. "Fear Itself: AIDS, Herpes and Public Health Decisions." *Yale Law and Policy Review* 3 (1985): 479–518.

D. TUBERCULOSIS

Gostin, Lawrence O. "The resurgent Tuberculosis Epidemic in the Era of AIDS." *Maryland Law Review* 54 (1995): 1–131.

Ball, Carlos A., and Mark Barnes. "Public Health and Individual Rights: Tuberculosis Control and Detention Procedures in New York City." *Yale Law and Policy Review* 12 (1994): 38–67.

Gittler, Josephine. "Controlling Resurgent Tuberculosis: Public Health Agencies, Public Health Policy, and Law." *Journal of Health Politics, Policy and Law* 19 (1994): 107–146.

Rothman, Sheila M. *Living in the Shadow of Death: Tuberculosis and the Social Experience of Illness in American History*. New York: Basic Books, 1994.

Gostin, Lawrence O. "Controlling the Resurgent Tuberculosis Epidemic: A Fifty State Survey of Tuberculosis Statutes and Proposals for Reform." *Journal of the American Medical Association* 269 (Jan. 13, 1993): 255–261.

Annas, George J. "Control of Tuberculosis—The Law and the Public's Health." *New England Journal of Medicine* 328 (Feb. 25, 1993): 585–588.

Reilly, Rosemary G. "Combating the Tuberculosis Epidemic: The Legality of Coercive Measures." *Columbia Journal of Law and Social Problems* 27 (1993): 101–149.

Dubler, Nancy Neveloff, Ronald Bayer, Sheldon Londesman, et al. *The Tuberculosis Revival: Individual Rights and Societal Obligations in a Time of AIDS.* New York: United Hospital Fund, 1992.

E. SEXUALLY TRANSMITTED DISEASES

National Conference of State Legislatures. *Sexually Transmitted Diseases: A Policymaker's Guide And Summary of State Laws.* Denver, Co: National Conference of State Legislatures, 1998.
Brandt, Allan M. *No Magic Bullet: A Social History of Venereal Disease in the United States since 1880.* New York: Oxford University Press, 1987.
Institute of Medicine *The Hidden Epidemic: Confronting Sexually Transmitted Diseases.* Edited by Thomas R. Eng, and William T. Butler. Washington, DC: National Academy Press, 1997.

F. TOBACCO

Hurt, Richard D., and Channing R. Robertson. "Prying Open the Door to the Tobacco Industry's Secrets about Nicotine." *Journal of the American Medical Association* 280 (Oct. 7, 1998): 1173–1181.
Jacobson, Peter D., Jeffrey Wasserman, and John Anderson. "Historical Overview of Tobacco Legislation and Regulation." *Journal of Social Issues* 53 (1997): 75–95.
Kelder, Graham E. Jr., and Richard A. Daynard. "The Role of Litigation in the Effective Control of the Sale and Use of Tobacco." *Stanford Law and Policy Review* 8 (1997): 63–87.
Glantz, Stanton A., Debrorah E. Barnes, Lisa Bero, et al. "Looking through a Keyhole at the Tobacco Industry: The Brown and Williamson Documents." *Journal of the American Medical Association* 274 (July 19, 1995): 219–224.
Jacobson, Peter D., Jeffrey Wasserman, and Kristiana Raube. "The Politics of Anti-Smoking Legislation: Lessons From Six States." *Journal of Health Politics, Policy and Law* 18 (1993): 787–819.
Rabin, Robert. "A Sociolegal History of the Tobacco Tort Litigation." *Stanford Law Review* 44 (1992): 853–878.
Warner, Kenneth E. *Selling Smoke: Cigarette Advertising and Public Health.* Washington, DC: American Public Health Institute, 1986.

G. FIREARMS

Vernick, Jon S., and Stephen P. Teret. "New Courtroom Strategies Regarding Firearms: Tort Litigation against Firearm Manufacturers and Constitutional Challenges to Gun Laws." *Houston Law Review* 36 (1999): 1713–1754.
Teret, Stephen P., Daniel W. Webster, and Jon S. Vernick. "Support for New Policies to Regulate Firearms: Results of Two National Surveys." *New England Journal of Medicine* 339 (1998): 813–818.

Polston, Mark D., and Douglas S. Weil. "Unsafe by Design: Using Tort Actions to Reduce Firearm-Related Injuries." *Stanford Law and Policy Review* 8 (1997): 13–21.

Robinson, Krista D. *Personalized Guns: Reducing Gun Deaths Through Design Changes.* 2nd ed. Baltimore: Johns Hopkins Center for Gun Policy and Research, 1997.

Vernick, Jon S., Stephen P. Teret, and Daniel W. Webster. "Regulating Firearm Advertisements That Promise Home Protection." *Journal of the American Medical Association* 277 (May 7, 1997): 1391–1397.

Table of Cases

468

Index

About the Author

Lawrence O. Gostin, an internationally recognized scholar in public health law, is Professor of Law at Georgetown University, Professor of Public Health at the Johns Hopkins University, and Co-Director of the Georgetown/Johns Hopkins University Program on Law and Public Health. Professor Gostin is also a member of the Institute of Medicine/National Academy of Sciences Board on Health Promotion and Disease Prevention. He works closely with national and international public health agencies, including the U.S. Centers for Disease Control and Prevention, the World Health Organization, and the Joint United Nations Programme on AIDS. Professor Gostin is the Editor of the Health Law and Ethics section of the *Journal of the American Medical Association (JAMA)* and holds several other editorial positions with scholarly journals. In the United Kingdom, while head of the National Council of Civil Liberties, he received the Delbridge Memorial Award for the person "who has most influenced Parliment and government to act for the welfare of society."

Compositor:	Publication Services, Inc.
Text:	10/13 Sabon
Display:	Sabon
Printer:	Friesens
Binder:	Friesens